NURSING ETHICS

Executive Editor: Richard A. Weimer
Production Editor: Michael J. Rogers
Art Director: Don Sellers, AMI
Printer: R. R. Donnelley Company, Harrisonburg, Virginia
Typesetting and pasteup: Bookmakers, Inc., Washington, D.C.
Typeface: Baskerville

NURSING ETHICS
Theories and Pragmatics

Leah Curtin
M. Josephine Flaherty

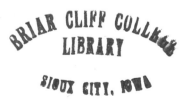
ROBERT J. BRADY CO.
A Prentice-Hall Publications and Communications Company
Bowie, Maryland 20715

Nursing Ethics: Theories and Pragmatics

Library of Congress Cataloging in Publication Data

Curtin, Leah.
    Nursing ethics.

    Bibliography: p.
    Includes index.
    1. Nursing ethics.   I. Flaherty, M. Josephine
    II. Title.
RT85.C87   174'.2   81-17962
ISBN 0-89303-051-1 (case)   AACR2
ISBN 0-89303-053-8 (pbk.)

RT
85
.C87

Prentice-Hall International, Inc., London
Prentice-Hall of Australia, Pty., Ltd., Sydney
Prentice-Hall of India Private Limited, New Delhi
Prentice-Hall of Japan, Inc., Tokyo
Prentice-Hall of Southeast Asia Pte. Ltd., Singapore
Whitehall Books, Limited, Petone, New Zealand

Printed in the United States of America

82 83 84 85 86 87 88 89 90 91 92   10 9 8 7 6 5 4 3 2 1

Dedication

To my family, friends, and colleagues whose patience, support, and guidance have made this book possible.

Leah Curtin

To my mother, Catherine Edna Flaherty, the first and still most influential nurse in my life, and

To my father, Richard Joseph Flaherty, who taught me the meaning of responsible membership.

M. Josephine Flaherty

Contents

Foreword

In the past decade increasing attention has been given to ethics in nursing and medicine, as reflected in professional literature, conferences, institutes, and even fellowships to enable health professionals to devote concentrated time to addressing ethical problems and dilemmas. This focus is understandable in view of the incredible scientific and medical advances and the resultant effects on medical and nursing practice and on the roles and responsibilities assumed by health professionals.

Nurses with advanced preparation are defining the nature of nursing knowledge, are identifying relevant questions about nursing practice that merit investigation, and are educating nursing students in a very different manner than has been traditional in nursing education. Nurses perceive themselves as advocates for patients and are determined in their efforts to recognize and uphold patients' rights to be involved in decisions about plans for their care and therapy and even to refuse prescribed therapy if they have been informed of the possible consequences. The question of rights and choices is made even more complicated in view of changes in society, in mores, in values, in roles and relationships, and in the aspirations and beliefs of young people entering the profession of nursing today.

Such changes in nurses may bring them into conflict with physicians, particularly physicians who have been accustomed to nurses who do not question, and who follow orders blindly. The strain on nurse–physician relationships is increased greatly in settings such as intensive care units, where nurses and physicians work in close contact under extremely stressful conditions which frequently involve ethical problems and dilemmas. Such ethical questions tend to arise also between nurses in practice who hold divergent ethical views and conflicting beliefs about patients' rights, the proper roles of nurses and physicians, and the appropriate relationships between them in practice settings.

Most nurses today view the institutions employing them quite differently than did nurses in the past. They hold expectations that a safe and supportive working environment will be provided to permit them to provide humane care and to be involved in decisions that affect their practice and lives. Such views may bring them into conflict with nurses and health care administrators who hold traditional values and believe they must accept conditions because that is the best the employer can provide.

As a consequence of such changes in society, in education, and in attitudes and values, nurses today face ethical issues and stresses and strains in intraprofessional and interprofessional relationships not envisioned in years past. Some are basic philosophical questions; some are issues and problems in working relationships; some are life and death issues; and some are problems that, if unresolved, influence all too many nurses to leave nursing.

This book offers a unique, thought-provoking, logical, and sensible approach to the whole question of ethics in nursing and health care. It presents a view of ethics as involved in all interactions between nurse and patient or client, not just those with tragic outcomes or those that present complex ethical problems. With such a pervasive concept of ethics as an integral part of all practice, the authors emphasize, as a basic expectation, recognition and respect of the rights of others—patients or clients, families, nurses, physicians—and the use of logical reasoning in addressing issues and conflicts in relationships between the nurse and recipients of care and in intraprofessional relationships.

Coauthored by an American nurse and a Canadian nurse who are widely recognized experts in the field of ethics in their own and each other's countries, the book provides a sound theoretical base and a philosophical approach for critical analysis of ethical problems and for developing wise strategies for addressing them. The authors' approaches are clearly those that could be formulated and articulated only by very knowledgeable and clinically competent nurses whose educational background has a firm base in philosophy and ethical inquiry which they apply skillfully to the practice of nursing and the delivery of health care. The scholarliness of the authors is reflected further in careful documentation of sources and an extensive bibliography at the conclusion of each chapter.

The fifteen case studies present a variety of ethical problems, some of which are encountered by nurses in daily practice while others are such complex dilemmas as abortion and euthanasia. Each case study is discussed by both authors presenting the most comprehensive and logical analysis yet to be found in the literature on ethics in nursing. It is clear that there are not answers to all of the ethical problems in nursing practice. There is a need, however, as Flaherty points out, for nurses "to keep nursing's ethical dimension under constant scrutiny—and to develop and apply it—as part of the profession's constant pursuit of optimal impact."

This book provides a rich resource for all practicing nurses, for nursing students and nurse educators, for nurse administrators, and indeed for physicians and health care administrators—all of whom should aim to render humane care, and to apply appropriate ethical concepts in the process of providing such care.

Jannetta MacPhail, Ph.D., F.A.A.N.
Dean and Professor of Nursing,
Case Western Reserve University
Cleveland, Ohio

Preface

Although we believe that the essence of human actions lies in the heart and soul found in them, actions are judged by the difference they make in the world. Effective nursing practice depends as much on the humanity of the nurse as it does on the nurse's knowledge and technical skill.

Nurses who recognize and respond to the human needs of patients discover a rich source of knowledge and understanding. Nurses who respect and collaborate with colleagues find strength and support. The professional roles of nurses and the human relationships inherent in them include specific responsibilities, privileges, and rights. These are the subject of this book.

In our own nursing practice and in our contacts with other nurses, we have been impressed with the depth of their concern about and their understanding of the importance of the ethical dimensions of nursing. This book is an attempt to share our experience and our reflections on some of the troublesome questions that nurses face in their day-to-day practice.

Leah Curtin

M. Josephine Flaherty

Section I

1

What Are Human Rights?

Leah Curtin

"When a right is maintained, human society is preserved,
but when it is neglected, society is corrupted."

Dante, *On Monarchy*

I would like to begin by challenging you to think about ethics in nursing—
not the fabulous life and death issues, but the day-to-day living actions that
make up the fabric of human life. The following true story has nothing of the
dramatic about it; rather, it represents the daily disrespect to which patients
are subject.

Some time ago, a six-year-old boy was playing in his backyard when he
tripped, fell, and hit his head on a sharp rock. Surveying the damage done to
the area above his right eye, his mother decided to take him to the local
emergency room to have the laceration stitched. On the way to the hospital
she tried to reassure her child by explaining what would be done to him,
by telling him that the nurses and doctors would "numb" the area before
they sewed it up and by assuring him that no one would hurt him deliberately.

When they arrived at the emergency room, there was another little boy
with a similar laceration already awaiting treatment. His father was trying
to comfort and calm him in much the same way as this woman had reassured her child. The child–parent couples were placed in side-by-side cubi-
cles and the curtain was left open. A nurse entered the cubicle next to my
friend's and, with no explanation, roughly cleansed the laceration above
the first little boy's eye. The little boy wriggled and cried out in pain. The
physician then entered the cubicle and sewed the laceration without benefit
of local anesthesia or even a comforting word. The child screamed in pain
and terror. My friend was horrified—and her child was very frightened.

However, when the same nurse approached her little boy, she was kind and gentle. The same physician entered and carefully injected a local anesthetic, waited for it to take effect, and only then stitched the laceration.

Why was there so great a difference in the handling of these two similar cases? Perhaps it was a difference in socioeconomic status. Perhaps it was the presence of a mother as opposed to a father. Perhaps it was because the first child was black and my friend is white. Whatever the reason, what was the essential difference between these children—a difference that would account for such divergence in treatment?

My first reaction to this story was anger at the injustice done, followed quickly by a feeling of shame (shame by association?) that my colleagues in the health profession would do such a thing. After a period of time, these reactions were augmented by an abiding sense of sorrow. Although feelings are by no means the most accurate indicators for action, the presence of these particular feelings requires explanation.

Was this case so important? No life and death decisions were made. The child was treated; his life and health were not threatened. No one died, but perhaps a little bit of our humanity was diminished. Let me explain. Although the specific actions seem relatively insignificant, the child's human rights were violated. What do I mean by this child's human rights? What is a human right? *A human right is a person's just due.* What is the source of human rights? What good are human rights if they can be violated with impunity? What is a person's just due? How is it determined?

RELATIONSHIP BETWEEN RIGHTS AND NEEDS

As we approach the concept of human rights, we must start simply, as beings whose knowledge begins with out senses. As human beings what do we *know* about human beings? One of our deepest convictions, confirmed by all our experience, is that we exist and we are one being. Moreover, we have certain needs that must be met if we are to continue to be. On the physiological level, we must have food, water, rest, shelter and protection from those elements (animate and inanimate) that could harm us. On the emotional, social, and intellectual levels we need to love and be loved, to learn and teach, to understand and be understood.

As we grow and mature, we come to realize that this unity of self is a part of another, greater unity. Although an individual is separate and distinct from all other human beings, he belongs to them and with them because he has grown from their growth, learned from their knowledge, and benefited from their sufferings. He is because they are; he can continue to be *only* because they are. Thus, awareness of one's own existence leads inevitably to a recognition of common human origins and interdependence.

If we have common origins, it is logical to conclude that we share certain common needs. Moreover, if we are interdependent, it is logical to conclude that the meeting of these needs is necessary to our mutual well being. If I must have food, other human beings also must have food. If I need rest, other humans also need rest. If I am hurt by the rough handling of a wound, others also are hurt. Because we are interdependent, the welfare of one is a concern for all.

Perceiving Others' Needs

There are those who claim that I really cannot know if someone else is tired, hungry, or in pain,[1] even though the data received daily by my senses confirm these observations. How can I be sure that the data are accurate?[2] I concede the point. One cannot *be* another person or experience the feelings and needs of another person. We are finite—limited by time, space, and the capacity of our brains. Whatever these limitations, we must acknowledge the fact that we have our senses alone to give us information. Moreover, as we have no way of confirming the validity of our senses, there is little point in our belaboring the obvious.[3] If I know anything at all, I know that I am. My senses tell me that others are. Although human beings differ in significant and interesting ways, my senses tell me that there are more similarities than differences.

In truth, some of our perceptions of the world vary greatly; beauty *is* in the mind of the beholder! That may be, but blood is not in the mind; rather, it is in the body and clearly recognized by all. If I am cut, I bleed. If others are cut, I can see that they bleed. If the bleeding is not stopped, I will die. I observe that others die when their bleeding is not stopped. Human perceptions on such points do not vary. Our brains organize these data and conclude that certain needs are inherent to the human condition.

These fundamental, shared needs form a foundation for a concept of universal human rights. That is, human rights belong to all human beings because fundamental human needs are found in all human beings. When we are very young people, our brains are not able to organize these data properly; hence, we do not recognize the needs of others. As our rational abilities develop, the needs of others are brought more sharply into focus. The ability to perceive the needs of others is, perhaps, the surest measure of our own maturity—our coming of age as *humane* beings.

Slowly and unevenly, most human beings come to recognize and to respect the needs of others. This ability to perceive and to honor the universality of human needs has led to a growing, maturing, continually evolving concept of human rights. Although progress has been slow, although there is little to keep us from backsliding, progress has been made.[4]

Having Rights and Exercising Rights

Just as there is a distinction between having a fundamental need (*e.g.,* needing food) and having that need filled (*e.g.,* eating food), so is there a distinction between having a right and exercising that right. Moreover, just as the denial of food does not remove the need for food, the denial of a right does not negate the right. It certainly interferes with the *exercise* of the right, but because there is a clear distinction between these two aspects of a right, the denial of a right does not eradicate the right. It exists. If fundamental or subsistence rights are founded in essential human need, they do exist just as need exists) whether or not they are respected (met).

As we approach human needs that are less easily observed and measured, it becomes more difficult to explicate the human rights involved. Indeed, most people can recognize readily the need for food; many rationally can derive from this observation a human right to at least adequate nourishment. However, what of the human need to learn, to understand and to share this knowledge with others? Again, we must fall back on our limited knowledge of ourselves and on the data collected by our senses. We know that we have learned. We observe the fact that others have learned. The briefest perusal of human history demonstrates the human striving *to know*. Moreover, we observe that those who do not or cannot learn fail to continue their development as rational beings.

Humans are not merely beings, but beings who know and who "know that they know." They laugh and cry and sometimes know why. Because we are distinguished from other beings by a superior ability to learn, to understand, and to apply what we have learned, anthropologists have named our species *Homo sapiens*. If, then, the ability to think is a distinguishing characteristic of human beings, the opportunity to develop thinking processes (however limited) can be seen clearly as a fundamental *human* need. As the needs that are essential to our humanity form the basic structure of human rights, the need for rational development becomes a right to learn. Not all human needs translate into human rights—only those needs do so that *must* be met if we are to be human beings. Thus, to lock an infant in a dark cellar, even though we would provide for all of his physiological needs, would be a fundamental violation of the child's human rights. Certainly, each member of our species has a natural right to develop as *Homo sapiens*. Although how much one *can* learn seems to vary significantly from person to person, as does the amount of food necessary to sustain life, the *need* to learn is as universal as is the need for food.

Human Wants Versus Human Needs

One must ask if there is any limit to human needs. The answer, of course, is yes. However, there seem to be no limits to human wants. Part of the problem is that we confuse what human beings need with what they want. So it is with human rights. Understandably, human beings want their desires fulfilled too. Thus, it has become quite popular to dress human wants in rights rhetoric and to claim them as fundamental human needs. The result is that the concept of human rights has been cheapened and subsequently too little respected.

There are moral and often legal obligations to fulfill fundamental human needs, but these obligations do not pertain to human wants, however understandable or even commendable these might be. This is why it is important to distinguish between human needs and human desires. Not everything that is claimed as a human right actually is a human right. Each claim must be examined carefully to determine if it is a just claim (*i.e.,* a right).

Even the most understandable and universal human desires are not seen as human rights. For example, although human beings avoid pain whenever possible, all human beings experience pain and often the experience of pain is an essential early warning system. We need to experience pain so that we can take action to protect ourselves. Because human beings cannot avoid pain entirely (however much they might wish to), freedom from pain cannot be a human right. However, to inflict unnecessary pain is to ignore a universal aspect of humankind. It is to fail to recognize the humanity of another person. *If human beings have any natural rights at all, they have the right to be recognized and respected as human beings.* To fail to respect the mutual humanity of another person is, in effect, to deny him his just due—to treat him as less than human.

To relate this to the situation presented at the beginning of this chapter, let us examine in which way the little boy's human rights were violated. The health professionals inflicted unnecessary pain. Even though freedom from pain is not a human right, all people have the right to be treated as human beings. In this case, the health professionals treated the child as less than human, as an object that does not share our universal human sensations. Clearly, this child *is* human, and thus we feel a sense of outrage at his treatment.

For at least three reasons, the concept of human rights must be limited to fundamental human needs only:

1. It is impossible to fulfill the unlimited desires of human beings.
2. It is inappropriate to predicate a *duty* to do the impossible.
3. The dilution of fundamental human needs with mere wants poses a threat to the most basic rights of all humans by expanding them beyond the limits of what reasonably can be provided.

The Limitations of Human Rights

We also must question whether fundamental human needs always have to be fulfilled. In short, can even the most fundamental human rights be limited? Each of us has a right to be and to remain alive, but how far does this right extend? For example, if I am starving, I justly may demand food from my neighbors who have plenty, but I may not demand food from them if they have only enough to feed themselves. How so? Is not my fundamental right violated? In the first instance, yes, because they have plenty. In the second instance, it would be more accurate to say that my right is inoperative: in effect, cancelled by the rights of others. That is, I may not demand of my neighbors the food they need to stay alive lest I violate their fundamental rights. It is in this sense that human rights, while universally applicable, are not absolute.

Human Rights, Human Freedom, and Human Values

Some modern philosophers assert that freedom is a precondition to all rights.[5] If the concept of human freedom means anything at all, it means that one should not be coerced unjustly. However, the rights we have been discussing—those founded on elemental human needs—undoubtedly contain an element of natural coercion. Human beings really are not free to decide that they do not need food or that they will not bleed if they are cut. These mundane particulars force certain conditions on human existence. Natural coercion is neither just nor unjust; it is simply fact; that is, universal and inherent requirements imposed on human life. Is it fair that I lose a limb to gangrene? Is it fair that others do not lose a limb to gangrene? Such things are neither fair nor unfair; they are nature's stipulations on human existence. Although there are few things in life as coercive as the threats of suffering and death, they cannot be unjust because they apply to everyone. Yet, they do not seem just because some suffer more than others. This universal, natural, and inherent coercion forms a recognizable foundation for a legitimate claim to the fulfillment of fundamental human needs.

However, an individual, for a variety of reasons, may choose *not* to fulfill a fundamental need. If he makes this choice, he will die. For example, I may choose to starve so that there will be enough food for my children to live. Although I can make this decision, I cannot make it with impunity because I must accept the consequences. Even in the face of elemental, natural coercion, I am free to make the choice. Human freedom at its most radical means that I am free to die for what I value more highly than my own life or free to continue living under execrable circumstances for something I value more highly than my own suffering.

As the concept of human freedom largely surrounds the concept of human values, it is essential to define values. By their very nature, values are both common and unique. That is, many values are held in common (civilization may be defined as values held in common) and are unique to each individual. Values are those assertions or statements that individuals make, either through their behavior, words, or actions, that define what they think is important and for which they are willing to suffer and even die—or perhaps to continue living. Each person's character is defined by the value choices he has made and, even though it is not explicated, he does have a value system. In like manner, a civilization is defined by the value choices made by those who constitute that civilization and society also has a value system (we may call them national priorities!).

Value choices constitute almost the whole of human freedom. Often I choose to do what I do because of the values I hold. This does not mean necessarily that I choose to do what I *want* to do, but rather what I think I *ought* to do, given those things that are important to me. Thus, although I want to go to sleep, I may choose to stay up with a sick friend who needs my help. When values conflict, I must choose which of them are most important to me. For example, if my mother is ill and needs my help and my child is ill and needs my help, which one shall I help? Of course, I may just go to bed and forget about both of them, but that also is a value choice.

Human beings are essentially free[6] but they are not free of nature's coercion. Rather they are free to accept or reject the consequences of this coercion. The right to be free is the "right to one's *domain,* whether it's one's body, one's life, one's property, or one's privacy."[7] The right to be free, to make decisions about one's self, is protection from the unjustified interference of any person. Interference in one's personal domain is justified only if someone else's fundamental natural rights are endangered. Thus, although I am free to do with my body what I will, I am not free to use my body to endanger the life of someone else. If I attempt to do so, others are justified in stopping me.

If there is such a thing as human freedom, it must include an option, a choice, to exercise rights or to refrain from exercising them. Thus, human freedom is absolute only in the sense that people have a right to choose a certain course of action in their own domain if they are willing to pay the price.

This discussion reminds me of two situations that on the surface are very different, but underneath are very similar.

The first case involves a 48-year-old man who was dying of oat-cell carcinoma of the lung. Although his prognosis was bleak (he had fewer than six months to live), he knew that he had to live for at least ten months to qualify under his employer's benefit plan for a pension that would provide for his family after his death. As the months wore on and the cancer spread, the pain became more acute; his sedation was increased and he often was confused. However, one thing remained clear in his mind: he had to live until a certain date. To the distress of his nurses and his family, he would ask what day it was every time he opened his eyes. When the landmark day finally arrived, he whispered, "Thank God." He died two days later. Against overwhelming odds, he continued to live until his obligation was fulfilled: he provided for his family.

The second situation involves a 42-year-old woman, a widow for many years. After her husband's death, she had worked as a cleaning lady and had taken in laundry to support herself and her only child, a daughter. When her daughter was four years old, their little flat caught fire and the child was trapped in her room. The woman ran through the flames, wrapped her daughter in a blanket to protect her from the fire, and managed to get her out safely. Unfortunately, the mother was burned around the face, neck, and arms. After extensive treatment, she recovered, but her face was severely scarred. She went back to her chores, but life was more difficult now because she could not "work out": people did not want such an ugly woman in their homes. Nevertheless, she scrimped and saved for her daughter's education so that she could have a better life. In her daughter's last year of college, this woman developed irreversible kidney failure. At that time, kidney dialysis units were very scarce and treatment costs were exorbitant. Special committees were established to decide who would receive the treatment. The committee decided in favor of this woman who was to return to the hospital twice weekly for treatment.

As a visiting nurse, I was assigned to her care. I was in her home one day when her daughter arrived with several of her friends. We were in another room discussing dietary restrictions. In the course of our conversation, she offered me a cup of coffee and we went to the kitchen to make it. When we entered the kitchen, one of her daughter's friends asked her who that *ugly* woman was. Her daughter responded, "Oh, that's just the cleaning lady. If she bothers you I'll tell her to leave." As long as I live, I shall never forget the pain in this woman's eyes. From that moment on, she refused further treatment. A psychiatric consult was sought, to no avail. She died three weeks later. Perhaps she saw no point in continuing her life, so she chose to die—an understandable choice for someone who must have constant treatment to live. Perhaps she thought that her obligations were over; her daughter was raised and educated. Perhaps she reconsidered because of the expense involved; the money could be spent instead to further her daughter's education. Perhaps not. The fact is that despite the efforts of a considerable number of health professionals, despite our earnest representations, she was free to make her own decision—and she did.

In the first case, the man decided to live. In the second case the woman decided to die. Both of them were making decisions *in their own domain*. Neither of them was transgressing or threatening the rights of other people. Both chose particular courses of action according to their values. However distressed the man's family and nurses were to witness his suffering, he was free to decide to live, and he did. However distressed the health professionals were about the woman's decision to refuse treatment, she was free to decide to die, and she did.

The Limits of Human Freedom

Human beings have the option of choosing not to exercise a given right. However, we are not free to make this decision for other human beings. Human rights are not dispensible merely because certain classes of human beings are not free to exercise them. If there were no other reasons, this alone should suffice as proof that freedom, while an essential aspect of the exercise of rights, cannot be a precondition to the existence of rights. In other words, infants, children, comatose persons, senile elderly persons and others do not lose their fundamental rights because they cannot exercise choice. In fact, their fundamental needs are magnified by these conditions; thus, exquisite care must be taken to protect their human rights.

Here, the idea of justice is paramount. According to Ramsey, a just society gives to each according to his need.[8] If society loses a sense of justice, whose rights are safe? To put it pragmatically, if our aged and senile parents can be killed for whatever reason, so can we, for "as they are now, we soon shall be."[9] If the youngest child can be killed with impunity, so could we, for "as they are now, we once were."[10] A sense of justice imposes a recognition and respect for the fundamental, shared needs of all humankind. Although we are free to abrogate our own rights, we are not free to negate the rights of others. It is in this sense that even a so-called absolute right to be free is limited by the rights of others.

In those cases where people cannot make their own decisions and, most particularly, when individuals' value systems either cannot be explicated or have not yet been formed, decisions regarding their treatment and well-being pose onerous burdens. Thus, throughout the decision-making process, we must be sensitive to the human rights involved, to the limits of human rights, to the demands of justice, and to the consequences of our decisions.

HUMAN RIGHTS AND THE LAW

As with all human endeavor, it must be recognized that the ability to govern the behavior of others is limited. Although laws can protect certain aspects of human rights, there is a vast area that laws cannot protect. For example, the law can restrain me from killing you, but it cannot require me to respect your humanity—to treat you with decency, kindness, or understanding. To a certain extent, law can control my behavior, but it cannot control my attitude. Perhaps this notion is expressed best in the New Testament: Jesus Christ called those persons "whited sepulchres" who obeyed the letter of the law while ignoring the spirit of the law.[11] Although outwardly just, they were inwardly corrupt. John Adams referred to this particular problem when he wrote: "Public virtue cannot exist in a nation without private, and public virtue is the only foundation of a republic."[12]

Perhaps the most significant aspects of human rights defy legal interpretation and application. Such things as the right to be respected as a human being, the right to be treated with dignity, and the right to be free of undue outside interference fall within this category. In these areas, the concept of human rights is particularly fragile. This vulnerability cannot be overcome *per se* by law. Even though these rights cannot be protected by law, they have a moral force derived from the common thread of our humanity. It is important to recognize that human rights, though violated, remain rights—just as human law, though transgressed, remains law.

Historical Perspective

The concept of natural or inherent human rights was entwined with law very early in human history. Cicero repeatedly exalted the superior position of human rights *vis-à-vis* human law.[13] (Today, however, we would disagree with him about who should be considered human!) Roman jurists, examining the laws of the known world, were able to compile the "Law of Nations," a system of law that incorporated the principles found in the laws of all nations that embodied the fundamental needs common to the human race.

During the Middle Ages, our duty to respect the human rights of others was summarized succinctly in the Golden Rule: Do unto others as you would have them do unto you. By and large, it would be fair to say philosophers during the Middle Ages equated respect for human rights with the Law of God.[14]

Following the Protestant Reformation, the concept of natural rights figured prominently in discussions of both general jurisprudence and international law. In fact, Hugo Grotius built a framework for international law on the concept of inherent, inviolable human rights. He held that no legitimate nation could establish laws that were contrary to the rights of man.[15]

Sir William Blackstone, in his *Commentaries on the Laws of England,* held that laws are invalid if they violate natural human rights and that such laws as are valid derive their force from the inherent rights of human beings. Both Locke and Rousseau identified natural human rights as the foundation of their political philosophy. Out of such philosophy came the American Declaration of Independence (1776), the French Declaration of the Rights of Man and Citizen (1789), and the United Nations Universal Declaration of Human Rights (1948).

Some legal savants and philosophers tend to take the position that not only must law fail to contravene human rights, but it must protect rights.[16] Others hold that human rights are meaningless apart from legal sanction; therefore, no right exists until it is recognized by law.[17]

Oliver Wendell Holmes, the famous American jurist and Supreme Court judge, defined a right as a permission secured and granted by positive legal act. According to Holmes, rights allow action without requiring it.[18] On the other hand, Thomas Holland defined a right as a power operating through the force of law to influence the acts of others.[19] In recent years, many American jurists have seen rights solely as whatever the Courts say they are.[20] Under such systems, human rights are placed beneath legal rights. Thus, all rights are perceived as having their origin and protection in the State. If the State can give individual rights, then the State also can remove rights.

However, John Salamond held that a right is an interest recognized and protected by law.[21] Paul Vinogradoff asserted that a right is more than an interest—it is a just claim.[22] Although both of these formulations allow for a pre-existing claim or interest (*i.e.*, something not already recognized by law), these respected legal scholars also held that all rights must be demanded actively before they become operative.[23] Thus, there is no particular obligation to respect a right unless it is claimed. Therefore, it can be concluded that those classes of persons who are unable to claim their rights in effect have no rights. Of course, others could act as advocates for them (*i.e.,* claim their rights on their behalf), but they have no duty to do so because rights are nonexistent until they are claimed. To reduce the human rights of these people to complete dependence on the good will of others is to vitiate any moral or legal force. Thus, unless others are willing to advocate for them, they may be killed, used for human experimentations, or simply left to die—and this is right, good, and proper because they have no rights. If the existence of human rights is totally dependent on the good will of fellow men, rights cease to be a force in society for any one other than the strong.

Discussion

When people claim human rights, they usually do so because they are aware of some political, social, or cultural force threatening to deny them their just due.[24] If human rights are equated solely with legal rights, how can citizens correct deficiencies or injustices inflicted by the State? If human rights depend on the good will of others, how can they be seen as an individual's just due?

Indeed, legal rights derive from the State and are ordered by law.[25] Thus, the State is the source as well as the protector of legal rights. As such, the State legitimately may add, remove or modify legal rights as it sees fit or necessary. However, if human rights derive essentially from fundamental human needs, they rest within individuals (singly and collectively). Moreover, they exist whether or not a given State (government) recognizes them, precisely because the human need exists whether or not the State recognizes it. Clearly, legal recognition and protection may be necessary for the exercise but not for the existence of human rights. For example, if the State promotes or even permits the killing of certain minority groups, it is likely that these groups will be decimated. The collective decision of society affects their ability to remain alive, but—and this is the crux—it does not affect their need to live.

Although many political realists claim that human rights unprotected by law are little more than pious platitudes, they are, perhaps, a bit hasty in their judgments. Although almost all theories of rights recognize the necessity for legal protection, it does not necessarily follow (1) that all rights have their origin in law and (2) that rights are of no use to individuals unless they are recognized by law.

Even though the proper exercise of human rights may depend on a combination of legal recognition and human good will, human rights exist apart from the law because they are derived from the fundamental needs of individual human beings. In fact, any justifiable claim against the power of the State entails the notion that one already has the right and is petitioning (or demanding) to have it recognized by law. The very notion of justice and justifiable claims suggests that human rights are philosophically prior to law and rest within individuals.

If individuals are the source and depository of human rights, it follows that the State derives its authority to rule from the collective consent of the people. In this view, the State retains the right to rule only to the extent that it protects the human rights of its citizens and arbitrates conflict in rights situations. Thus, no law is legitimate if it violates human rights and no State is legitimate if it passes such laws. An appeal to human rights carries with it great force because it claims an authority higher than the State, an authority founded on essential and universal human need. The concept of human rights has served a very useful function for humanity, for not only is it the source of rebellion against an oppressive State, but it also serves as a clarion call for social change.

Human Rights and the Collectivity

In the modern democratic republic, the concept of human rights faces yet another challenge. The "father" of existentialism, Soren Kierkegaard, succinctly summarized this threat when he expressed the fear that ethics would become a branch of statistics.[26] He meant that human rights could become a matter for opinion poll. It would appear that he was not far wrong. The concepts of rights, duties, good, and bad often are presented today as "most people think this" or "most people would do that." The implication, of course, is that the existence of these concepts depends on collective opinion. For example, if the majority of the people in a given society think that mentally retarded people have no rights, then they have no rights—and this is just, good, and proper because "most people" agree.

At this point, we will recall a few facts. The first is that human need exists whether or not others recognize this need. If I am starving, I am not made less hungry because you refuse to recognize my need for food. Second, statistical data (*e.g.,* opinion polls) consist of numbers. Numbers are mental constructs intended to describe, not rule. Third, people are real. Fourth, decisions made about what we may or may not do to people translate into very real action.

Even though the majority of the members of a society chooses to ignore or even destroy a minority group, can this be seen as right, good, and proper because the majority agrees? Do the fundamental needs of the minority cease to exist because the majority denies their existence? Indeed, they do not. Although human history is replete with examples of the enslavement, torture, and decimation of peoples, this proves only that human rights can, have been, and continue to be violated—not that human rights do not exist.

It is only because human rights exist independently of either law or public opinion that blacks *justly* can claim equal rights with whites, that women *justly* can claim equal rights with men, and that the weak *justly* can claim equal rights with the strong.

CONCLUSION

It is not in the exciting and dramatic areas of health care that nurses are most likely to transgress the human rights of patients, clients, and their families. Because decisions made in these areas are somewhat out of the ordinary, they are more obvious; we are acutely aware of their importance. It is not because our decisions in these areas are always right (should I initiate CPR?), but because we clearly recognize their significance that we tend to think more carefully about them.

It is in our ordinary, day-to-day contacts with patients or clients that we are most likely to fail to respect them as human beings. We are too busy or too caught up in "important" technicalities to take time to discover and respect the humanity of each individual. Respecting persons in small matters requires sensitivity to their human needs and presents a tremendous challenge for nurses.

NOTES

1. Berkley, George. "A Treatise Concerning the Principles of Human Knowledge," in A. C. Fraser, ed. *The Works of George Berkley* (Clarendon Press, Oxford, 1901) Vol. 1, Part 1, p. 1r.
2. *Ibid.*
3. Descartes, Rene. "Principles of Philosophy," in *The Philosophical Works of Descartes,* translated by E. S. Haldane and G. R. T. Ross (Cambridge University Press, 1938) Vol. 1, pp. 239–240.
4. Dubos, Rene. *So Human An Animal* (Charles Scribner's Sons, New York, 1968) p. 67.
5. Hart, H. L. A. "Are There Any Natural Rights?" in A. I. Melden. *Human Rights* (Wadsworth Publishing Company, Belmont, California, 1970).
6. Kant, Immanuel. "Introduction to the Elements of Justice," in *The Metaphysical Elements of Justice,* translated by John Ladd (Bobbs-Merrill, Indianapolis, Indiana, 1965).

7. Bandman, Bertram. "Option Rights and Subsistence Rights," in Elsie L. Bandman and Bertram Bandman, eds. *Bioethics and Human Rights* (Little, Brown, Boston, 1978) p. 51.

8. Ramsey, Paul. *The Patient as Person* (Yale University Press, New Haven, 1970) p. 133.

9. Anonymous, "Epitaph," in Louis Untermeyer, ed. *A Concise Treasury of Great Poems* (Perma Books, New York, 1953).

10. *Ibid.*

11. Kung, Hans. *On Being a Christian,* translated by Edward Quinn (Doubleday, New York, 1976) p. 181.

12. Adams, John, in a letter to Mary Warren, April 16, 1776.

13. *De Republica,* III, 22.23.

14. *Concordia Discordantium Canonum,* I.D., 1, praef.

15. *De Jure Belli et Pacis,* II, 3.6.

16. Wellman, Carl. *Morals and Ethics* (Scott, Foresman, Glenville, Illinois, 1975) p. 240.

17. *Ibid.*

18. Holmes, Oliver Wendell. *The Common Law* (Little, Brown, Boston, 1881) Chapter 6.

19. Holland, Thomas. *Elements of Jurisprudence* (Clarendon Press, Oxford, 1924) Chapters 7 and 8.

20. Llewellyn, Karl. *Jurisprudence* (University of Chicago Press, Illinois, 1962).

21. Salamond, John. *Jurisprudence* (Sweet and Maxwell, London, 1920) 6th Edition, Chapter X.

22. Vinogradoff, Paul. *Collected Papers* (Clarendon Press, Oxford, 1928) Vol. II, Chapter 20.

23. *Ibid.*

24. May, William F. "The Right to Die and the Obligation to Care," in David H. Smith, ed. *No Rush to Judgment* (Poynter Center, Indiana University, 1977) p. 68.

25. Davis, Anne and Mila Aroskar. *Ethical Dilemmas and Nursing Practice* (Appleton-Century-Crofts, New York, 1978) p. 46.

26. Kierkegaard, Soren. "Attack Upon 'Christendom'." in *A Kierkegaard Anthology,* translated and edited by Robert Bretall (The Modern Library, New York, 1946) p. 446.

2

The Commitment of Rights: Responsibility

Leah Curtin

*"As if it harmed me, giving others the same chances and rights
as myself . . . As if it were not indispensable to my own
rights that others possess the same."*

Walt Whitman, *Thought*

In an ideal world, all people's rights are respected. Whatever your age, status, race, occupation or religion, your rights are respected simply because you are a human being. This is what our forefathers meant when they wrote, "We hold these truths to be self-evident, that all men are created equal . . .".

However, in the real world some people are more respected, some are less respected, and some are not respected at all. Does this mean that some humans do not have rights or does it mean that we do not respect the rights of some humans? Respecting rights means that we assume certain obligations toward other human beings: the mirror image of rights is duties. Just as the image in the mirror is not the person but a reflection of the person, so a duty is not a right but a reflection of what a right entails. If people do not like what they see in the mirror, they may avoid mirrors or even break them. However, this behavior will not change what is. So it is with rights. We all want them for ourselves but we are afraid to take a good look at their mirror image, duties. We might not like what we see. Whether we like it or not, every right has its price.[1]

LOGICAL AND MORAL CORRELATIVITY

Each fundamental right carries with it corollary duties that impinge on one's self as well as on others. That is, when claiming the right to life, I am saying that others have a duty to respect my life and that I have a duty to

17

respect my own life. Such formulations involve the concepts of logical and moral correlativity.[2]

Logical correlativity refers to those obligations imposed on others by my right. That is, if I have a right to be alive, it is logical to hold that others have a duty at least to refrain from killing me.

On the other hand, *moral correlativity* refers to my responsibilities as a right holder. That is, if I claim the right to be and to remain alive, I impose a duty on myself to take reasonable precautions to protect and preserve my own life. I cannot both claim and negate a right at the same time.

Balancing Logical and Moral Correlativity

As we have come to understand the needs of human beings, so we have come to understand the demands of human rights. That is, as our knowledge grows, we are more capable of understanding human needs, of predicating fundamental rights, and of understanding the duties these rights entail.

For example, if I have a right to life, then I clearly have a right to at least enough food to keep me alive. If I have a right to adequate nourishment, others not only have a duty to refrain from starving me, but also may have a duty to provide at least enough food to keep me alive. However, this extension of the duties of others (logical correlativity) is contingent on at least four factors:

1. *The degree to which individuals are capable of providing for their own needs* (moral correlativity), in this case, food. That is, you have no obligation to provide for me what I can provide for myself. If I can provide for myself and refuse to do so, you are not violating my right: I am negating my own claim. However, to the degree that I cannot provide for myself, your obligations toward me increase.

2. *The degree to which others are able to fulfill these obligations without violating their own rights.* That is, you are not obliged to provide for me what you need for yourself. You may *choose* to sacrifice your life for mine, but you have no obligation to do so.

3. *The existence of claims prior to this claim.* That is, if two people who are in equal need of food and who are equally incapable of providing their own food, come to you and you have enough food to feed only one of them without starving yourself, the one who comes to you first has the prior claim.

4. *The presence of a duty that is higher than the duty to fulfill this need.* For example, you not only have no obligation to give me the food your children need to live, but you have a duty to refrain from doing so. That is, you have a greater duty to your children than you do to a stranger.

DUTIES IN PERSONUM AND DUTIES IN REM

Although human rights impose duties on all human beings, certain persons have higher claims on other persons according to the relationships between them as determined by the requirements of roles assumed in life. For example, all adults have responsibilities to all human beings, but they have a greater obligation to children because, to some extent, children are incapable of exercising the duties of moral correlativity. For example, although all drivers are required to exercise prudence in driving, they are required to take special precautions around school buses.

Although I have a general duty to provide, to the extent that I reasonably can, for the welfare of all children, I have a specific duty to care for my own children. My duty to care for my own children is a duty of me in particular to provide for my children.[3] It is my obligation and this duty does not fall on others or on society unless I am incapable of fulfilling it.

General duties, that is, the duties of all human beings toward all other human beings, are called duties *in rem*.[4] Specific duties, that is, the duties of a particular person to another identifiable person or group of persons, are called duties *in personum*.[5]

The various roles one assumes in life increase one's duties and they may raise the level of one's duties. For example, although all citizens may have a general duty to provide health care in the proportion necessary to the life and well-being of others (this duty may be discharged through public funding of educational programs, hospitals, clinics, and home care agencies), they have no personal duty to provide nusing services. Nurses in general assume a personal duty to provide nursing services to the public. As an individual nurse, I have a duty *in personum* to provide nursing care to a particular patient or group of patients by virtue of the direct relationship between us. My duty to this patient or group of patients is of a higher order than is my duty to the general public because it is a duty of me in particular to these specific, identifiable persons. Thus, for example, the head nurse on a hospital floor legitimately may refuse to accept more patients if she cannot care for them properly: her general duty to the incoming patients is not yet a duty *in personum*.

Although a personal duty usually is of a higher order than is a general duty (it takes precedence in decision making), this is not always the case.[6] The decisive factor is the importance or rank of the rights involved. For example, an emergency room nurse caring for a violent patient who has taken PCP (angel dust) is justified in taking action to prevent this patient from returning to the public streets until his behavior is nonviolent. Even though the patient insists on leaving, and even though the nurse has a duty *in personum* to respect the human rights of this particular, identifiable person, and even though the nurse's duty is to provide direct care to him, her duty *in rem* to the welfare of the general public takes precedence. Why? Because the rights to life and bodily integrity of unspecified members of the general public is of a higher order than is this particular patient's right to freedom of action. However, one must take great care when exercising such discretionary judgment and always be aware of the fact that it involves transgressing this patient's rights: that is, one must have good reason to so act and one may not violate any other of his rights.[7]

Discussion

The concept of human rights comes alive only when it is applied to specific people and specific situations. It is very easy, and sounds quite noble, to espouse the concept of human rights in general—probably because it is quite easy to ignore the general duties attached to these rights. In the past, it was easier to identify duties toward specific individuals because access to information about the needs and sufferings of all humanity was limited. Today, the news media bring such information to us in our homes, our workplaces and even in our cars. Moreover, human misery is reported on such a vast scale that we are overwhelmed by its magnitude. Even when we recognize a duty to help, and we sincerely want to fulfill that duty, we are stymied by the size, complexity, and number of human needs.

Such massive claims are beyond the capacity of any one person to fulfill. Thus, a just society, one that values human rights, responds to such needs collectively by establishing organized methods for dealing with human need on a grand scale, for example, through public welfare and disaster relief agencies. If a problem is such that even the collective efforts of an entire nation are insufficient to meet the needs, nations band together in international efforts through such bodies as the United Nations and the International Red Cross.

These efforts are right, good, proper, and necessary. However, we have a tendency to regard them as sufficient to human need. Because we have fulfilled our duty *in rem,* we tend to feel a reduced responsibility to meet our duties *in personum.* In other words, "let someone else do it," or "society will take care of them." For some reason, we often think that our inability personally to relieve the victims of famine in India is just cause for our ignoring the needs of our next door neighbor.

Sometimes we carry this line of thinking farther, expecting society to assume all of our personal duties. For example, "Social Security will meet my parents' needs" or "Aid to Dependent Children will meet my children's needs." We forget that this is an obligation of me in particular to specific, identifiable persons. Others are obliged only to the extent that I am truly incapable of fulfilling my obligations and then only to the extent that they reasonably can fulfill these obligations in light of the prior or higher claims on them.

Unfortunately, one of the results of an increased understanding of the dynamics of human behavior is an increased tendency to deny personal responsibility. In his recent book, *Whatever Became of Sin?,* psychiatrist Karl Menninger explores this phenomenon and, in effect, concludes that an understanding of the factors we *cannot* control has led us to deny our responsibility to control the factors we *can* control.[8] In more scientific language, Dr. Menninger expressed the sentiment of a song made famous by Anna Russell in the 1930s:

> At three I had a feeling of
> Ambivalence toward my brothers.
> And so it follows naturally
> I poisoned all my lovers.
> But now I'm happy; I have learned
> The lesson this has taught;
> That everything I do that's wrong
> Is someone else's fault.[9]

This hardening of our personal moral sense (personal response to duty) can have calamitous results: because people become frustrated with irresponsibility, even justifiable needs can be ignored. Only as each individual meets personal obligations can respect for human rights (our own and others') be preserved.

BALANCING RIGHTS AND DUTIES

At times, we protect our own rights inappropriately at the expense of the rights of others. However, some of us have too little regard for our own rights—those things that are our just due. For example, a very young nurse who had worked 16 hours at a local hospital was asked by her supervisor to remain for yet another shift. It was not an emergency situation, but the supervisor needed someone to fill in for a nurse who was ill. The young nurse was exhausted, functioning at a very low level, and knew this. She justly deserved some sleep; the patients justly deserved good nursing care. The nurse's right to adequate rest and the patients' rights to adequate care are of a higher order than is the right of the employer to the young nurse's services. In this particular situation, some other nurse (perhaps one on vacation or one on a day off) had a greater obligation to care for the patients than did the young nurse. The supervisor was obliged to find that other nurse.

On the other hand, even though recreation is recognized as a human need, a nurse justly may be called in to work on a day off if the situation warrants her presence. A nurse freely has assumed the role of nurse and has assumed obligations to meet certain fundamental human needs. Although a nurse has a right to adequate recreation, the needs of patients and the rights of her employer to her services are paramount under some conditions, certainly under disaster or emergency conditions. If a need is acute, lesser needs are secondary. Hence, if patient acuity is high, staffing is poor, and nurses are in short supply, the nurse has a duty *in personum* to those patients and to that hospital; her plans for recreation will have to be put off for another day.

To extend the discussion of balancing rights and duties, and to understand why some rights take precedence over others, let us examine the following situation reported in the news media. A young boy living in Florida was injured in a minor accident; his forearm was lacerated. His mother, even though she did not have the money to pay for treatment, took him to the closest physician's office for medical care. In due course, the physician cleansed the wound and stitched the laceration. When the physician demanded immediate payment, the mother was unable to pay. The physician, therefore, removed the stitches from the child's arm and sent mother and child away. The boy was treated later in an emergency room, and the physician's conduct was censured by his local medical society as a breach of professional ethics.[10]

Was the medical society justified in its censure of this physician's conduct? As a human being, is the physician not free to choose his own course of action? Do health professionals not have a right to just recompense for their labors? Although this physician's measures were drastic, were they wrong?

Analysis

This child's right to bodily integrity conflicted with the physician's right to just recompense for his services. This was not a matter of life and death; the physician could have referred the patient to a clinic or emergency room for treatment. He did not do so, presumably because he did not know the mother had no money.

When people present themselves at a place of business, they have a duty to pay a reasonable amount for the service they desire or need. By presenting herself and her child at the physician's office, the woman entered into an implied contract with this physician. Moreover, this physician's office was not the only place where medical services could be obtained; the community provided and paid for health care services through free clinics and through a general hospital emergency room. However, for unknown reasons, the mother did not use these facilities.

The fact is that the woman did present her child for treatment and the physician did treat the child. If the woman had gone to a department store to buy a television set on credit and had not been able to pay for it, the owner of the store would have been justified in repossessing the television set. Can medical care be seen in the same light? Apparently the physician thought it could. He "repossessed" his services.

A physician, however, by virtue of the role he has chosen freely, assumes certain duties, among which is the duty to refrain from harming a patient. By removing the stitches from this boy's arm, the doctor increased the child's pain, further aggravated the wound, and subjected the boy to a greater risk of infection, not to mention the mental trauma he inflicted on both mother and child.

Moreover, the physician had a duty *in personum* to respect the humanity of this child. In this case, he treated the child like an object and his body like a television set that could be repossessed. The right of a laborer to his wages is not on the same level as a person's right to bodily integrity. Moreover, the right to just recompense is not on a par with the right to be treated as a human being. Because other medical services were available, the physician might have been justified in referring this patient to another source. The physician failed in his duty as a human being and in his duty as a physician.

Professions in general hold privileged places in society by virtue of the special knowledge possessed by their members and the value of this knowledge to the welfare of the public. With membership in a profession come certain privileges and responsibilities, among which are public trust and the duty to protect the public's interest.[11] If a member of a profession acts at variance with the welfare of either the general public or of a particular member of the public who seeks services, the entire profession is affected by a diminution of public trust and respect. This physician did not act in the best interest of the patient; hence, the medical society not only was justified but was obliged to censure his conduct.

CONCLUSION

Each person has rights; for these rights to be operative, the duties of logical and moral correlativity must be fulfilled. Duties assume two forms: general and personal. Hence, all persons have obligations to one another (duties *in rem*); these duties become personal duties according to particular individuals' just and direct claims on other persons (duties *in personum*). A society is a collection of individuals; its value system is a reflection of values held by its members. Each citizen's response to personal duties affects the value that a nation places on human beings.

Health professionals freely assume additional duties toward others when they enter their professions. All duties, including these special duties, are created and surrounded by the rights of human beings. Although human rights provide the foundation for the patient–professional relationship, duties provide form for this relationship.

NOTES

1. Bandman, Bertram. "Option Rights and Subsistence Rights," in Elsie and Bertram Bandman, eds. *Bioethics and Human Rights* (Little, Brown, Boston, 1978) p. 53.

2. Bandman, Bertram. "Some Legal, Moral, and Intellectual Rights of Children," *Educational Theory* (Summer 1977) Vol. 27, p. 169.

3. Wellman, Carl. *Morals and Ethics* (Scott, Foresman, Glenview, Illinois, 1975) p. 249.

4. Austin, John. *Lectures in Jurisprudence* (John Murray Company, London, 1885) Vol. 1, Lectures 12, 15 and 17. It must be noted that Mr. Austin equated rights with relative

duties. Therefore, he spoke of *rights in rem* and *rights in personum.* I have borrowed his notion of relative duties and his nomenclature, but I consider rights and duties to be separate entities.

5. *Ibid.*

6. London, Perry. "The Ethics of Behavior Control," in Richard Wertz, ed. *Ethical and Social Issues in Biomedicine* (Prentice-Hall, Englewood Cliffs, New Jersey, 1973) p. 162.

7. *Ibid.*

8. Menninger, Karl. *Whatever Became of Sin?* (Hawthorne Books, New York, 1973).

9. Levenstein, Aaron. "Days of Stress," *Supervisor Nurse* (September 1979) Vol. 10, No. 9, p. 69.

10. "Doctor Censured," news story in *The Cincinnati Enquirer,* February 9, 1979.

11. Hauerwas, Stanley. "Medicine as a Tragic Profession," in David Smith, ed. *No Rush to Judgment* (Indiana University Foundation, Bloomington, Indiana, 1978) pp. 62–63.

3

Is Health Care a Right?

Sr. Francesca Lumpp

"The Lord leads the just through right paths."

Psalm 92

There are three necessary parts to a thorough ethical study of the question, "Is health care a right?" The first involves a distinction between rights *to* health care services and human rights *in* health care.[1] The second requires an exploration of the notion that while some health care services may be a right, health itself is more a duty than a right.[2] The third consideration includes the rights of persons already under treatment to services adequate to meet their needs.

A Right to Health Care Services

Considerations of a right to health care services generally involve questions of access to the health care system[3] and may include access to some of the highly sophisticated medical–technological advances.[4] Although largely a function of social policy,[5] it involves significant obligations for the various health professions.[6]

The Function of Justice

In his book, *Who Shall Live?*, Victor Fuchs contends that everyone cannot have all of the health or all of the medical care he wants or even needs. "Highest quality care for all is 'pie in the sky.' We have to choose."[7] When we affirm a certain value in society (health) and try to assure it through policy decisions regarding allocation of resources, we inevitably come into conflict

25

with other needs and values.[8] Thus, Fuchs concludes that we, as a nation and as individuals, have to choose between health care services and other desirable goals. That is, we must decide where to put most of our money—in health, education, welfare, urban renewal, the arts, defense, and so forth.[9]

To the extent that the provision of health care services is seen as a function of social policy, it behooves us to examine public policy choices regarding the allocation of resources to health care. Essentially, "public policy is whatever governments choose to do or not to do."[10] What has the United States government done or failed to do to provide health care services to its populace?

To a certain extent, the government has tried to guarantee all of its citizens some degree of protection from certain health hazards. Among our earliest laws are statutes regarding quarantine and immunization. During the Roosevelt era (the 1930s and 1940s), the scope of government involvement in health broadened. Phrases such as "the right to adequate medical care" and "the opportunity to achieve and enjoy good health" were articulated and designated as governmental responsibilities. Subsequently, each president and Congress has explored health care issues until, in the 1960s, significant legislation, in the form of Medicare and Medicaid, was passed. Although this legislation greatly increased governmental involvement and, indeed, provided many health care benefits for certain groups of citizens, a comprehensive, government-paid health care program has yet to be enacted. Thus, it seems that certain classes of citizens in specific circumstances have a qualified right to health care services.

Joel Feinberg, in his article on the nature and value of rights, asserts that "having rights enables us to 'stand up like men,' to look others in the eye and feel in some fundamental way the equal of everyone."[11] Although illness challenges a person's physical and emotional freedom, it should not make an economic or psychological beggar of the individual. However, our means of helping the sick are not unlimited; they are relatively costly and compete with other goods.[12]

"Hegel spoke of tragedy as the conflict of right with right; what makes any protagonist's situation tragic is that he inevitably has to choose between wrong and wrong."[13] The problems presented by the allocation of health resources at the expense of other social goods are so difficult that they are "almost, if not completely incorrigible to moral reasoning" or "to rational determination."[14] Moreover, the health needs of a population are served better by good sanitation, decent housing, adequate nutrition, and public education than by the provision of either preventive or illness care.[15] In addition, it is known that the quality of the environment has a direct impact on the health of the public. Thus, to provide health care services at the expense of programs of social welfare or environmental protection would be counterproductive.

Nonetheless, health care services are valuable and essential to most, if not all people at some point in their lives. They are not purchased as luxuries and they are not desirable in themselves (who really wants an injection of a vaccine or an operation in the sense of what he prefers to do?); rather, health care services are seen as necessary to the continued life and well-being of individuals.[16] The principle of distributive justice demands the delivery of valuable and essential services to the whole community. Thus, it is necessary to define and limit those health care services essential to the welfare of individuals and to determine how they can be distributed most equitably.

When ethicists speak of distributing a scarce resource, they refer to the requirements of justice. Perelman enumerates six approaches to the principle of distributive justice: (1) to each the same thing; (2) to each according to his merits; (3) to each according to his works; (4) to each according to his needs; (5) to each according to his rank; and (6) to each according to his legal entitlement.[17] Let us expand on each of these approaches to determine which one is most appropriate when consideration is given to the distribution of health resources.

Justice renders to each the same thing. This approach requires that all people be treated the same way without regard to distinguishing particulars. We know that different people, often because of circumstances beyond their control, are at high risk of disease and are exposed to serious health hazards. For example, at high risk are elderly persons, people who live in areas of high pollution, the poor, and so forth. Moreover, some diseases are more life-threatening than others and some chronic disabilities require more resources for their treatment than others. If we accept the case for equal access to health care services while recognizing that such services are not unlimited, it seems only fair to discriminate according to categories of illness, risks to health, and basic needs for care.[18]

Justice renders to each according to his merits. This approach to justice does not demand universal equality; rather it bases access to care on the personal merit of individuals. That is, it uses as a criterion personal excellence. This approach may be appropriate in some areas (*e.g.,* excellence in education is rewarded with higher grades), but its merit in health care is problematic. Precisely how would we go about correlating demonstrated virtue with the receipt of privileged medical treatment as a reward?[19] On the social level, it could mean allocation of resources for the care of lung cancer victims only to those who do not smoke . . . or treatment of accident victims only if they were not the cause of an accident (*e.g.,* the drunken driver would not be treated). Shall we withhold treatment for syphilis from those who are promiscuous? Clearly, on this level alone, the difficulties are enormous, not to mention impractical. On the individual level, the problems are even greater. How could a health professional judge the personal merit of an individual needing his or her services? According to whose values? By what authority shall a health professional become the arbiter of personal excellence or virtue among those needing care? If it were possible to conceive of an individual who would be a perfectly just judge,[20] it is extremely unlikely that any or all health professionals would come up to this standard.

Justice renders to each according to his works. This approach does not call for equal treatment, but rather proportional treatment according to one's social utility. The application of a canon of social productivity assumes, *a priori*, that individual citizens merely are means or instruments to the welfare of society. It ignores a concern for merit (*e.g.*, the elderly may not be productive anymore even though they contributed work and taxes for fifty or more years) or for need (*e.g.*, the "useful" person with a broken finger would be treated while the elderly man with pneumonia would be abandoned). These obvious inequities, among others, lead us to reject the notion of social utility as a criterion for access to health services.

Justice renders to each according to his legal entitlement. Such a formulation presupposes that law is just—a dangerous assumption. If, indeed, the laws of a country are so formulated as to protect the rights of individual citizens, and provided that these laws assure similar treatment for similar problems regardless of patients' socioeconomic status, and provided that a just judge could be found to determine that this utopia exists, only then could one rely on legal entitlement alone to determine a person's right to access to the health care system. As this world is imperfect at best, we can reject this approach to social justice.

Justice renders to each according to his need. This approach comes closest to meeting the demands of human rights. For example, it recognizes the social imperative inherent in the articulation of a right to life. Although individuals are expected to take reasonable precautions to protect and preserve their own rights (moral correlativity), others in society are seen as having a duty to protect the lives of others insofar as the individuals themselves no longer can do so. It implies that a basic minimum of resources must be assured to each person according to his need.

Gene Outka, in his article "Social Justice and Equal Access to Health Care," elaborates on the concept of justice that renders to each person according to his needs. He puts the need for health care in this category and refers to it as an essential need, one that is arbitrarily given rather than acquired.[21] Moreover, the term "natural lottery" often is applied to the distribution of essential needs. Why is one child born sighted and another blind? Why does one neighbor have cancer and another not? An unknown fate, a natural lottery, puts some persons in a state of having essential needs that must be met, while other persons may never have these needs.[22]

Outka differentiates between having universal basic needs met (*e.g.*, food, shelter, *etc.*) and having essential health needs met. He claims that basic, universal needs can be planned for appropriately while essential health needs are arbitrary—they arrive unplanned for and uninvited. Lastly, Outka suggests that the concepts of justice and charity overlap. He refers to charity as *agape*; it urges us to give equal consideration to the essential needs of each member of the human community.[22]

Distribution of Scarce Medical Resources

In the determination of public policy about health care, the principles of justice are helpful. To a certain extent, they already have proven useful to those involved in and concerned about the equitable distribution of scarce, life-saving medical resources, particularly in the area of renal disease.

However, let us consider the following situation. A nurse visited a well-known university medical center to tour the kidney dialysis and transplant unit. Her tour was conducted by the head nurse of the unit. "How do you know who is next in line for a kidney transplant?" asked the visitor. "I just call the next name on the list," the head nurse replied. The following dialogue ensued:

Visitor: "Who makes up the list?"

Head Nurse: "The physician in charge of the unit."

Visitor: "How is the list compiled?"

Head Nurse: "I don't know."

Visitor: "If the next person can't be reached, what do you do?"

Head Nurse: "Call the next name."

Visitor: "Do you ever question how the list is drawn up?"

Head Nurse: "No, I just follow doctor's orders."

Is it a good thing for the head nurse to be so uninvolved in the part she plays in the distribution of this scarce medical resource? Perhaps it is, because then she can be totally impartial. On the other hand, it may not be a good idea, for then she would be more concerned about the justice of trying to reach the person who is next in line: she would try harder before skipping over this person and proceeding to the following name.

James Childress in his article, "Who Shall Live When Not All Can Live?" suggested that two factors be considered. Given that each person under consideration is in equal need of a kidney transplant, those who are the best medical risks (i.e., who are most likely to be able to survive the operation and in whom the transplantation is most likely to be successful) should be given first consideration. Among those who are medically acceptable, each should be given equal consideration by means of a lottery.[23] Childress warns against social criteria or wealth entering the process and goes on to explain that "first-come-first-served" is a form of the natural lottery discussed earlier. To preserve justice, he would allow no deviation from this order.[24]

Would such considerations be helpful to the head nurse of the dialysis unit? If she seriously were concerned, the following would occur: (1) the nurse would question the compilation of the list to assure herself that it had been drawn up on a first-come-first-served basis (given that the medical criteria were met); (2) she would try conscientiously to reach the person next in line on the list; (3) she would realize the injustice of favoritism, wealth and power insidiously entering the selection process and do what was within her power to avoid them.

Albert Jonsen reported the findings of a panel of experts who were considering the ethical problems involved in the selection of patients to receive a totally implantable artificial heart (TIAH). Two major conclusions were reached. First, as substantial amounts of public funds have been used in development of TIAH, it should be broadly available. Its availability should not be based on the person's ability to pay. Second, after the medical criteria have been satisfied, random selection by some form of lottery should be strictly enforced.[25]

Health as a Duty

Even with acknowledgment that some health care services meet the essential needs of people, determination that all persons have a right to them and provision for the equitable distribution of scarce resources, all the demands of justice are not met. To meet these demands, we must approach the concept of preventive care from the perspective of enabling persons to care for themselves. If "having rights enables us . . . to look others in the eye and feel in some fundamental way the equal of everyone,"[26] it follows that exercising rights means that we know we have some measure of control over our destiny.

If we fail to make serious attempts to educate the public about health hazards and health promoting behaviors, we are keeping people from fulfilling their own responsibilities for their personal health. The words of Ivan Illich clearly demonstrate this concern: "Once a society is so organized that medicine can transform people into patients because they are unborn, newborn, menopausal, or at some 'age of risk,' the population inevitably loses some of its autonomy to its healers."[27]

There is mounting evidence that people's life styles are one of the key determinants of their health status. People who eat regularly, sleep at least seven hours a night, keep their weight down, do not smoke, do not drink excessively, and exercise daily will live longer, healthier lives.[28] Moreover, significant data have been amassed that indicate an improved health status among those who marry, do not divorce, have about two children and who are geographically stable.[29] Although people generally are unlikely to place health at the top of their priority list (unless, of course, they are ill), they must know what can promote and protect their health before they can or will choose to act accordingly.

As we articulate a right to at least a decent minimum of health services, it becomes abundantly clear that the feasibility of the right will depend greatly on individual citizens accepting a large amount of responsibility for their own health status. We must recognize that along with an increase in governmental spending in this area, there is likely to be an increased demand for individuals to assume more responsibility for their own health precisely because tax payers may object to paying for the avoidable afflictions of others.*

Only a certain percentage of ill health is a result of chance; the rest is the result of choice—choice for which each individual is responsible.

The Right to Adequate Nursing Care

Nurses offer essential health care services, and nursing, like health care generally, suffers distribution problems throughout the country. In addressing the overall problem, we must emphasize the ideal of justice and equality in distribution of nursing care. Although all people in need of nursing care have an equal right to it, the pragmatics of meeting multiple and competing needs can place nurses in difficult situations. For example, let us consider the following situation.

A weary night nurse entered the hospital cafeteria one morning, weighed down from physical work, worry, and the responsibility of having cared for a group of very ill patients. Before she left the nursing unit, she telephoned a former teacher and asked her to meet her for coffee. After a brief greeting, she told her friend this story. "During shift report last night, I was made aware of how many very ill patients were on the unit. One was a dying man who had orders that read, 'suction q 15 min'. When I assessed the needs of other patients, I knew I couldn't possibly suction the dying man every 15 minutes. However, I arranged my work so that I could be with him every hour to suction him, position him, and try to be present to his wife. About five-thirty this morning, his wife came to the nursing desk sobbing 'He's gone, he's gone!' She was alone with him when he died. I tried to comfort her, but now I wonder if I gave him the best care I could have given him. Had I suctioned him every 15 minutes, would he have lived longer? Would his wife have been more prepared for his death? I know I didn't waste a minute last night. It was a question of priorities."

Did this dying man have a right to the nurse's almost continuous presence during his last hours? What about the needs and rights of the other patients? In the face of a nursing shortage, nurses must learn early to set priorities fairly in rendering care so they can make decisions without guilt. We must recognize the fact that the demand for nursing care makes it impossible for us to render a constant ministry to all who need us. Whenever appropriate, we must use "nurse-extending" concepts. That is, whenever possible we must promote self-care or enlist the aid of families and significant others in caring for their

---

*See, for example, Marc Lalonde, *A New Perspective on the Health of Canadians,* a Government of Canada Green Paper, 1974. Lalonde, who was Minister of National Health and Welfare, received the Dana Award in recognition of his work on this internationally acclaimed document.

loved ones. Staffing, scheduling, and budgeting procedures must be examined carefully to avoid understaffing in a unit with many acutely ill patients.

A study of the principles of justice can help us recognize the needs of all but it also should help us realize that those with the greatest needs take precedence. Among those who have equal needs, the first-come-first-served approach can help us survive to function another day. An appreciation of justice will help us realize the dangers of favoritism or socioeconomic criteria in the delivery of our own services to specified groups of patients. In accepting our limitations, we can find solace in the Book of Micah: "This is what Yahweh asks of you, only this: to act justly, to love tenderly, and to walk humbly with your God."[30]

Suggestion for Improving Health Care Distribution

Over the years, the greatest opposition to any type of government provision and, thus, control of health care has come from those in the ranks of the health professions, most notably from the American Medical Association. The A.M.A. opposes (1) any interference with the fee-for-service form of payment; (2) the establishment of a system of payment that would allot a certain amount of money for the care of a defined population; and (3) the establishment of a system of salaried physicians in institutions (beyond the specialties of x-ray, laboratory, and emergency room). By and large, this opposition is based on the physicians' legal right to market their services for a fee that they determine is fair and to determine their own work schedule.

Moreover, some prominent ethicists have argued that the onus to deliver health care services rests solely on society; professionals *per se* have no particular obligation to meet the needs of the community. It is contradictory to claim that society must provide health care services if professionals have no particular obligation to meet the need for their services. Health professionals must share this responsibility because, quite simply put, they are the only ones who actually can provide these services.

Clearly, to begin to meet the needs of the whole public, institutional reorganization and reform are necessary. Gene Outka suggests three such institutional reforms:

1. The problem of geographic maldistribution could be solved in part by the offering of incentive subsidies to health professionals and hospitals to provide service in poverty and underserved areas. Physicians' licensing could be controlled so that an overabundance of physicians would not occur in certain areas.

2. Provision must be made in any national health plan to meet the special needs of those who require more services than the specified limit.

3. The entry points to the health care system should be more flexible. The present fee-for-service, physician-only entry point does not meet the essential needs of the whole populace. Although health maintenance organizations are

struggling, we need an organized system of care to deliver services to a defined population for a fixed amount of payment per person per family.[31]

Another author, Charles Fried, suggests the following:

1. There should be a positive approach to maternal–infant care; a child should have a chance for a strong beginning.

2. There should be more reasonable and humane limits for the care of the dying. Emphasis should be placed on worthy surroundings rather than technological intervention.

3. The agreed-upon limit to services should be flexible.

4. Problems not strictly within the scope of the health professions, for example, alcohol and drug addiction, obesity, and smoking, should be viewed as social in nature and the problems handled on a society-wide basis.

5. We should increase the supply of competent, qualified physicians.[32]

Although there also is a shortage of professional nurses, nurses today are better prepared than they have ever been. If nurses and physicians could begin seriously to cooperate and to coordinate their efforts, radical changes could be made in the "entry point" to the health care system. Nurses could do initial screening and see sick persons themselves and refer them to hospitals and physicians as necessary. Broadening the entry point would make care available to more people and it would offer people more options for care.

Simple answers are not to be found to the complex problems posed by a right to health care services. Most probably, we never will solve all the problems involved in the distribution of scarce resources. However, a strict regard for justice accompanied by a willingness to work together as a community will help us come close to meeting this goal.

NOTES

1. McGarvey, Michael. "Some Considerations Regarding Ethics and the Right to Health Care," in Elsie Bandman and Bertram Bandman, eds. *Bioethics and Human Rights* (Little, Brown, Boston, 1978), p. 363.

2. Kass, Leon. "Regarding the End of Medicine and the Pursuit of Health," *The Public Interest* (Summer 1975) No. 40, p. 39.

3. Kuskey, Garvan F. "Health Care, Human Rights and Government Interventions: A Critical Appraisal," in Robert Hunt and John Arras, eds. *Ethical Issues in Modern Medicine* (Mayfield Publishing Company, Palo Alto, California, 1977) p. 466.

4. Rescher, Nicholas. "The Allocation of Exotic Lifesaving Therapy," *Ethics* (April 1969) Vol. 79.

5. McGarvey, *op. cit.,* p. 364.

6. Curtin, Leah. "Is There a Right to Health Care?" *American Journal of Nursing* (March 1980) Vol. 90, No. 3, p. 464.

7. Fuchs, Victor R. *Who Shall Live?* (Basic Books, New York, 1974) p. 7.

8. Curtin, *op. cit.,* p. 463.

9. Fuchs, *op. cit.,* p. 17.

10. Dye, Thomas R. *Understanding Public Policy,* 2nd Edition (Prentice-Hall, Englewood Cliffs, New Jersey, 1975) p. 1.

11. Feinberg, Joel. "The Nature and Value of Rights," *The Journal of Value Inquiry,* 1970, Vol. 4, pp. 243–257.

12. Jonsen, Albert R. "Right to Health Care Services," in Warren T. Reich, ed. *The Encyclopedia of Bioethics* (The Free Press, New York, 1978) p. 629.

13. MacIntyre, Alastair. "How Virtues Become Vices: Values, Medicine and the Social Context," in H. Tristan Englehardt and Stuart Spicker, eds. *Evaluation and Explanation in the Biomedical Sciences* (D. Reidel Publishing Company, Dordrecht, 1975) p. 110.

14. Ramsey, Paul. *The Patient as Person* (Yale University Press, New Haven, 1970) pp. 240, 268.

15. *Cf.* Ginzberg, Eli. "Health, Medicine and Economic Welfare," *Journal of the Mount Sinai Hospital,* Vol. 19, No. 6 (March–April 1953) p. 734.

Lees, D. S. *Health Through Choice* (Institute of Economic Affairs, London, 1961) pp. 55 and 941.

Groves, Harold M. "Economic and Public Finance Aspects of the Medical Care Program," in *Financing a Health Program for America,* Volume 4 of President's Commission on Health Needs of the Nation, *Building America's Health* (Washington, D.C., Superintendent of Documents) p. 143.

16. Klarman, Herbert E. *The Economics of Health* (Columbia University Press, New York, 1965) p. 176.

17. Perelman, Charles. *The Idea of Justice and the Problem of Argument,* translated by John Petrie (Routledge and Kegan Paul, London, 1963).

18. McGarvey, *op. cit.,* p. 365.

19. Outka, Gene. "Social Justice and Equal Access to Health Care," in Thomas Shannon, ed. *Bioethics* (Paulist Press, Ramsey, New Jersey, 1976) p. 380.

20. Firth, R. "Ethical Absolutism and the Ideal Observer," *Philosophy and Phenomenological Research,* Vol. 12 (1952) pp. 317–345.

21. Outka, *op. cit.,* p. 385.

22. *Ibid.,* pp. 373–395.

23. Childress, James. "Who Shall Live When Not All Can Live?" *Soundings,* Vol. LIII (Winter 1970) pp. 339–362.

24. *Ibid.*

25. Jonsen, Albert. "The Totally Implantable Artificial Heart," *Hastings Center Report,* Vol. 3, No. 5 (November 1973) pp. 1–4.

26. Feinberg, *op. cit.,* p. 243.

27. Illich, Ivan. "Excerpts from Medical Nemesis," in Robert Hunt and John Arras, eds. *Ethical Issues in Modern Medicine* (Mayfield Publishing Company, Palo Alto, California, 1977) p. 474.

28. Belloc, Nadia, and Lester Buslow. "Relationship and Physical Status and Health Practices," *Preventive Medicine,* Vol. 1 (March 1972) pp. 409–421.

29. Fuchs, Victor. *Who Shall Live: Health, Economics and Social Choice* (Basic Books, New York, 1975) p. 52.

30. Micah 6:8.

31. Outka, *op. cit.,* pp. 389–392.

32. Fried, Charles. "Equality of Rights in Medicine," in Stanley Reiser, Arthur Dyke, and William Curran, eds. *Ethics in Medicine* (The MIT Press, Cambridge, Massachusetts, 1977) pp. 582–583.

Section II

4

Human Problems: Human Beings

Leah Curtin

"A man is but what he knoweth."

Francis Bacon

Albert Schweitzer once remarked that "good is to know pity, to help others conserve their life, and to spare their suffering . . . [it occurs when] we reach true understanding of ourselves."[1] The Lebanese philosopher, Kahlil Gibran, echoed this thought when he wrote, "You are good when you are one with yourself."[2]

A human being's direct, personal encounters with himself, others and the world constitute what he knows; for him it is reality. Human beings are bombarded continually with sensations; their brains constantly are receiving information from their senses. Both consciously and unconsciously, people choose from among these bits of information those data they think are important.[3] These facts are valued (*i.e.,* assimilated by the knower–valuer) or disvalued (*i.e.,* discarded by the knower–valuer). No particular datum is any more important than any other except to the extent that human beings assign value to it. If the person thinks something is important enough (*i.e.,* if he values it highly), he will investigate it further.[4] This information becomes a part of him. That is, it creates and extends his consciousness, his awareness of his own being and his relationship with the objects and beings in the world.

Human beings, then, perceive, value, investigate, assimilate, and implement knowledge. Although the acts of perceiving, valuing, and knowing are conceptually distinct, they are related in the person. Rational choices are based on factual information, but they always retain a subjective component, that is, choices always involve a value judgment. The concept of choice necessarily involves freedom (the ability to make a choice) and with it, human responsibility for right and wrong action. It is not the faculty of reason alone that is engaged when one is faced with a decision, but the whole being—the unity of knowing and valuing that comprises an individual—is put to the test when human beings make choices, most particularly when they make difficult ethical choices.

HOW TO DISTINGUISH AN ETHICAL PROBLEM

Human beings face many problems and make many choices in their lives, but all the problems are not ethical problems and all the choices are not moral choices. How does one go about distinguishing an ethical problem from any other problem? Perhaps the best way to approach this question is to propose an ethical problem and to identify its unique characteristics.

Let us consider the question, "Should a person with two healthy kidneys be forced to donate one of them to an otherwise healthy person who is in irreversible kidney failure?" Which branch of science is competent to answer this question? Many of the sciences may contribute information, but the answer to the question is not strictly within the competence of the scientific disciplines. Therefore, one of the distinguishing characteristics of an ethical problem is that it cannot be resolved solely through an appeal to empirical data.

Any person seriously approaching the problem of whether a healthy person should be forced to donate a kidney will be puzzled. How much information and what kind of information can support a claim, *pro* or *con?* To save a life is a "good" thing to do. To force surgery on an unwilling and healthy individual is a "bad" thing to do. The person who is ill has a right to life. The person who is healthy has a right to bodily integrity. Conflicts of values and uncertainty about the amount or type of information needed to make a decision are typical of ethical problems. Hence, a second characteristic of an ethical problem is that it is inherently perplexing.

Another quality of an ethical problem is that the answer reached will have a profound and far-reaching effect on one's perception of (1) human beings, (2) relationships among human beings, (3) the relationship of human beings to society, and/or (4) the relationship of human beings to the world.

For example, if the choice is made to force an individual to donate his kidney to another, this choice entails, among other things, the notions that (a) an individual's right to bodily integrity may be violated if another person can benefit from it; (b) an individual's right to life includes the right to require others to undergo painful surgery, some degree of risk and permanent loss of a body part; and (c) health professionals or others in authority can force one person to sacrifice his bodily integrity for the well-being of another person. This one choice involves the concept of human rights, the limits of benevolence and the power of those in authority. It follows that the third identifying characteristic of an ethical problem is that the answer will have profound relevance for several areas of human concern. Moreover, each such decision tends to establish precedent and justification for future activity; it serves as a model for future behavior.

When approaching a particular problem, one can decide whether or not it is an ethical problem by determining whether it has (or lacks) the following characteristics: (1) it does not fall strictly within any one or all of the sciences; (2) it is inherently perplexing (how much and what type of information is needed and which value should be maximized?) and (3) the answer reached will have profound relevance for several areas of human concern.

A DILEMMA DEFINED

Every problem is not an ethical problem and every ethical problem is not a dilemma. *A dilemma is a choice between equally undesirable alternatives.* If the choice is between what one *ought* to do and what one *wants* to do, the person has a problem for which there is an answer. If the choice is between the greater of two goods or the lesser of two evils, one still has only a problem and an answer can be found. In a true dilemma, however, any action taken will result in an unfavorable outcome and/or will constitute a breach of one's duty to another. Some philosophers have referred to dilemma situations as incorrigible to moral reasoning.

A dilemma may not be solvable, but it is resolvable. Even though there is no right or wrong when one is dealing with a choice between two *equally* unfavorable actions, taking no action may be even worse than making the choice.

For example, let us consider a situation for a nurse in an emergency room. The nurse is alone, no other professional is on duty, and no one else is immediately available. If two patients arrive at the same time, one who has severed a major artery and one who has had a heart attack, the nurse has a problem. Both patients are in imminent danger, but only one is in immediate danger. In this case, the nurse stops the hemorrhage from the severed artery before attending to the needs of the heart attack victim. Moreover, she will call for assistance so that both patients can be cared for properly.

However, what will this nurse do if two patients arrive at the same time and each of the patients has severed a major artery, both of them are in shock, and both are in equal need of attention? Each of these patients has equal claim on the nurse and the nurse's clear duty to each patient is to stop the bleeding. No matter what she does, she will fail in her duty to one of them. However, if she fails to act at all, she will violate both patients' rights; she must act—and quickly.

If the patients are conscious and one of them says, "Take care of the other fellow first," the nurse has a way out because this person has chosen to sacrifice himself for another. Should both patients be unconscious, the nurse would know nothing about either one's value system, responsibilities in life, or reasons for living. She knows only that each of them has a vital and pressing need that *must* be met if each is to continue living. What should the nurse do?

She must do the best she can. Although there is no personal right or wrong in the nurse choosing to care for one over the other, a wrong is done. If she refuses to make a choice, both patients will die. By acting to save one of the patients, the nurse will act rightly, but this is little consolation to the patient who dies as a result.

Fortunately, a true dilemma is relatively rare. Ordinarily, one is faced with problems that are difficult, perplexing, often seemingly unresolvable, but actually solvable. The time factors in this case precluded both alternative actions and the gathering and consideration of relevant information. For example, had the nurse had time to call for assistance she would have had a potential solution to the problem. Had the nurse had more information (*e.g.,* that one patient was suffering from an unrelated terminal disease), she could have chosen what she perceived to be the lesser of two evils. The amount of time available can create a dilemma where none would exist otherwise.

LEVELS OF DECISION MAKING

Having the time available to make a decision increases one's responsibility to gather information, to weigh the values involved and to ascertain the possible results of each alternative course of action. People must guard against a tendency to avoid making a choice where one is necessary. Although people should not procrastinate (a mechanism used to avoid responsibility), they also should not be hasty in their judgments (a mechanism to avoid careful reflection). There are levels of immediacy in decision making; however, the fact that decisions must be made immediately in some situations cannot be used to excuse rash actions in other situations. For example, it is justifiable to give treatment in an emergency situation (*i.e.,* when a person is in immediate danger of death) without the patient's informed consent. However, it is not justifiable to do so in situations in which some time (however little) is available. In such cases, the need may be imminent but not immediate. Therefore, time must be taken to explain what could be done, to explore alternative choices with the person, and to discover which alternative most nearly conforms to the person's value system. For example, there are many people who would prefer not to have a hemicorporectomy even though it might prolong their lives and prevent greater suffering.

In general, there are three levels of decision making: (1) *the immediate level,* in which there is no time for reflection; (2) *the intermediate level,* in which there is some time for exploration and reflection; and (3) *the deliberate level,* in which there is adequate time to explore, examine, and reflect in order to reach a rational, thoughtful decision. Although often inadvertently or even purposely circumvented, the deliberate level of decision making is by far the most common. Some people try to avoid making difficult ethical decisions because they are personally taxing, entail great responsibility and require a profound sensitivity to the human rights and values of others.

CONCLUSION

All decisions, including ethical decisions, occur in a context that consists of an inner and outer environment. An inner environment consists of the sum total of one's experiences. A decision reached tomorrow will have behind it more experience than will a decision made today; in particular, it will have behind it the experience of yesterday's decision. In short, people are not fixed; they are enlarged constantly by their own experiences, that is, the limits of their experience are extended daily. Although persons may share the same experiences, their inner environments differ. This difference is derived from the way in which each individual translates experience into readiness for action. However, similar experiences and backgrounds tend to enable persons to understand each other's decisions more fully.

One's outer environment consists of those factors that are extrinsic to the person: the actions and reactions of others, time constraints, material resources. It is improbable that one's external environment will repeat itself exactly. Therefore, the events that modify the setting of a decision are unlikely to be repeated and the operational self brought to decision making cannot be repeated. In this sense, all decisions are unique, but not necessarily unrelated.

Knowledge of one's self arises from experience gained from observation of the world and from experience gained from interaction with other living beings. In relationships with other people, one perceives and identifies their actions and feelings because one has experienced them; one knows them from the inside. That is, one can identify pain, anger, or fear in another person because one has experienced them. One learns the value of such things as compassion by entering the experience directly or, possibly, by identifying with the experience of others. People enlarge their knowledge of themselves and of others through such experiences.

The human ability to organize, translate, and generalize experiences enables people to form and to share general concepts—to postulate scientific theories or to propose ethical norms. That is, the ability to form general concepts enables humans to analyze their world—the world of fact and the world of experience—and to use this analysis to try to improve the conditions of life. The struggle to improve the conditions of life is the driving force behind humanity's search for the right thing to do. To succeed in this search, the ethic developed must link social duty with a sense of each person's individuality. A viable ethic recognizes the social nature of human behavior and provides for individual freedom.

NOTES

1. Schweitzer, Albert, quoted in Erica Anderson, *The Schweitzer Album* (Harper and Row, New York, 1965) p. 43.

2. Gibran, Kahlil. *The Prophet* (Alfred A. Knopf, New York, 1966) p. 64.
3. *Summa Theologica,* 1a–2ae, XXVII, 2, ad2.
4. *Ibid.*

BIBLIOGRAPHY

Bronowski, J. *The Identity of Man.* The Natural History Press, Garden City, New York, 1965.

Camus, Albert. *The Myth of Sisyphus.* Vintage Books, New York, 1955.

Camus, Albert. *The Rebel.* Vintage Books, New York, 1956.

Carnap, Rudolph. "The Rejection of Metaphysics," in Morris Weitz (ed.). *20th Century Philosophy: The Analytic Tradition.* The Free Press, New York, 1966, pp. 206–219.

Dewey, John. *Reconstruction in Philosophy.* Henry Holt and Company, New York, 1942.

Dubos, Rene. *So Human An Animal.* Scribners and Sons, New York, 1968.

Fletcher, Joseph. *Situation Ethics.* Westminster Press, Philadelphia, Pennsylvania, 1966, Chapter 3.

Frankl, Viktor. *Man's Search for Meaning: An Introduction to Logotherapy.* Pocket Books, New York, 1959.

Francoeur, R. T. *Utopian Motherhood.* A. S. Barnes Company, New York, 1972.

Hospers, John. *Human Problems: Problems of Ethics.* Harcourt and Brace, New York, 1972.

Williams, James, "The Moral Philosophers and the Moral Life," in Jesse A. Mann and Gerald F. Kreyche (eds.). *Approaches to Morality.* Harcourt, Brace and World, New York, 1966, pp. 308–325.

Menninger, Karl. *Whatever Happened to Sin?* Hawthorne Books, New York, 1979.

Moore, G. E., "A Defense of Common Sense," in J. H. Muirhead (ed.). *Contemporary British Philosophy,* 2nd ed. The Macmillan Company, London, 1925.

Skinner, B. F. *Beyond Freedom and Dignity.* Alfred A. Knopf, New York, 1971.

Stevenson, C. L., "The Emotive Meaning of Ethical Terms," in Morris Weitz (ed.). *20th Century Philosophy: The Analytic Tradition.* The Free Press, New York, 1966, pp. 236–253.

5

Conscience: Right and Wrong

Leah Curtin

"How shall I go in peace and without sorrow?"

Kahlil Gibran, *The Prophet*

Ethical problems raise two questions for a person: "How can I find an answer that will allow me to be at peace with myself?" and "How can I find an answer that will allow me to be at peace with others?" The answers to these questions are related but distinct. To answer the first question, a person tries to determine the degree of congruity between a particular choice or action and his own perceptions of right and wrong. The criteria used to judge them are internal. That is, the analysis is purely subjective.

However, the answer to the second question is not purely subjective. It involves either a consideration of the duties one person owes another by virtue of commitments made and roles assumed, or a consideration of the effects that a choice of action could have on the lives of others. Although the consideration of both duties and outcomes is an internal function, the criteria used to judge them are external. In this sense, the analysis of the second question is objective.

In relation to the first of the two questions, no one outside the person can know what will bring him peace. However, the second question involves peace with others and someone outside the person can know the answer, that is, other people can know what duties are involved and what effects a choice or action could have on them or others. As the philosopher Albert Camus put it: "It is probably true that a man remains forever unknown to us and that there is in him something irreducible that escapes us. But practically, I know men and recognize them by their behavior, by the totality of their deeds, by the consequences caused in life by their presence."[1] The distinction between judging human actions and judging human beings may be the most difficult distinction to convey.

All people must live together in the world; therefore, they necessarily are concerned with the relationship of human actions to their own welfare and/or the welfare of others, to the actions and reactions of other human beings, and to the consequences or results produced in the world by those actions. Thus, human interdependence imposes conditions that compel individuals to judge the rightness or wrongness of their own actions and those of others.

Ethics proposes to identify, organize, examine, and justify human acts by applying certain principles to determine the right thing to do in specific situations.[2] The subject matter of ethics is not involuntary human behavior but human acts—that is, those actions that are chosen freely and intentionally.[3]

Because ethics is an ancient discipline, it is not surprising that a number of proposals have been made regarding how one can approach an ethical problem. Generally, these many propositions fall into two categories of outlook: normative and non-normative. Normative ethical thinkers seek universally understood principles to guide human conduct. Non-normative ethical thinkers deny that universal principles exist, although some try to discern orderly processes for decision making. Both approaches have strengths and weaknesses that deserve careful scrutiny.

NON-NORMATIVE THEORIES

There are three major approaches to non-normative ethics: ethical emotivism, ethical skepticism and ethical relativism. Although there are many variations in each category, all non-normative systems of ethics fall into one of them.

Ethical Emotivism

The emotivists assert that statements about right and wrong express or evoke emotion, but do not state facts. Therefore, they conclude that moral judgments have no basis in fact. People use such statements as "Murder is wrong." to express negative emotions aroused in them by this action. That is, the statement "Murder is wrong." can be equated with the statement "I don't like murder." A person also may use this term (and others like it) to try to evoke the same feelings in others and, thus, to compel them to modify their behavior or to share the speaker's interests. Presumably, listeners will not engage in murder if a speaker can arouse the same negative emotions in them.

Although ethical emotivism seems to explain the emotions often aroused in debate over ethical issues, it fails to account for why ethical terms elicit emotion. In addition, the emotivists' claim that ethical judgments have no basis in reality strains credibility. Actions that bring pain or death to others have an existence separate from emotions. Even if such actions evoked no emotions, they still would exist and a rational judgment that they are wrong could be made.

Ethical Skepticism

The ethical skeptic does not deny the existence of right and wrong; he merely claims that human beings cannot know the difference between right and wrong. The skeptic supports his claim by pointing out that people often disagree about ethical issues. Clearly, two opposing opinions can not be correct. Therefore, the skeptic concludes that humans cannot know right from wrong.

Although this approach recognizes differences of opinions among people, it assigns equal weight to opposing opinions without exception. The amount of information gathered to support an opinion and the possible outcomes of an action are not considered. One is required to believe that in every situation of choice, judgments of right and wrong are equally valid. Is not an informed judgment supported by adequate data more believable than an uninformed opinion unsupported by data? Are the results of one action (at least in some circumstances) never more desirable than the results of another action? People must and will act, and the results of their actions will make a difference at least to themselves and to some other human beings. Hence, people can and will try to determine how to control that difference.

Ethical Relativism

Some non-normative ethicians do not deny the existence of right and wrong; they claim that the rightness or wrongness of an action is determined by a specific context. However, relativists disagree about the nature of this context. Some relativists claim that determinations of right and wrong are relative to the individual; others relate them to the culture; still others relate them to the situation. Each claim warrants separate consideration.

1. *Right and wrong are relative to the individual.* If determinations of the rightness or wrongness of an action rest solely with the individual making a decision, absolute authority is vested in him. He cannot act wrongly because the only criterion for his decision is his own value system. Thus, the effects of this person's choice on others and the commitments or responsibilities he has to others may be unimportant. For example, if Nurse X decides to abandon his patients in mid-shift because he wants to shop for a new car, this decision would be right, good, and proper simply because Nurse X has decided that this is what he will do. The needs of the patients, the contract he has with his employer, the results of his action (even the death of a patient) would be important factors in his decision only if Nurse X valued them.

The strength of this approach to decision making is its recognition of the relationship between personal values and a choice of action. Its greatest weaknesses are that it equates personal values with right and wrong action, it fails to recognize limits of personal experience and perspective and it implies that a person's moral judgments are infallible.

2. *Right and wrong are relative to the culture.* Some relativists claim that right and wrong are determined by the culture of a particular social group.

Therefore, the rightness or wrongness of a particular action is determined by whether or not it conforms to societal norms or expectations.

The greatest strength of this approach is that it promotes understanding of the differing values held by people in other cultures. For example, it helps individuals to understand why people in one culture may regard with approval the practice of exposing their elderly members to the elements, while people in other cultures may abhor such a practice.

Its greatest weakness is that it forces one to assume that all actions required by the customs or mores of a society are right and that those that diverge are wrong. Therefore, according to this approach, if one lives in a society in which slavery is the custom, and the buying and selling of human beings are in keeping with the mores, any opposition to slavery would be seen as wrong and actions that encourage and advance slavery would be seen as right. Cultural relativism places personal conscience in an inferior position to tradition and social custom. Under this system, one must conclude that any action to change society is wrong. Thus, a social reformer's actions are wrong unless the majority of the people in that society approve of them. One might be willing to take the position that his efforts are unlikely to succeed until others agree with him, but can one honestly take the position that his actions are wrong? Although cultural relativism helps one to understand the relationships among cultural mores, social custom and ethical choice, it alone cannot justify human actions.

3. *Right and wrong are relative to the situation.* A popular form of ethical relativism is situationism. The situationist recognizes guides for conduct that may be helpful in decision making, but denies that these guides may be universally applicable.

The situationists claim that there are no rules that must not be broken. Each situation gives rise to its own principles of right or wrong and decisions reached cannot be generalized to any other situation. There is a big difference between claiming that right and wrong arise only in a context (situation) and holding that the context (situation) gives rise to the right and wrong. The greatest strength of this form of relativism is that it seems to be in accord with how people actually make decisions. Its greatest weakness is that it seems to equate personal responsibility for actions taken with rightness or wrongness of an action. The following example may help to clarify this distinction.

Ms. M, a 42-year-old head nurse employed in a large hospital, was assigned to manage a most difficult ward. She also had a number of personal problems: she was divorcing her husband, her two teenage sons were rebelling, and she recently had been told that she had a chronic, painful, increasingly debilitating disease.

This nurse did a fine job of organizing the ward; patient care and staff morale improved dramatically. Everyone in the hospital admired Ms. M—she practically had performed a miracle.

As time went on, her improvements in the ward became accepted practice. Ms. M was not less admired, but her excellence was accepted as the rule rather than the exception. Meanwhile, her personal problems grew more severe, particularly as the disease progressed and her pain increased. Her medication no longer satisfactorily eased her pain; when she asked for more, her physician would not prescribe a heavier dose for two reasons: (1) hers was a progressive, long-term, increasingly painful disease; if he gave her too much pain medicine too soon, the medication would not relieve the greater pain to come; and (2) if she wanted to continue working (and she did), she could not practice nursing safely under the influence of heavy doses of narcotics.

One day, when Ms. M opened the narcotic cupboard to give 50 mg. of Demerol to a patient, there were no 50 mg. doses available, but there were some tubexes of 100 mg. She was about to "waste" half of the 100 mg. tubex when she thought, "Why waste it?" She gave the patient his 50 mg., took 50 mg. herself, and noted on the narcotics record that 50 mg. of Demerol were wasted. The Demerol helped her so much that she continued this practice whenever the opportunity presented itself. Soon, the occasional injections of Demerol were not enough. When Demerol was ordered for any of the patients, she began taking it herself if the patients did not ask for it. However, she noted on the patients' charts and in the narcotic record that the patients had received the pain killer.

Within 6 weeks, even this amount of Demerol was not sufficient. She began diluting the doses given to patients and eventually gave some of the patients a saline injection and saved the Demerol for herself. Ms. M tried to justify her actions by taking the Demerol of only those patients who "really didn't need it."

Although understandable, were Ms. M's actions right? Was it right for Ms. M to steal, to lie, to endanger patients by working while under the effects of narcotics and to increase the suffering of others because she was suffering? Could Ms. M's past excellence make her present behavior acceptable? What factors in this situation could make Ms. M's actions right?

Does understanding why a person chooses a certain course of action change the rightness or wrongness of the actions? Although one might understand Ms. M, have a great deal of compassion for her, and in no way condemn her as a morally corrupt person, does this mean that her actions were right?

Clearly, the rightness or wrongness of an action is not determined solely by the situation, although personal responsibility for an action taken may be reduced by situations. Situations do not create their own moral principles; rather the principles are applied to situations. One's personal responsibility for an action may be contextual, but right and wrong are not purely contextual. *Right and wrong actions are determined within situations, not by situations.*

While non-normative theories increase understanding and tolerance, both of which are important in decision making, they are not sufficient to determine right and wrong.

NORMATIVE THEORIES

Normative ethicians assert that there are universally applicable principles of right and wrong. That is, there are rules that should not be broken. However, normative ethicians agree that honest people presented with the same problem may hold opposing views of the right thing to do in a particular situation. General principles are interpreted differently by different people. In addition, there are several moral principles, and their relevance for and importance in a specific situation vary. Thus, universal principles can differ in their applicability to a discrete ethical problem.

Moreover, a moral rule or norm can guide us to right action in the majority of cases, but fail in a few. This does not mean that the rule is invalid, but merely that there may be an exception to the rule. In fact, a normative ethician may claim that exceptions prove that the norm exists. For example, the prohibition against killing is a universal moral norm. Any exceptions to this rule must be justified and fortified by a strong reason (such as killing in self-defense). The fact that one must justify the action proves that the norm exists. Only if one can prove that indiscriminate killing, on no provocation and for no good reason, is appropriate human conduct can one claim correctly that there is no norm. The rule has been broken, but it must exist or it could not be broken.

Although all normative ethicians hold that there are universally applicable principles of right and wrong, their positions differ on the derivation of the norms and sometimes on the content of the norms. Most normative approaches to ethics can be classified into two broad categories. The first, *deontology,* derives norms or rules from the duties human beings owe one another by virtue of commitments made and roles assumed. The second approach, *teleology,* derives norms or rules for conduct from the consequences of actions. There are many variations of both approaches; some of these will be discussed briefly.

Deontological Theories

Generally, deontologists hold that a sense of duty consists of a rational respect for the fulfilling of one's obligations to other human beings. These obligations arise from commitments made and roles assumed and from consideration of the fundamental rights of other persons. According to this approach, any act congruent with one's duties is right. Conversely, any act contrary to one's duties is wrong. However, how people determine what their duties are is a point of disagreement among deontologists.

Kantian theory. Immanuel Kant, the famous eighteenth century deontologist, asserted that respect for persons is the primary test of one's duties. Kant held that people always must be treated as ends, not means only. There are three components to this imperative:

1. All persons must be respected as persons. Respect for persons consists of recognition of their humanity and honoring of their rationality. That is, one

respects the autonomy of persons by not interfering with the choices another person makes in his own sphere.

2. A person must respect his own humanity. If all persons must be treated as ends, an individual should not use himself solely as the means to an end. Thus, a Kantian probably would disapprove of the actions of those who volunteer for a suicide mission, because such people use themselves solely as a means to an end: they do not respect themselves as persons.

3. Persons must never be treated solely as the means to an end. Kant does not forbid the use of people as means; what is forbidden is their use as means *only*. For example, it is not wrong for a person to earn a living by nursing the sick (using patients as a means of earning a livelihood), provided that he treats them as human beings with goals, values, and purposes of their own. A Kantian would not approve of any type of exploitation—even mutual exploitation. For example, a Kantian would disapprove of prostitution if the prostitute used the consumer of her services solely as a means of earning a living, and if the consumer of a prostitute's services used her solely as a means to an end. If neither one of the parties to a transaction exhibits respect for the humanity of the other, the action is wrong.

According to Kant, every consciously controlled human action is morally relevant: persons are responsible for any freely chosen action, whether or not they planned it in advance, and even if they do not recall making a deliberate choice to do it. For this reason, Kant holds that a maxim (norm) is implicit in every conscious human act. Moreover, he holds that one can test the rightness or wrongness of an action by generalizing the norm implicit in any act. Kant called this test the *principle of universalizability,* that is, one always should choose to act as all human beings should choose to act in a similar situation. Actions that can be universalized are right; those that cannot be universalized are wrong. Actions can fail the test if, when generalized, they become self-contradictory or unacceptable to most rational persons. Perhaps an example would help to clarify the application of the principle of universalizability.

A nursing student had great difficulty learning the material presented in her physiology class; she simply could not understand it. Therefore, she cheated on her final examination. The maxim implicit in her action is that "all nursing students who do not understand physiology should cheat on their final examinations." However, if all nursing students cheated on their final examinations in physiology, a student would gain no advantage by cheating. Therefore, a student does not want others to cheat; she wants only herself to cheat. To predicate a universal norm that applies to all except one's self is inconsistent, or self-contradictory. Moreover, if all nursing students who could not grasp physiology cheated on their final examinations, a significant number could graduate who do not have sufficient knowledge of physiology to practice nursing safely. Nurses who do not practice safely could endanger the lives of patients. Most rational persons would agree that nurses should not endanger the lives of patients. Therefore, they would find this situation unacceptable. The student's maxim, "All nursing students who do not understand physiology should cheat on their final examinations" does not pass the test: it is both self-contradictory and unacceptable to most rational persons. Therefore, the student acted wrongly when she cheated on her final examination in physiology.

The greatest strengths of this theory are its emphasis on human responsibility for action and its emphasis on the dignity of human beings. The major problems of this approach are: it does not account for how one can know what all human beings should do in a given situation, and it does not address the problems presented by conflicting duties.

Human nature. Some deontologists hold that people have an obligation to act as though they are human. That is, the rightness or wrongness of an action is related directly to its conformity with human nature. Proponents of this approach attempt to identify the elements that comprise a human being and determine the relationship that ideally should obtain among them. An element unique to human nature is the ability to think, to reason, and to understand. Human actions are thought to be influenced by two general inclinations: self-love and benevolence. The relationship between the inclinations is controlled by conscience. That is, any particular choice of action is right if it can be justified rationally and wrong if it cannot be justified rationally.

One strength of this approach is that it recognizes human complexity and the conflict that can exist between self-interest and the interests of others. The greatest problems with this approach are that no act performed by a human being can be outside human nature entirely, and that an act may be rationally defensible but emotionally indefensible. For example, one can defend rationally the notion that unproductive members of a society should be destroyed. One even might present benevolent reasons for their destruction; for example, it could eliminate the misery of those who are hungry, suffering from disease or disability, and those who are burdens on others. Does the rational defense make the act right?

The Law of God. Some ethical theorists hold that human beings have a duty to act in accord with the Will of their Creator. Knowledge of the Will and Word of God is derived from careful study of and reflection on the sacred writings preserved and promulgated by the various religions through the centuries. Thus, the thinking of good and wise people spanning many centuries can be brought to bear on a difficult problem. The authority to interpret God's Will usually is vested in a religion or in the representatives of a religion (minister, priest, rabbi).

The greatest strength of this approach is that it recognizes human finitude and fallibility. Its principal difficulty lies in conflicting interpretations of the inspired word of God. How can one know which of the proclaimed versions is correct? Moreover, there are many contemporary problems that simply are not covered in the sacred writings (*e.g.*, recombinant DNA, 'n-vitro fertilization, overpopulation). To complicate matters further, human beings have done a great deal of harm in the name of God (religious wars, persecutions, inquisitions). It is paradoxical to fulfill one's duty to God by destroying others who see their duty to God somewhat differently. Although the inspired Word of God as interpreted by various religions can assist greatly in decision making, critical thinking and rational analysis are not precluded; they are demanded.

Compliance with duties (derived from whatever source) is important in decision making, but is it alone sufficient for decision making? The results of one's actions (whether or not they are in accord with duty) also are significant and consequential approaches to ethics merit careful study.

Teleological Theories

Generally, teleological theories are straightforward; right consists of actions that have good consequences and wrong consists of actions that have bad consequences. Teleologists disagree, however, about how to determine the goodness or badness of the consequences of actions. Some hold that right actions produce the greatest amount of good or the least amount of bad for the most people (utilitarianism). Others claim that the rightness or wrongness of an action relates to the degree of its congruence with the function or purpose of human life (natural law). Recently, some behavioral and biological scientists have advanced the notion that right action consists of conformity to known scientific truths (scientism). Each of these three claims will be examined briefly and some of their strengths and weaknesses will be identified.

Utilitarianism. All utilitarians hold that what makes an act right or wrong is its utility or inutility. Useful acts bring the greatest amount of good into existence. Inutile acts produce harmful effects. That is, acts are judged according to their instrumental value. For example, telling the truth is considered useful (right) because it promotes trust in human relationships and enables a society to function more efficiently. Clearly, if people could not believe what anyone else said without first verifying it for themselves, everyone's life would be made far more difficult. Therefore, lying is not useful (wrong).

One master utilitarian, Jeremy Bentham, held that the usefulness of an act was determined by the amount of happiness it produced. By happiness, Bentham meant pleasure and the absence of pain. He believed that the search for pleasure characterized all human endeavor. He also thought that pleasure could be measured in terms of quality and quantity. Therefore, Bentham argued that all people should act to maximize pleasure and minimize pain.

Although John Stuart Mill, a superb utilitarian theorist, gave qualified approval to the principle of the greatest happiness for the greatest number, he held that "happiness" must be defined as *social* utility. Happiness for an individual is something bound to the common good; it is not selfish concern for one's personal pleasure. For this reason, Mill attached great importance to education. He believed that only through the education of the human intellect could the human race rid itself of the selfishness that interferes with progress in human affairs. He rejected Bentham's hedonistic man and sought to replace him with a man who had learned to identify his own happiness with that of the good of society as a whole.

The problems presented by utilitarianism are (1) the difficulties involved in defining "the good" for all people, (2) the injustices to individuals that are engendered when the benefit of the majority is placed always in a superior position to the benefit of the minority, (3) the questions raised by the adoption of a philosophy that entails the notion that the end justifies the means, and (4) the classic problems one encounters when attempting to measure the quantity, quality, or social utility of any action.

Natural law. Natural law theorists hold that human beings are capable of establishing a standard of morality based on human nature. According to Aristotle, everything strives to fulfill its potential. The natural imperative, then, is for each thing to strive to be all that it can be. Acts are seen as right to the extent that they actualize human potential or advance the struggle to attain the "fullness of humanhood." Actions contrary to this purpose are seen as wrong. To determine what constitutes the ideal human, one must undertake a logical study of the ends of human existence and the best means to accomplish those ends. Fulfilling the purpose of human existence leads to the ultimate end of human striving: happiness.

This approach has many strengths, among which are its recognition of the changing, maturing aspects of human beings, its emphasis on human responsibility, the dignity and importance that it places on human choice, and its requirement that all facets of human character be considered in determination of a course of action. One of the problems of this approach is that it requires a vision of the ideal human being. Moreover, people differ about what they think are the ideal ends of human existence. Until there is agreement on the purpose of human striving, there will be great differences of opinion about what humans should be (end) and how (means) they are to accomplish that end.

Scientism. A small but increasing number of scientists espouse to varying degrees a system of beliefs based on science, utilitarianism, and legalism. In the extreme of this view, individuals are seen as biological entities all of whose actions are determined by environment and heredity. What people call "choice" is an as yet unexplained chemical/physiological reaction. Concepts such as human rights and human freedom are myths devised by human beings in an attempt to explain what they cannot understand.

Although human beings cannot be seen as either good or bad, right consists of conformity to known scientific truths. Only through the appropriate application of scientific knowledge can undesirable human conduct be controlled and war, crime, poverty, and disease be subjugated and ultimately eliminated. As the mechanisms determining human behavior and human health become more clearly understood, law must provide for their implementation. According to this approach, what is right (scientifically grounded and proven) must become law (that which will be enforced) to the good of humankind.

The chief strength of this approach is its reliance on known scientific data and technological advances. It recognizes human interdependence and emphasizes human responsibility for the welfare (present and future) of the human race. Moreover, its goals are laudable: health of mind and body, peace, social equality, and elimination of poverty.

However, it has many problems. Its proponents fail to recognize that in denying the existence of choice, they deny humans the ability to make a free decision to do anything. What will be is controlled by biological or social determinants; humans have no control over this "chemical/physiological" reaction and, thus, they can do nothing to alter their destiny. Moreover, humans cannot be responsible for either the genetic heritage or the environmental factors that determine their behavior.

Those who espouse scientism seem to think that their chemical/physiological reactions (choices) are superior to those of others—so much so that they want them to be made law and enforced. Those who hold that humans must control through science and deny the existence of human choice create a paradox: humans cannot control if they are unable to make a choice to control. If facts control humans, how could humans control facts? It is useless to claim that humans must control through the application of scientific data if the data determine themselves.

CONCLUSION

This chapter presents an overview of some of the major approaches to ethical decision making that have been developed over the centuries. It is by no means either inclusive or exhaustive. Interested readers are urged to examine the bibliography and to read the original works if possible.

In summary, approaches to ethics can be characterized as normative and non-normative. Non-normative approaches fall within three major traditions: ethical emotivism, ethical skepticism, and ethical relativism. Normative approaches can be divided into two general categories: deontology (duties) and teleology (results). Each approach to the determination of right and wrong has strengths and weaknesses. Each offers insights into how and why people engage in ethical decision making. Different theories emphasize different aspects of decision making, some to the exclusion of all others. In its pure form, none of these theories is adequate.

Therefore, it would be useful to develop a model for decision making that will incorporate as many of the strengths of each approach as possible and eliminate as many of the weaknesses as possible. While such a model cannot assure that the right decision will be reached, it could reduce the margin of error.

NOTES

1. Camus, Albert. *The Myth of Sisyphus* (Vintage Books, New York, 1955) p. 9.
2. Wellman, Carl. *Morals and Ethics* (Scott, Foresman, Glenview, Illinois, 1975) p. 317.
3. *Ibid.,* pp. 29–50.

BIBLIOGRAPHY

Aquinas, St. Thomas. *Basic Writings of Saint Thomas Aquinas.* Edited by Anton C. Begis, Random House, New York, 1945.

Aristotle. *Complete Works,* Vol. 19. The Lobb Classical Library, Harvard University Press, Cambridge, Massachusetts. The important works of Aristotle for the study of Ethics are *Eudemian Ethics, Nichomachean Ethics, Magna Moralia, Politics and Rhetoric.* Translated by H. Rockham, 1962.

Ayer, Alfred. *Language, Truth and Logic,* 2nd ed., Chapter 6. Victor Gollancz Ltd., London, 1936.

Barnes, W. H. F., "Intention, Motive and Responsibility," in *Aristotelian Society,* Sup. Vol. 19 (1945), pp. 230–248.

Beadle, George W. and M. Beadle. *The Language of Life.* Doubleday, New York, 1966.

Bentham, Jeremy. *An Introduction to the Principles of Morals and Legislation.* Edited by J. H. Burns and H. L. A. Hart. Atheone Press, London, 1970.

Bergsma, Daniel (ed.), "Advances in Human Genetics and Their Impact on Society." *Birth Defects Original Article Series* 8(4), July, 1972, The National Science Foundation, Washington, D.C.

Bronowski, J. *The Identity of Man.* The Natural History Press, Garden City, New York, 1966.

Camus, Albert. *The Rebel.* Vintage Books, New York, 1956.

Carritt, Edgar F. *Theory of Morals.* Oxford University Press, New York, 1928.

Cassirer, Ernst. *Rousseau, Kant and Goethe.* Harper and Row, New York, 1963.

Clarke, Arthur C. *Profiles of the Future.* Harper and Row, New York, 1973.

deBeauvoir, Simone. *The Ethics of Ambiguity.* Philosophical Library, New York, 1948.

Dewey, John. *Experience and Nature.* Open Court Publishing Company, LaSalle, Illinois, 1925.

Dewey, John. *Political Power and Personal Freedom.* Collier Books, New York, 1962.

Ebersole, F. B., "Free Choice and The Demands of Morals," *Mind.* LXI (1952), pp. 234–257.

Ellery, John B. *John Stuart Mill.* Grosset and Dunlap, New York, 1964.

Empericus, Sextus. *Skepticism, Man and God.* Wesleyan University Press, Middleton, Connecticut, 1964, pp. 31–87.

Fletcher, Joseph. *Situation Ethics.* Westminster Press, Philadelphia, 1966.

Francoeur, R. T. *Utopian Motherhood.* A. S. Barnes Company, New York, 1972.

"Genetic Science and Man." *Theological Studies* 33(3), September, 1972. (Complete issue on ethical and philosophical considerations of human genetics.)

Hamilton, Michael (ed.). *The New Genetics and The Future of Man.* William B. Eardmans, Grand Rapids, Michigan, 1972.

Hegel, G. W. F. *Philosophy of Right.* Translated by T. M. Knox. Clarendon Press, Oxford, 1942.

Herskovits, Melville. *Man and His Works: The Science of Cultural Anthropology,* Chapter 5. Alfred J. Knopf, New York, 1947.

Hunt, Robert and John Arras. *Ethical Issues in Modern Medicine,* Chapters 1 and 2. Mayfield Publishing Company, Palo Alto, California, 1977.

Kant, Immanuel. *Foundations of the Metaphysics of Morals.* Translated and edited by Lewis W. Beck. University of Chicago Press, Chicago, 1949.

Kant, Immanuel. *The Fundamental Principles of the Metaphysics of Ethics.* Translated by Otto Manthey Zorn. Appleton-Century-Crofts, New York, 1938.

Katz, Jay. *Experimentation With Human Beings.* Russell Sage Foundation, New York, 1972.

Kierkegaard, Sören. *A Kierkegaard Anthology.* Edited by Robert Bretall. Princeton University Press, Princeton, 1951.

Kohlberg, Lawrence, "The Child as a Moral Philosopher," *Psychology Today,* Vol. 7, September, 1968, pp. 25–30.

Mann, Jerse and Gerald Kreyche. *Approaches to Morality.* Harcourt, Brace and World, New York, 1966.

Marcel, Gabriel. *Man Against Mass Society.* Translated by G. S. Fraser. Henz Regnery Company, LaSalle, Illinois, 1962.

Maritain, Jacques. *Moral Philosophy: An Historical and Critical Survey of the Great Systems.* Chas. Scribner and Sons, New York, 1964.

Mead, Margaret, E. Mesthene, P. Ramsey, P. Drinan, J. Fletcher, H. Thieliche. *Who Shall Live?* Fortress Press, Philadelphia, 1970.

Meyeroff, Milton. *On Caring,* Chapters 2, 3, 4 and 5. Harper and Row, New York, 1971.

Mill, John Stuart. *On Bentham and Coleridge.* Harper Brothers, New York, 1950.

Moore, G. E. *Ethics.* Henry Holt and Company, New York, 1912.

Moore, G. E. *Principia Ethica.* Cambridge University Press, Cambridge, England, 1903.

Moore, G. E., "The Subject Matter of Ethics," in Morris Weitz (ed.). *20th Century Philosophy: The Analytic Tradition.* The Free Press, New York, 1966.

Nietzsche, F. *The Birth of Tragedy and the Geneology of Morals.* Doubleday, New York, 1956.

Perry, Ralph B. *General Theory of Value,* Chapter 5. Harvard University Press, Cambridge, Massachusetts, 1926.

Plato. *The Republic.* Translated and edited by Francis MacDonald Corkford. Oxford University Press, New York, 1945.

Ramsey, Paul. *Basic Christian Ethics,* Chapter 2. Chas. Scribner and Sons, New York, 1950.

Ramsey, Paul. *Fabricated Man.* Yale University Press, New Haven and London, 1970.

Rawls, John. *A Theory of Justice.* Belknap Press of Harvard University Press, Cambridge, Massachusetts, 1971.

Ross, William David. *The Right and The Good.* Clarendon Press, Oxford, England, 1930.

Rousseau, Jean Jacques. *The Social Contract and Discourses.* Translated by G. D. H. Cole. E. P. Dutton, New York, 1950.

Skinner, B. F. *Beyond Freedom and Dignity.* Alfred A. Knopf, New York, 1971.

Stevenson, C. L. *Ethics and Language.* Yale University Press, New Haven, Connecticut, 1960.

Stevenson, C. L., "The Emotive Meaning of Ethical Terms," in Morris Weitz (ed.). *20th Century Philosophy: The Analytic Tradition.* The Free Press, New York, 1966, pp. 236–253.

Wellman, Carl. *The Language of Ethics,* Chapter 10. Harvard University Press, Cambridge, Massachusetts, 1961.

N.B.   This is only a small selection of possible resources, but it represents a wide range of approaches.

6

No Rush to Judgment*

Leah Curtin

"The quality of the beer doesn't matter if there is a hole in the barrel!"

A Russian Proverb

Sometimes the most common human activities are the most difficult to understand. They seem to be so much a part of life that little thought is given them. Human beings make decisions about themselves, about how they are going to treat other people and about their relationships with the world every single day and, most of the time, do not give these decisions a thought. Only when faced with something clearly labelled "important" do people pause to reflect. For example, while health professionals may agonize over whether they should "pull the plug" on one patient's respirator, they may give no thought to the person in the bed next to him and of what it does to him to be placed in the same room with a patient on full life-support equipment. The following situation illustrates this point.

Sixty-eight-year-old Mr. X was brought to the hospital with a bowel obstruction. On admission, he was placed in a room with a man who was comatose and who had a tracheostomy, a respirator, a monitor—everything. Mr. X took one look at this man and said, "Don't ever do that to me!" The nurse smiled, murmured a few comforting words, and left. A few moments later, a young resident came in, asked him a few questions, examined him, and left. Before Mr. X knew what was happening, the nurse returned and

---

*This chapter was adapted from the article, "A Proposed Model for Critical Ethical Analysis," *Nursing Forum,* Vol. XVII, No. 1, 1978, pp. 12–17. It is used here with the permission of the publisher.

inserted a Levin tube and someone else started an intravenous feeding. Mr. X tried to ask questions but no one seemed to hear him. People were not unkind precisely, but no one bothered to tell him what was going on or why the staff members were doing the things they were doing. Meanwhile, Mr. X was watching the man in the bed next to him; people turned him, washed him, cleaned him up as necessary, suctioned him, adjusted his I.V. fluids and checked the machines, but the man could not talk, move, eat, laugh, or cry. Mr. X thought, "Never, never, are they going to do this to me!"

After several days of mysterious and sometimes painful tests, an unknown man in a white coat came into Mr. X's room and said something about pneumonia; a moment later, someone else put an oxygen mask over Mr. X's face. Within a few hours, a technician came in and put him on a monitor—just like the one on the man in the next bed. Mr. X was having difficulty breathing, his throat hurt from the Levin tube, his arm hurt from the I.V., he could not eat, he could not talk, and he even had to press the call button when he had to urinate. A few hours later, Mr. X had so much difficulty breathing that someone decided that he needed "assisted" respirations; he was placed on a respirator—just like the one on the man in the bed next to him.

No one really told Mr. X anything, but everyone assured him with a smile and a perfunctory pat that he was going to be "all right." It certainly did not look that way to him. As a matter of fact, he felt a great deal worse than when he came in. Moreover, he was beginning to look frighteningly like the man in the bed next to him. Sometime during the night, Mr. X unhooked everything and left the hospital without permission or detection. He was found two blocks away—dead.

This was an unusual and dramatic end to a common problem: insensitivity in daily decision making. No thought was given to the collective impact of multiple daily decisions probably because none of them seemed important enough to the health professionals to warrant an explanation; each decision was *routine.* How was Mr. X to know that his problem was in no way similar to the man's in the next bed? How was he to know that his major problem was pneumonia, that his bowel obstruction was not cancer and that the monitor was attached for precautionary reasons only? How was he to know that the intravenous feedings and assisted respirations were temporary measures? People treated his room as though it were their own and his person as though it were an object. For forty years, strangers had called him Mr. X; now people younger than his granddaughter called him by his first name and did whatever they chose to do to him without as much as a "by your leave." Perhaps these actions and decisions were common, everyday occurrences to the efficient youngsters scurrying around Mr. X, but they were not common to him.

The purpose of this case presentation is not to discuss whether or not Mr. X had a right to refuse treatment, or even to discuss the facts surrounding his death. It is to point out the importance of the decisions health professionals make every day in their interactions with people. Why do they make the decisions they make? What is the data base? What ethical principles are involved? What do human rights mean in the everyday context? What are their duties and how are they determined?

INTEGRATION OF THEORIES

Each ethical theory emphasizes certain aspects of decisions or decision making. Some are suited to decision making on a grand scale, others to the more modest scale demanded in daily life. Some are personalistic and others require impartiality.

However, the gathering of information is important in all decision making. Recognition of the emotional impact that difficult situations have on the human beings involved in them can lend valuable insight to ethical determinations (situational and emotive approaches). It also seems true that the customs and mores of society are important factors to consider in determination of courses of action (cultural relativism). The responsibilities attached to roles assumed in life cannot be discounted in any serious decision (deontologic approaches). Moreover, one cannot avoid consideration of the impact that actions may have on others (teleological approaches). There is no doubt that consulting an authority should improve the quality of one's decisions. It is true also that in some circumstances, one instinctively seems to know the right thing to do and that experience is an excellent teacher.

The application of general ethical principles to a specific situation can help to clarify what is the ethical problem and these principles can act as guides in decision making (normative). However, general principles are so amorphous that they must be brought sharply into focus according to the demands and needs of the people and problems involved. In all decision making, one is a finite being with limited capabilities (natural law). A person could be wrong (skepticism) but must act with integrity (conscience) according to the knowledge he possesses in keeping with his obligations (deontology), in the search for a satisfactory outcome (teleology). If there is one absolute, it is that human beings must never judge the moral worth of other persons, even during attempts to determine the rightness or wrongness of their actions.

To add order and structure to ethical deliberations, it is helpful to construct a model for critical ethical analysis. Such a model should incorporate each of the major approaches to ethical analysis in order that the strengths of one will offset weaknesses of others. In the course of various analyses, one will encounter some situations in which one value conflicts with another, other situations in which duties conflict and, not infrequently, some in which duties conflict with desired outcomes. Often what a person wants to do will conflict with what he thinks he ought to do. However, the most common problem is that a person does not realize he is making an ethical choice; he does not think about what he is doing, why he is doing it, or whom it may affect.

The following proposal for critical ethical analysis (see Figure 6-1) attempts to incorporate the strengths of each major approach to decision making.

Background Information or Data Base

Not every factor in a situation will have relevance for an ethical decision, but one cannot understand fully or appraise correctly the rightness or wrongness of an action without first knowing as much about the circumstances as possible. Who is involved in the situation? What information is available (scientific, cultural, sociological, psychological)? Information should be gathered, organized, and ranked according to its *direct relevance for the decision at hand.* When the information has been gathered, organized, and ranked, one can determine more precisely what the problem is.

Identification of Ethical Components

Once any problem has been defined clearly, one can examine it to determine whether it has the following characteristics of an ethical problem: it does not belong solely within science, it is perplexing, and the answer has implications that touch many areas of human concern.

If a specific problem meets these criteria, the type of ethical problem involved should be identified. Is it a case of conflicting rights? Are duties conflicting with outcomes? Is the problem one of lying or withholding the truth and obtaining informed consent? Is it a case of powerlessness *versus* authority? Freedom *versus* submission? It is not uncommon for one situation to have a number of ethical components. Most of the normative theories emphasize the identification of components to enable one to determine the principles that are involved, such as respect for persons, prohibitions against killing, lying, or stealing, and so forth. The clearer the definitions, the more precise the analysis.

Common sense and a measure of perspective help tremendously at this stage of the analysis. On the one hand, people may think that they are faced with an ethical problem when it is not a moral one at all. For example, the controversy over the definition of death* may be couched in moral terms, but it is not a matter of ethics—it is a matter of fact: either a person is dead or he is not. On the other hand, one may fail to recognize the ethical components of a situation and act as though the problem is purely technical or requires nothing more than discretion. For example, a decision to put a patient on a respirator involves more than a technical option, but this often may be the only apparent consideration.

---

*Heart–lung criteria versus brain death criteria.

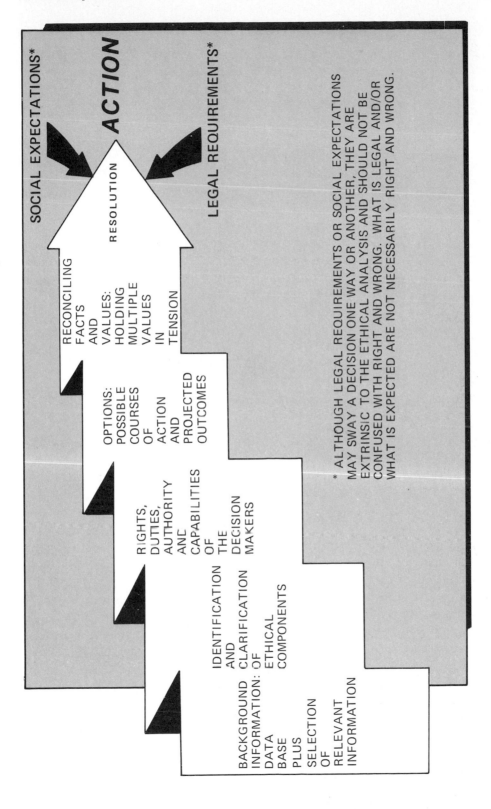

ACTION

SOCIAL EXPECTATIONS*

LEGAL REQUIREMENTS*

RESOLUTION

RECONCILING FACTS AND VALUES: HOLDING MULTIPLE VALUES IN TENSION

OPTIONS: POSSIBLE COURSES OF ACTION AND PROJECTED OUTCOMES

RIGHTS, DUTIES, AUTHORITY AND CAPABILITIES OF THE DECISION MAKERS

IDENTIFICATION AND CLARIFICATION OF ETHICAL COMPONENTS

BACKGROUND INFORMATION: DATA BASE PLUS SELECTION OF RELEVANT INFORMATION

* ALTHOUGH LEGAL REQUIREMENTS OR SOCIAL EXPECTATIONS MAY SWAY A DECISION ONE WAY OR ANOTHER, THEY ARE EXTRINSIC TO THE ETHICAL ANALYSIS AND SHOULD NOT BE CONFUSED WITH RIGHT AND WRONG. WHAT IS LEGAL AND/OR WHAT IS EXPECTED ARE NOT NECESSARILY RIGHT AND WRONG.

Individuals Involved in Decision Making

All persons involved in a particular decision must be identified, together with how they are involved. What is the scope of their authority and responsibility? On what foundation are their duties predicated? Lines of authority and responsibility should be determined as clearly as possible. The human rights that may conflict in a situation (*i.e.,* rights to life, to bodily integrity, to liberty, to privacy, and so on) must be identified and ranked. If rights and duties are not ranked according to their importance, resolution of a problem may not be possible. Moreover, one must consider how free each person is to make a decision. Is a patient's intellect clouded by excessive pain, drugs, or trauma? Is the professional facing a conflict of duties? Is the family laboring under excessive emotional strain?

If rights, responsibilities, and scope of authority are not identified and the factors that impinge upon a person's ability to make a decision are not assessed, one is likely to err in decision making—perhaps quite seriously. It is the failure to deal carefully with this component of ethical analysis that often leads to the wrong person making the wrong decision for the wrong reasons. Guidance and counsel may help the right person to avoid the wrong decision, but whose decision it is must be known. In short, it is careful analysis in this area that will help to identify who should be making the decision and why he or she should be making it.

There are times when more than one person is involved in particular aspects of a decision. In this step of the analysis, one can determine why certain people should be involved and which persons should be deciding what about whom. Only through identification of the rights and responsibilities of each ethical agent can confusing, overlapping, or contradictory conclusions and intrusive conflict be avoided.

Options or Possible Courses of Action

In any given situation, there are at least two (and usually quite a few more) courses of action available. One must project as accurately as possible the consequences of each course of action and identify the good and/or the harm that can result. Occasionally, none of the projected results is desirable, but usually one can find an option that will produce more good or less harm than others. Some options may be rejected immediately because their outcomes are disastrous, they involve the transgression of a moral norm or they conflict with important duties.

Reconciling Facts and Principles

Generally, ethicists are concerned only with actions that are intentional and freely chosen. Some theories (*e.g.,* those based on an analysis of human nature) hold some actions to be wrong in themselves because they either debase the human being or frustrate human nature. Other actions will be seen as right in themselves because they respect or enhance human nature. The deontologist holds that actions in keeping with duties are right in themselves and that actions contrary to duty are wrong in themselves. The teleologist holds that any action that produces more harm than good is wrong in itself and should be avoided.

All these values must be held in creative tension as one proceeds toward the resolution of a problem. At times, one norm may take precedence over another in accord with the rank of the rights and duties (*e.g.,* human freedom, justice, compassion) involved in a situation. The situation may determine the ranking of the norms but not their existence. The reasons for the ranking and ultimately the decision itself must be articulated rationally and defended.

SHARED DECISIONS

If there are conflicting conclusions among various participants in a shared decision, one may have to defer to the person who is affected most directly by the decision. Although people never should undertake an action they sincerely believe to be wrong (for that is the definition of immorality), they should weigh all factors carefully before withdrawing or blocking decision making. There are times when both of these activities are appropriate, but sometimes acquiescing to the will of the majority is the best course of action. Where is the greater good or the lesser harm? Is the problem better served by one's withdrawal or participation? Is the situation best handled by submission to the authority of the group? Sometimes a person may have to stand alone. On no account should dissenters be forced to comply against their will or be denigrated in any way. Even when the group members cannot agree with a dissenter, they can understand how and why the person dissents. No matter what decision must be made, it cannot assume more importance than the people making it, lest people be sacrificed for the principles designed to protect them. Even if they cannot agree with a group's decision, dissenters can come to understand how and why the group reached a particular decision.

RESOLUTION

The adoption of this approach to the analysis of an ethical phenomenon cannot guarantee that one will determine the right thing to do in every situation, but it does offer some assistance—as a tool—to those who must make very difficult choices. There are times when either legal requirements or social expectations (or both) will sway the final decision. However, neither law nor social custom should be confused with what is right or wrong.

Health professionals are involved frequently in making or helping to make decisions, not only for themselves but also for others. However, as much as possible, they must refrain from making decisions for others and, in fact, must do all in their power to help others make their own decisions.

Section III

7

Nursing's Contract With Society

M. Josephine Flaherty

"Nursing as an art to be cultivated, as a profession to be followed, is modern; nursing as a practice originated in the dim past, where some mother among the cave-dwellers cooled the forehead of her sick child with water from the brook . . ."[1]

Sir William Osler

HISTORICAL EVOLUTION OF NURSING

Nursing exists in response to a need of society and holds ideals related to man's health throughout his life span. As nursing's body of knowledge has increased and as members of the public have become more aware of their health needs, nurses' responsibilities have changed markedly. As a result, the nursing profession is attempting to identify and to clarify nursing's unique role in society.

Such activity is not confined to this one profession, for today's society as a whole is characterized by a wide-spread search for meaning and identity, the result of a belief that each person is free and responsible for the development of his own self through use of his own will. This drives people to seek means of self-development, self-realization, and a unity with the essence of the universe. Hence, the eighties are witnessing the overt striving of many heretofore suppressed and oppressed individuals, groups, and nations to attain recognition and status. Nursing, representing a significant group in society, is part of this movement as it seeks to establish itself as an identifiable profession that makes important contributions to the promotion of health and to the cure of illness.[2]

A conviction that the discipline of nursing is a theory-based field of inquiry is a phenomenon of the last two decades that is growing in scope and depth.

Scrutiny of it has suggested to some observers that "nurse researchers seem to function primarily on tacit rather than explicit knowledge of the broad conceptualizations unique to nursing."[3] Aydelotte noted that a great part of nursing knowledge consists simply of a record of "unrationalized experiences" and that although nurses use knowledge from the physical and social sciences, "a large portion of it has not been studied . . . [for] its relevance to nursing phenomena."[4] Stinson maintains that the uniqueness of methods of inquiry in nursing "lies not so much in the *kinds* of descriptors used but in the *combinations*" and in the use of instruments from general research literature together with instruments developed specifically for nursing, with the result that nurses often use creative approaches to the development of nursing knowledge.[5]

Nursing has acquired from history at least three images that have tended to inhibit its progress toward self-determined professionalization.[6] The first of these, dating from primitive times, is the folk image of the nurse as mother with the biological function of suckling and taking charge of an infant. Later, this function was broadened to include care of young and the sick, injured, aged, and weak. How to perform the tasks was instinctive, was learned by chance, or was common knowledge.

The image of the nurse as a nurturer was positive in one sense because the work of nursing was viewed as useful and people were glad to receive nursing services. At the same time, however, nursing skills were seen as experientially derived and somewhat unrationalized because it was believed that nursing was not based on a body of knowledge and that no critical thought was required in the exercise of nursing. Its outcome was enhancement of the well being of the recipient of nurses' ministrations. Although this was welcomed by the receivers, it was an intangible commodity and a nurse's position in life was not perceived to be a particularly high estate. This early folk image of the nurse as a simple, mothering care-giver has persisted to some extent to the present.

The nurse's second image, from medieval times, is the religious image of the nurse as a care-giver for the sick, who fulfilled her function as a Christian duty and a means to salvation. This image tended to fit nicely with the earlier image of nursing care being given for love, without pay or formal learning; the absence of temptations of worldly concerns and a high level of discipline were additional and significant dimensions of this image. This was a positive image of nursing as an honorable and high estate that was a vocation rather than a profession or a service that was worthy of significant economic rewards. Even today, this image of nursing as charitable work is in the minds of many people.

The third image of the nurse as servant emerged in Europe and Great Britain between the sixteenth and nineteenth centuries with the development of the Protestant–capitalist ethic that was derived from the new philosophies and the scientific principles of men such as Galileo and Newton. It was believed that the universe was ruled by immutable laws of God; nursing entered its "Dark Ages," as ignorant and ill-paid women, unlike the inspired religious sisters of the earlier time, accepted work as nurses as a last resort. In Canada and in the United States, perhaps because they were new countries with a pioneer ethic, a large measure of the religious tradition persisted for a longer time than was the case in Europe and Great Britain. This served to preserve the tradition of honor in the care of the sick; however, it did little to remove the servant role and to promote the development of the current sought-after image of the nurse as a learned professional, adequately paid and independent in much of her practice.

During the nineteenth and twentieth centuries, certain social factors contributed to the development of nursing as a profession; these included unprecedented growth of science and technology, the development of humanitarian philosophies, several great wars, and major changes in the social structure. Man achieved greater control over the environment, and the size of the middle class increased while that of the lower class decreased. These phenomena, together with a reaction against the cold scientific philosophies of the time, helped to pave the way for the rise of a new romantic and emotional spirit of humanitarianism.[7] Standards of living improved; medicine learned more about cause, effect, treatment, cure, and prevention of certain diseases; hospitals moved toward becoming scientifically oriented; a work ethic flowered; people became sensitive to and aware of the sufferings of others; and demographic changes helped to provide a pool of women in the work force. Women played significant roles in wars, both in and outside nursing, and had major impacts on post-war societies. These changes prepared the way for the women's emancipation movement that affected women from all sectors of society, including the one in which Florence Nightingale lived.

Her early work in nursing laid a foundation for the profession that included militaristic discipline, long hours of devoted work, and a measure of isolation from the mainstream of society as even living arrangements for nurses consisted of tightly controlled residences. Nightingale saw the need for two types of nurses—the well educated, leader nurses who would supervise and teach the work of the other, larger group of trained nurses who did the bulk of the work in hospital settings. Although Nightingale wanted to "open a career, highly paid,"[8] the "respectful, obedient handmaiden" image of the nurse has persisted in the minds of many members of society, and of many members of the nursing profession, to this day. Although Nightingale specified the need for the two types of nurses, society today, well over a century later, is observing the profession, still debating the pros and cons of various levels and types of nurses, the role of nurses in the health care system and the relationship of nurses to other health professionals.

It is little wonder that both nurses and non-nurses are still asking: Exactly what is nursing? How does it fit into society and into the health care system? What is a nurse's responsibility to society? What should society be able to expect from nurses and nursing? Is the situation that does exist the one that should exist? Why or why not? What should nursing do about this? What should society do about this?

WHAT IS NURSING?

Although nursing is discussed a great deal by many people, it is neither well-known nor well understood even by nurses. Whenever members of the profession meet, they express concern about the character of nursing care that is available and about the quality and quantity of their own professional practice. Discussion of nursing involves a wide variety of ideas and points of view. A concern of the profession is the need to articulate nursing's unique contribution to society. Today, nurses want to transform nursing knowledge from a record of unrationalized experiences to a logical organization of relevant phenomena. Indeed, there have been many statements about nursing that have been offered as definitions of it. Most of these, however, have said *what nurses do* rather than *what nursing is.*

Florence Nightingale was the first (and perhaps the last!) person to believe that she had done this and to be sure of what nursing is. She noted, "And what nursing has to do . . . , is to put the patient in the best condition for nature to act upon him."[9] Her *Notes on Nursing* were "by no means intended as a rule of thought by which nurses can teach themselves to nurse, still less a manual to teach nurses to nurse. They are meant simply to give hints for thought to women who have personal charge of the health of others. . . . [These hints for thought were] "the knowledge of nursing, or in other words, of how to put the constitution in such a state as that it will have no disease, or that it can recover from disease. . . . " Nightingale recognized it as "the knowledge which everyone ought to have—distinct from medical knowledge, which only a profession can have."[10] Here Nightingale was distinguishing nursing from medicine, a profession, but she valued nursing highly when she noted ". . . how immense and how valuable would be the produce of her united experience if every woman would think how to nurse."[11]

A couple of decades ago, Virginia Henderson defined nursing for the International Council of Nurses as "to assist the individual, sick or well, in the performance of those activities contributing to health or its recovery (or to a peaceful death) that he would perform unaided if he had the necessary strength, will or knowledge. And to do this in such a way as to help him gain independence as rapidly as possible."[12] This statement, that has been used widely in nursing, is another significant contribution to the description of *what nurses do.*

In the eighties, the scope of nursing is regarded as falling within and being an essential part, but not all, of health care, in the broad sense, as opposed to strictly illness care. Since its goal is to help people attain, retain and regain health, the phenomena with which nurses are concerned are man's health seeking and coping behaviors as he strives to attain health.[13] Today's nurses are committed—through practice according to nursing models, that lend themselves to change and to adaptation to many venues (as opposed to medical or other models), to assess the functional or coping levels of individuals and families in the light of their biology, their environment, their lifestyle, the health care system and the interactions among these, to plan and implement proactive and reactive nursing interventions and to evaluate the effectiveness of these. This lends further clarification to what nurses do.

Today, examination of definitions of nursing reveals that there is a wide variety of philosophical, conceptual, and theoretical models under consideration. Each model contains common threads such as patients, environmental factors, adaptation factors, and professional interventions and most describe what nurses do.

One Canadian nurse works with a statement about nursing that constitutes a definition of it. McGee describes nursing as a process of nurse–patient interaction that stems from the assessment of a patient's needs and levels of functioning and that is designed to optimize the patient's adaptability through modification and/or reinforcement of the environment, modification and/or reinforcement of behavior, and biological care and maintenance. The process can be accomplished through the use of nursing care strategies in appropriate measure.[14] This definition says what nursing is and what nurses do. It incorporates the notion that nursing practice focuses on the promotion of optimal health for individuals and families. Health is a manifestation of the competence with which individuals and families function. States of health vary according to the efficiency and effectiveness with which individuals and families interact with their environments. Hence, health states are measures of functional competence. It follows that if the aim of nursing is to promote functional competence, nurses in various settings must be well versed in the knowledges, the techniques, and the conceptual and theoretical rationales that underlie nursing practice. What are the characteristics that qualify nurses for their work?

CHARACTERISTICS OF PROFESSIONAL NURSES

Nurses of the eighties have declared that they are professional and that they want to embrace the privileges and responsibilities of professional status. Nurses, like other health care workers, are faced daily with complex issues and are called upon to make far-reaching decisions. Members of our society believe that professional nurses possess certain characteristics[15] that have prepared them to exercise their proper roles as citizens and as health care professionals.

The first of these is education, both general and specific. General education equips nurses to think and reason with accuracy and to appreciate the world in which they live and work; specific education gives them a theoretical framework for their practice. Nursing education programs are designed to meet the needs of students in light of the professional demands that are expected to be placed upon them in the health field.

A second characteristic of professional nurses is acceptance of a code of ethics. The high value that nurses place on the worth and dignity of human beings directs them in their practice. As certain elements and characteristics of society change and as roles of people, including professionals, are altered, ethical codes may be subject to modification. The basic quality demanded by a code of ethics is integrity; that means "doing what one believes to be right, regardless of the cost."[16] Belief in something implies that a person has given careful thought to the information at his or her disposal and has arrived at a logical conclusion. Beliefs may be modified in the light of new evidence and the nurse with integrity has the courage to change his or her mind. "But this change of opinion must proceed only from a certain persuasion, as of what is just or of common advantage, and the like, not because it appears pleasant or brings reputation."[17]

A third characteristic of nurses is dedication to the ideal of master craftsmanship in their work. ". . . the master craftsmen are superior in wisdom, not because they can do things, but because they possess a theory and know the causes."[18] True mastery of nursing is not something that is acquired suddenly; rather, it is an ongoing process that demands of nurses that they strive constantly to add to personal knowledge, to perfect professional skills and to enlarge the body of knowledge for the discipline. Florence Nightingale is said to have stated that "Nursing is a progressive art in which to stand still is to have gone back. . . . Progress can never end but with a nurse's life."[19] The hallmark of a master craftsman in nursing is an inquiring mind and a commitment to continuous learning.

A fourth characteristic of professional nurses is informed membership and involvement in the organized profession. Nurses who are intellectually self-employed think and speak for themselves and act according to their own decisions rather than according to what someone else has told them to do. Nurses with inquiring minds know what is going on in the profession and are involved in the development of new patterns. They will not tolerate the absolutism that could result if, as members of a "tired democracy," they fail to participate.

The final characteristic of professional nurses, that subsumes the other four, is accountability or the taking of responsibility for one's own behavior. Nurses do not blame others for what is done or not done in the profession and in the society in which they live and work. Rather they participate in decision making and live with the decisions. They accept the fact that, over time, they will experience both failures and successes, but believe that if they act responsibly, the successes will outnumber by far the failures. These nurses strive constantly to practice in a diligent, reasonable, and justifiable manner, they document their rationales and they are willing to subject their practice to the scrutiny of their peers. Feeling no obligation to shoulder the burden of omniscience, they develop and apply strategies to deal with the almost instant obsolescence of knowledge and professional practice and achieve the "Maturity: that means among other things—not to hide one's strength out of fear and, consequently, live below one's best."[20] The ethical nurse's "best" involves exercise of professional practice, through application of the nursing process, at the highest level of which that nurse is capable.

The nursing process, for which professional nurses are responsible according to national, state, and provincial standards of nursing practice,[21,22,23] is composed of at least four dimensions: planning, implementation, evaluation, and research.[24] Careful attention must be given to these, each of which can be affected markedly by the far-reaching scientific and technological advances of our age and by actual and hoped-for changes in delivery of health care. *Planning* involves recognition of real or potential problems or needs of patients and the identification of strategies for coping with these. Planning may be narrowed to one or more individuals or broadened to a department, an institution or a community. *Implementation* involves decisive action toward a defined goal. It can become routinized, cold, almost mechanical, but it has the potential to be the most creative, communicative and satisfying component of the nursing role. It is the "art of nursing" to which Florence Nightingale made reference when she said, "The art is that of nursing the sick. Please mark, not nursing sickness. . . ."[25] *Evaluation* is the process of determining the significance of worth of nursing action by careful appraisal and study. It should involve also the determination of appropriateness. It takes place concurrently with and retrospectively to implementation, as well as prior to new planning. One of the marks of a profession is that it monitors its own practitioners; thus, accountable nurses must be prepared for peer review as well as self-evaluation. *Research* involves disciplined study of the effects of nursing actions that will lead to the development of nonarbitrary standards for nursing practice, standards that are developed by specialists in nursing rather than by administrative or organizational tradition or convenience.

In our society, health care is provided, in a variety of venues, by the members of a number of professions of which nursing is but one. Like other health care professionals, nurses function in several dimensions. The first of these is the *independent* dimension, in which nurses make judgments that are based on education and experience and that depend on sound theoretical knowledge. The second is the *dependent* function, in which nurses act according to the directions of physicians or other health professionals and according to the policies of health care agencies. Professional nurses in Canada and in the United States are obliged by ethics, by law, and by professional standards to question those directions and policies about which they have concern. The third is the collaborative or *interdependent* function, in which nurses work with patients, families, and other members of the health care team in the effort to meet patients' needs. This requires mutual respect and cooperation among health care workers and health care recipients. Nursing, then, like the other health care professions, has its own distinctive characteristics, identifiable functions, and significant contributions to the health care enterprise. Nursing practice has undergone change, and will continue to do so, in response to society's needs and demands. From time to time, nursing practice functions overlap with the activities of other health professionals. An ethical imperative for nurses is to recognize when it is appropriate for them to engage in expansion and/or contraction of the scope of their functions in the attempt to refine nursing practice such that health care consumers will be assisted to achieve optimal health states. As collaborative health care practitioners, nurses are recognized[26,27,28,29,30] as *accountable for* their behavior, rather than simply *accountable to* someone in a hierarchy. Hence, every registered nurse is obliged to exercise judgment in accepting and in delegating responsibility. The acts of registered nurses require substantial knowledge, skill, and judgment and are performed either independently or in cooperation with other health care professionals.

In some states, provinces, and territories, recognition of the autonomy of the nursing profession and of its responsibility for self-regulation may be explicit in the statutes,[31,32] whereas in others, this acknowledgment may be implicit. There is general agreement, however, that nursing is a distinct profession that involves the three dimensions of the nursing function.

The ethical implication of this for nurses, whether they are engaged in practice, education, administration, research, or consultation, is that they are responsible and accountable for professional behavior that involves application of the nursing process and cooperation with appropriate others, within current legislation affecting the practice of nursing, according to the profession's codes of ethics and of practice, within the context of the policies and practices of the employing agency and within the customs and values of the society in which the nursing care is being provided. This requires nurses to practice with competence and to exercise judgment in the preservation of the safety, dignity, and autonomy of patients. While factors that promote safety and dignity can be recognized fairly easily, nurses must guard constantly against slipping into habits of practice in which goals are defined *for* patients rather than *with* them. Current recommended nursing practice models do not direct nurses to sustain hope in patients by promising survival or cure of disease that both patients and nurses often know to be impossible. Rather, such models prompt nurses to keep patients as much in command of themselves, their symptoms, and their situations as possible[33] and thus preserve patient autonomy. This calls for a measure of independence or freedom of choice and requires for the patient knowledge, ability to reason, and ability to act in a way that is true to his own nature. Thus would nurses work with patients toward optimization of their functional competence with the least possible interference from the disease or therapeutic regime.[34]

BEYOND DIRECT PATIENT CARE

In the eighties, perhaps more than ever before, ethical nurses will be expected to go beyond direct patient care to consider and act on factors associated with the nature and shape of the health care system, the responsibilities and practice of various members of the health care team, and the changing roles of consumers in the maintenance of their own health. Nursing will continue to promote the adaptation of patients in situations where changes in health status (including but not restricted to illness) place new demands on those patients.

Nurses appreciate that what they observe about their patients, and how the patients perceive what is happening to them, will be influenced by the setting in which it occurs and by the forces, obvious and subtle, that the setting contains. Nurses' education and experience prepare them to subject all nursing phenomena to the analytic scrutiny that is part of the nursing process. Although Florence Nightingale identified observation as a nurse's most necessary skill, she noted that "merely looking at the sick is not observing. To look is not always to see. It needs a high degree of training to look so that looking shall tell the nurse aright. . . . A conscientious nurse is not necessarily an observing nurse, and life or death may lie with the good observer."[35] This component of excellent nursing practice goes beyond the mere counting and recording of the results of observation that " . . . tells us the fact; reflection [allows one to discern] the meaning of the fact. Reflection needs training as much as observation."[36] This implies a subjective determination—the putting together of all parts to form the meaningful whole that theoretically and technically skilled and personally and socially perceptive health care practitioners formulate as they make clinical judgments.[37]

As society evolves and changes and as biological, medical and technical knowledge expands, nurses will examine information that may shake, if not shatter completely, certain personal and professional beliefs that they value highly, such as convictions about the dignity of human life, the uniqueness of each human being and the freedom of every individual to control his life and his lifestyle. As members of society and as health care professionals and practitioners, nurses may have to re-think and re-define their purposes, nature, and value systems. To do this, they will require personal philosophies that are meaningful to them, explicit definitions of their ethical beliefs, identification of their own personal–professional conflicts and acknowledgment of the extent to which they are imposing these on others and to which such conflicts affect the health care being provided.[38]

Nurses, who are the largest group of health care professionals, have the potential to influence very strongly the health care system, its practitioners, and its consumers. Nurses who are professionally accountable recognize that the direction of scientific discovery and its application to mankind are not out of their hands. They have personal, professional, and legal responsibilities to ask probing questions about scientific and technical research and its application (or lack of it) in practice. Each health professional and each patient must be given the right to hear a different drumbeat and to be accepted for what he is, regardless of his social values and capacity for achievement. Care is developed out of the patient's needs, health problems, the family and community and their resources, the character of the health care system, and the resources of the health care workers who are available.

Society has the right to expect professional nurses to be guided by the words of Socrates in Plato's *Apology:* "The unexamined life is not worth living."[39] as those nurses question the prevailing customs and taboos of the situations in which they find themselves, including their own behavior, to identify whether what they see is consistent with the standards of practice for which they stand accountable.

In *The Present Crisis,* James Russell Lowell warned:

"New occasions teach new duties; Time makes ancient good uncouth;
They must upward still, and onward, who would keep abreast of Truth."[40]

This challenges accountable nurses to subject established methods, policies and institutions, including codes of ethics and of practice and tried and proven methods of acting, to constructive criticism to determine the need to transform the old order into a new and better one. This will not provide solutions for all of the dilemmas of professional practice but it can stimulate nurses to strive for excellence, to apply appropriate ethical concepts to the cultures in which they work and to be sensitive to the need for thoughtful and sound decision making in the face of ethical dilemmas.

NOTES

1. Osler, Sir William. "Nurse and Patient," Address at Johns Hopkins Hospital, 1897, in *Aequanimitas (with other Addresses to Medical Students, Nurses and Practitioners of Medicine),* by Sir William Osler (H. K. Lewis and Co. Ltd., London, 1920) pp. 153–166.
2. Uprichard, Muriel. "Ferment in Nursing," *International Nursing Review,* Vol. xvi, No. 3 (1969) p. 222.
3. Donaldson, Sue K. and Dorothy M. Crowley. "The Discipline of Nursing," *Nursing Outlook* 26 (February 1978) p. 113.
4. Aydelotte, Myrtle K. "Clinical Investigation and the Structure of Knowledge," in *Current Perspectives in Nursing.* N. H. Miller and B. C. Flynn, eds. (C. V. Mosby, St. Louis, 1977) p. 46.
5. Stinson, Shirley M. "Nursing Research: The State of the Art," in *Ph.D. (Nursing).* Proceedings of the Kellogg National Seminar on Doctoral Preparation for Canadian Nurses. Glennis Zilm *et al.*, eds. (Canadian Nurses Association, Ottawa, 1979) p. 14.
6. *Ibid.,* pp. 222–224.

7. Waelder, R. *Progress and Revolution,* Chapters I to IV (International University Press, New York, 1967) cited by Uprichard, p. 225.

8. Woodham-Smith, Cecil. *Florence Nightingale 1820–1910* (Collins (Fontana Books), London, 1951) p. 361.

9. Nightingale, Florence. *Notes on Nursing for the Labouring Classes.* New edition, abridged edition of *Notes on Nursing: What It Is And What It Is Not* (Harrison, London, 1868) p. 113.

10. *Ibid.*, p. 3.

11. *Ibid.*, p. 4.

12. Henderson, Virginia. *Basic Principles of Nursing Care* (International Council of Nurses, London, 1961) p. 42.

13. Schlotfeldt, Rozella. "This I Believe . . . Nursing Is Health Care," *Nursing Outlook,* Vol. xx, No. 4 (1972) p. 245.

14. Adaptation of definition after personal communication with Dr. Marian McGee (University of Western Ontario, London, Ontario, 1975).

15. Flaherty, M. Josephine. "Professional Obligations with Effective Rewards," *Alberta Association of Registered Nurses Newsletter* (June, 1975) n.p.

16. Adaptation of definition after personal communication with Dr. Peter Moloney (Connaught Medical Research Laboratories, Toronto, Ontario, 1962).

17. Aurelius, Marcus. *The Meditations,* IV, 12 (trans., George Long) (Doubleday, Garden City, New York, 1960) p. 37.

18. Aristotle. *The Metaphysics Book I,* 1, 11–12 (trans., Hugh Tredennick) (Heinemann, London, 1933) p. 7.

19. Dolan, Josephine A. *Nursing in Society—A Historical Perspective,* 13th edition (W. B. Saunders, Philadelphia, 1973) p. 175.

20. Hammarskjold, Dag. *Markings* (Faber and Faber, London, 1966) p. 87.

21. American Nurses' Association. *Standards of Nursing Practice* (American Nurses' Association, Kansas City, Mo., 1973).

22. College of Nurses of Ontario. *Standards of Nursing Practice: for Registered Nurses and Registered Nursing Assistants, Revised, May 1979* (College of Nurses of Ontario, Toronto, 1979).

23. Canadian Nurses Association. *Definition of Nursing Practice and Standards for Nursing Practice* (Canadian Nurses Association, Ottawa, 1980).

24. Flaherty, M. Josephine, "Accountability in Health Care Practice: Ethical Implications for Nurses," Chapter 23 in *Contemporary Issues in Biomedical Ethics,* John W. Davis *et al.*, eds. (The Humana Press, Clifton, New Jersey, 1979) pp. 267–276.

25. Nightingale, Florence. *Paper contributed to Nursing Section of Congress on Hospitals, Dispensaries and Nursing.* World's Fair, Chicago, 1893. Cited by Goodnow, Minnie. *Outlines of Nursing History, 2nd ed., revised* (W. B. Saunders, Philadelphia, 1921) p. 79.

26. International Council of Nurses, *I.C.N. Code for Nurses—Ethical Concepts Applied to Nursing* (International Council of Nurses, Geneva, 1973).

27. American Nurses' Association. *Code for Nurses With Interpretative Statements* (American Nurses' Association, Kansas City, Missouri, 1975).

28. College of Nurses of Ontario, 1979, *op. cit.*

29. Canadian Nurses Association. *Definition of Nursing Practice and Standards for Nursing Practice* (1980) *op. cit.*

30. Canadian Nurses Association. *CNA Code of Ethics: An Ethical Basis for Nursing in Canada* (Canadian Nurses Association, Ottawa, 1980).

31. *The Health Disciplines Act, 1974, Part IV, Nursing.* Statutes of Ontario, 1974, Chapter 47, as amended by 1975, Chap. 63 (Queen's Printer, Toronto, 1975).

32. *Bill 273, Nurses Act.* National Assembly of Quebec, Fourth Session, Twenty-Ninth Legislature (Quebec, 1973).

33. Cassell, Eric J., "Autonomy and Ethics in Action," *New England Journal of Medicine,* 297 (1977) pp. 333–334.

34. *Ibid.*

35. Goodnow, Minnie. *Outlines of Nursing History, 2nd ed. revised* (W. B. Saunders, Philadelphia, 1921) pp. 78–79.

36. *Florence Nightingale–Her Wit and Wisdom.* Compiled and edited by Evelyn Barritt (Peter Pauper Press, Mount Vernon, New York, 1975) p. 33.

37. Lewis, Edith P., "Quantifying the Unquantifiable." Editorial, *Nursing Outlook,* Vol. 24, No. 3 (March, 1976) p. 147.

38. Flaherty, 1979, *op. cit.*, p. 274.

39. Cited by Romanell, Patrick, "Ethics, Moral Conflicts and Choice," *American Journal of Nursing,* Vol. 77, No. 5 (May, 1977) p. 850.

40. Lowell, James Russell, "The Present Crisis," dated December, 1844, in *The Complete Poetical Works of James Russell Lowell,* Cambridge Edition (Houghton Mifflin, Boston, 1897) p. 68.

8

The Nurse–Patient Relationship: Foundation, Purposes, Responsibilities, and Rights*

Leah Curtin

"Your friend is your needs answered."

Kahlil Gibran, *The Prophet*

It is a mistake to think that all ethical concern in nursing revolves around ethical issues. It does not. Moreover, it should not. Certainly, ethical issues surround and impinge on nursing practice, but until we explore the ethical dimensions of practice, we have no direction from which to approach the ethical issues. The profession of nursing and professional nurses have the privilege of serving human beings in need. Nursing is a *service* profession. Because service is its reason for being, all that nurses do—each concern that they have—must be contemplated in its light. At the crux of this service is the relationship that develops or fails to develop between nurses and patients or clients.[1] Because health professionals almost always are involved with significant, personal concerns of other human beings,[2] the foundation, form, and balance of values within the relationship are of great importance.

HISTORY

The sociocultural and historical roots of health care professionals' relationships to and with patients or clients are centuries old and in the Western tradition are derived from the Hippocratic corpus. The Hippocratic

---

*This chapter is an expansion, adaptation and interpretation of the article, "The Nurse as Advocate: A Philosophical Foundation for Nursing," *Advances in Nursing Science,* April 1979, pp. 1–10. It is used here with the permission of the publisher.

corpus is a collection of seventy-two works representing various points of view about medicine, only four of which are deontological, that is, containing prescriptions and proscriptions about the relationship of the physician with the patient.[3] The whole spirit of this corpus ascribes to the physician (and by derivation to other health professionals) an authoritarian and paternal position that provides for no options on the part of those being served. This position is neither a Western peculiarity nor an inevitable outgrowth of the Judeo–Christian culture. As a matter of fact, the Chinese Code of the First Century A.D. was equally authoritarian in its ethos.[4] Moreover, the Indian Code (the *Charaka Samhita*) of approximately the same time was even more definitive in its declaration of the power of the physician. It prohibited the treatment of those who were unclean or immoral, and it was the physician who made this determination.[5]

Many early writers on ethics for nurses stressed obedience to the physician, even to the point of lying to the patient if the physician so desired.[6] Although the nurses' duty to be loyal to the physician often appeared to be the sole focus of ethical concern in nursing, nurses always were enjoined to act in the best interests of patients (as defined by the physician) and to care for patients in such manner as to hasten recovery and/or bring them comfort.[7] Thus, nurses' relationships to patients or clients were founded in and formed by the physician, and not by the nurse and the patient.

These historical perspectives are significant because they represent historically "proper" views of physician–patient and nurse–patient relationships. This view has some validity in that *medical* authority, by and large, rests with physicians. Points at issue today are (1) whether physicians have *moral* authority to make decisions for patients or nurses in the realm of values; (2) whether physicians have *technical nursing* authority to make decisions for nurses about nursing care; and (3) whether physicians have moral and professional authority to control nurse–patient relationships.

In the past, respect for the singular identity of human beings has not been of major concern to health professionals.[8] This grew out of a tradition of elitism (reinforced by time and habit)[9] rather than insensitivity to human beings. However, the individual who has been damaged by injury or disease is in an exquisitely vulnerable state; the protection and fostering of his or her human rights require special attention.

FACTORS CALLING FOR CHANGE

Sociological phenomena have emerged in our contemporary society that challenge significantly the traditional approaches. Among these are:

1. *The capabilities of modern medicine.* Brought about by our expanding knowledge and technological development, these advances have increased greatly medicine's ability to intervene in an individual's life. Through the use of such developments as psychotropic drugs, implants, transplants, and

artificial respirators, the power to sustain, expand, and modify the lives of humans has weighted the relationship between the provider and receiver of health services even more heavily in favor of the provider.[10] Among the questions growing out of these advances are: to what use will this knowledge be put as far as society is concerned, and as far as individuals are concerned?[11] Do people want their lives modified? If so, to what extent?

2. *The increasing institutionalization and bureaucratization of health care.* In today's health care system, individuals often cannot find a locus of authority. Today's patient must find a way of dealing with teams, groups, institutions, and even provincial, state, and federal governments.[12] Placed in a society of strangers, he is expected to conform to rules that are applied impersonally and uniformly.[13] Decision making and an individual's ability to participate in it are made difficult by these developments. People are questioning the absolute authority frequently exercised by persons whom they do not know and whom they may never see.

Does satisfaction for both patients and professionals lie in the traditional security of authority, that is, an apparently simple, unified, absolute response? Or is satisfaction to be found in the more humble provision of assistance, that is, the helping that results from communication of concern, information, support, and guidance?

How is the sufferer best relieved of his suffering? By submission to the command of traditional authority—absolute and unified in formula, total in general application, and inflexible in demanding obedience? Undoubtedly there are advantages to this approach; unilateral decisions are firm, quick, and simple and responsibility is located easily.

In eras of few options, man-powered techniques, short time spans, immobile capital resources, and limited access to knowledge, command ethics worked well. However, those epochs have passed. Burgeoning technology, multiple options, and diffusion of knowledge have rendered the command ethic obsolete. Many people are involved in critical health care decisions—patients, families, health professionals, and institutions—and each must bear responsibility for his own decisions if each is to maintain integrity. Thus, an adult relationship is called for—one that maximizes the contributions each partner in this relationship has to offer and emphasizes mutual guidance, support, and shared decision making.

3. *The increasing sophistication and activism of the consuming public.* With the rapid diffusion of knowledge to members of the public who are in highly diverse states of intellectual and psychological development, the traditional elitism of the health care professions has come under severe attack. Many individuals no longer are content to be the objects of someone else's actions. They are demanding a share in decisions regarding their own care and, at times, the care of others.

The rising cost of health care, coupled with an understanding that to a large extent an individual's health status is determined by personal choices in life style, is partially responsible for a shift in public attitudes toward funding of care of the sick. It is not that the public is unwilling to underwrite the cost of caring for those who are unavoidably ill, but rather that many citizens are beginning to resent paying for the avoidable afflictions of others.[14]

This factor alone could have tremendous impact on the patient–professional relationship. Given that the establishment of such a relationship requires the health professional to act in the best interests of the patient,[15] what will the professional do when the welfare of the patient conflicts with the interests of society? Will our society maintain an ethos that is sufficient to support the commitment of health professionals to the welfare of individuals whose continued existence may pose a threat to the economic or social well-being of the community?[16] If it does not, it is quite possible that professionals will shift the major focus of their concern to the welfare of society as a whole—a shift that will affect dramatically (and to some extent already has affected)[17] the patient–professional relationship. Even more suspicion will enter the relationship and with it will come increased demand for control over what is or what is not done.

4. *The changing image of health professionals.* To an alarming degree, health professionals no longer are seen as benign and humanitarian dispensers of care. Health professionals are seen as people who can provide health care—even save lives—but for a price. This factor, coupled with media reports of unnecessary surgery, chicanery, waste, and money-grubbing, has led to an erosion of trust in health professionals that has had profound impact on the relationship between the consumers and providers of health care services.[18] This is not to say that the public does not think that professionals should be paid for their services; rather, it points out that yet another element of suspicion has entered the relationship, particularly when performance does not match expectations.[19]

As health care increasingly is pictured as a money-making industry, people are demanding greater value for money paid. Moreover, they expect their purchase of services to result in the satisfaction of their needs. Errors, pomposity, and general uncertainty regarding the results of medical intervention are tolerated less frequently. The gap between what is demanded and what generally can be achieved further threatens the credibility of health care providers and health care institutions. This strain reveals itself in a growing, debilitating network of fear. In the past, people were afraid of what they did not know. Today, they fear what they do know. Patients fear overtreatment or undertreatment. They fear death and they fear a damaged life. Professionals fear failure and they fear doing more harm than good. They also fear legal liability, loss of income, and loss of prestige.[20]

If health practitioners are to deal with this fear-breeding spirit of the times, they can start by reminding themselves of what their scientific and ethical commitments imply and promise. Scientific advances increase our range of options and, at the same time, uncover new limits to experience and technique. Uncertainty about the nature of these limits creates pressure that demands a modest, systematic, compassionate sharing of decision making and underscores the need for rational guidelines and mutual emotional support.[21]

5. *The impact of moral pluralism.* In the past, it was possible to grant health professionals moral authority because there was more agreement about personal values.[22] Today, there are debates about individual rights, societal rights, and the responsibilities attached to those rights. Men and women of undoubted good will and scholarship disagree profoundly, and the resolution of the conflicts is impeded by increasing technological power and the ramifications of the application of that power.

Today, members of society seem to be saying that freedom and self-determination are higher values than are health and even life. For example, an individual can refuse a blood transfusion for reasons of religious belief, even though it may mean that he will die. A woman can refuse to have a cancerous breast removed, even though she may die as a result. Many people are refusing genetic screening and counseling, even though it could lead to a healthier populace. Moreover, people generally are refusing to adjust their life styles to conform to what health professionals define as healthier modes of living. The clash between what health professionals want others to do and the amount of personal freedom people are willing to relinquish is bound to lead to even more conflict unless information and decision making are shared freely.

6. *Changes in nursing.* Before we can consider a more humane concept of the nurse–patient relationship, we must determine how free the nurse is to act in a responsible and ethical fashion. The first obligation of any nurse to any patient is to provide excellent nursing care through the application of the nursing process. The patient has a right to expect and demand this from the nurse by virtue of the role the nurse has assumed, the education she has acquired, the experience she has amassed and the duties inherent in the patient–professional relationship.

As recently as 1949, Moore, in the book *Principles of Ethics,* held that the nurse as "a faithful servant to a master" has a primary duty of loyalty to the physician and to his good name.[23] McAllister, writing some years later, also claimed that loyalty to the physician is the primary duty of any nurse.[24] Moreover, although every approach to ethics presupposes that the moral agent is free of coercion, at least three contemporary philosophers hold that not only are nurses not free, but they ought not to be free to make decisions.

One such example is Langham's article in *Nursing Forum* in which he claims that "whether nurses should or should not participate in a morally controversial medical procedure should *not* be a personal decision because it may by implication mean that there is no difference between right and wrong."[25] That is, if nurses are allowed to make moral decisions about their participation in controversial procedures, there will be no moral standards! What Langham seems to fear is that if individuals do not follow group decisions, each person eventually will be considered the sole arbiter of right and wrong. Although one may sympathize with Langham's position regarding pure subjectivism in ethics, his arbitrary denial of conscientious objection for nurses is a contradiction of every established ethical approach.

An even more blatant example of the denial of the moral responsibility of nurses appeared in the Summer 1973 issue of *Perspectives in Biology and Medicine.* In an article discussing the deliberate starvation of an infant born with Down's Syndrome and duodenal atresia, the author stated that the nurses' duties were " . . . to carry out the order of the physician. Even if they conscientiously believed that the orders they were executing were immoral, they could not radically reverse the order of events; they could not perform surgery. It was their lot to be the immediate participants in a sad event but to be powerless to alter its course. *They are the instruments of the orders of the physicians.* They have no right of conscientious objection, at least not in this set of circumstances."[26] [Emphasis added.]

May one assume, then, that the welfare of patients or clients is, at best, a secondary consideration for nurses? These particular views of nursing have been challenged by nursing leaders from the beginning of modern nursing to the present day. The Florence Nightingale Pledge contains the proviso that nurses will not "knowingly administer harmful drugs"; it safely can be assumed that this prohibition included deleterious drugs ordered by physicians. Moreover, the American Nurses' Association's *Code for Nurses* (Article Three) asserts, "The nurse [must] act to safeguard the client and the public when health care and safety are affected by the incompetent, unethical or illegal practice of any person."[27] Thus, according to the profession of nursing, nurses not only must refrain from doing that which is deleterious or harmful, they also must *act* to safeguard the patient.

These clearly conflicting views of the moral responsibilities of nurses indicate that the study of ethics in the context of nursing cannot be limited either to analysis of particular sets of problems and issues or to explorations of the ethical dimensions of the nurse–patient relationship as an isolated entity. Nursing practice occurs within a context that involves a complex interaction of social and political values and certain relationships in society. Because of the particular mix of obligations impinging on nurses (as employees, employers, independent practitioners, patient advocates, physician extenders), nurses frequently are placed in paradoxical situations. That is, nurses know that even when (or most particularly when) they practice their profession responsibly in accord with established standards of practice, they may suffer recriminations, job loss or, in some circumstances, even loss of their licenses to practice. However, the ANA *Code for Nurses with Interpretive Statements* (1976) asserts: "Neither physicians' orders nor the employing agency's policies relieve the nurse of ethical or legal accountability for actions taken and judgments made."

What the profession is saying is that the conflicting values and obligations inherent in nursing's multiple roles must not be taken to mean that any specific duty or value is any less a duty because nurses cannot fulfill it. Nurses may have conflicting obligations, one of which they cannot fulfill, but each of these may be necessary for the moral direction of the profession.[28] Although the nurse's primary moral commitment is to the patient, nurses are bound by the same obligations other persons have as human beings, as employees, as employers, and so forth. For example, the nurse's duty to carry out a legitimate direction from a physician regarding the medical treatment of a patient ("do not resuscitate") may conflict with the nurse's duty as an employee to carry out the legitimate policies of the institution ("resuscitate"). Either of these duties may conflict with the nurse's duty to act in the best interests of the patient. These contingent incompatibilities create conflict but they do not mean that any of these obligations is inappropriate or invalid, even when the fulfillment of one necessarily means that the others cannot be fulfilled.

John Ladd makes a helpful distinction between contingent and logical incompatibility that is relevant to this situation: "Generally, contingent incompatibility obtains when two [or more] states of affairs [or actions] that are desired or desirable cannot, for contingent reasons, coexist. . . . Logical incompatibility . . . holds between the assertion of a value and the denial of that value."[29] Ladd argues that logical incompatibility cannot derive from contingent incompatibility. Simply put, this means that nurses have moral obligations even when they cannot fulfill or are prevented from fulfilling them.

The provision of nursing care is the primary obligation of any nurse. Unwarranted outside interference often prevents nurses from fulfilling this duty. As a result, the most pervasive ethical dilemma in nursing is that nurses are not free to practice nursing. That is, nurses are obligated to provide nursing care and that duty pertains even though they may be prevented from fulfilling it. The expanding education of nurses, the professionalization of nursing, the rapid advance of technology, the emergence of feminism, and significant changes in the character of the public increase the intensity of these conflicts.

DEVELOPING A NEW APPROACH

Nursing, then, and the relationship of nurse and patient or client are being reexamined in light of these sociological phenomena and the conflicting values they represent. Nurses no longer can accept (if they ever did) the physician as the initiator and controller of their relationships to and with patients. Both as individuals and as members of a profession, nurses are seeking fundamental clarifications and asking radical questions.

In light of all of these changes, what is the role of the nurse? What is nursing? What is it that makes a nurse a nurse? What kind of relationship should exist between nurse and patient? What is the foundation for this relationship (if it is not the physician and it is not the institution)? Anyone who is familiar with the history of nursing is acquainted with the various roles proposed for nursing, that is, the nurse as physician assistant (extender, surrogate), the nurse as care-taker, the nurse as parent surrogate, the nurse as champion of the sick, the nurse as healer, and the nurse as health educator. None of these seems adequate. Perhaps the major problem is that nurses have permitted nursing to be defined sociologically and have tried to limit nursing to a specific set of functions.[30]

Nurses fill so many different roles and perform such radically different functions that a sociological definition of the profession is not possible. However, nursing can, should be, and is distinguished by its philosophy of care, its point of view and its particular approach to patients or clients.

A PHILOSOPHICAL DEFINITION

The end or purpose of nursing is the well-being of other people. This end is not a scientific end; it is a moral end. That is, it involves the seeking of a good and it involves relationships with other human beings. The science learned and the technological skills developed are designed and shaped by this moral end. The wise and humane application of knowledge and skill comprises the art of nursing. *Therefore, nursing is a moral art.*[31] Nursing science serves this art and nursing would not be possible without this science.

A PHILOSOPHICAL FOUNDATION

The practice of nursing involves a nurse–patient relationship that includes the "diagnosis and treatment of *human responses* [emphasis added] to actual or potential health problems."[32] Therefore, nurses must view patients in their wholeness—their completeness as human beings. In this sense, person does not mean body alone; rather, it means the intangible union of those physiological, psychological, and subjective elements that comprise the human *dasein* (the human being in the world). The point of view brought to health care by the physician is directed primarily toward discovery of the cause of disease and application of scientific principles to the prevention or cure of disease. The pharmacist, the physical therapist and others are concerned with specific and circumscribed needs of patients or clients. The nurse is not as circumscribed.

It is for this reason that nurses must learn and adapt knowledge from many disciplines (psychology, medicine, sociology, pharmacology, epidemiology, physiology, *etc.*) in the practice of nursing. A unique feature of nursing is its ability to adapt and blend knowledge from many disciplines with specific nursing skills in order to identify and meet individual needs of patients or clients. Nursing science involves the discovery of how best to apply the blend of knowledge and skill that is the hallmark of nursing. Nurses may specialize in specific areas in which their functions vary radically. However, their philosophy—their point of view—remains the same. That is, nursing's philosophy of care distinguishes nurses from other health professionals; it is what makes a nurse a nurse.

THE FOUNDATION OF NURSING—THE NURSE–PATIENT RELATIONSHIP

Because the humanity of the patient is at the core of nursing's philosophy, the unique needs of patients or clients as persons are the central focus of ethical concern in nursing. The foundation of the nurse–patient relationship is the mutual humanity of the participants. The nature of the nurse–patient relationship is determined by the patient's human needs and the nurse's responses to them. On this natural foundation, the nurse and the patient in any given encounter structure the particular features of their relationship. However, the nature of the relationship is dynamic, that is, at any time, the relationship may exhibit the characteristics of one or all of the following types of relationships: child and parent, client and counselor, teacher and student, friend and friend, colleague and colleague, and so forth, through a wide range of possibilities. The common humanity of nurse and patient is philosophically prior to any one relationship and the particular mix of needs and obligations gives structure and content to a relationship. It follows that the features of a relationship will change as needs change.

HUMAN NEEDS

To begin to comprehend the human relationship in the professional context, one must understand that disease magnifies universal human needs, creates new needs, and renders an individual vulnerable to abuse. Therefore, nurses not only must identify the specific physiological damage caused by disease or injury, but also must discover how illness has disrupted the humanity of sufferers (*i.e.,* impinged on their integrity as human beings). The damage produced by illness stretches far beyond the physiological, and even the psychological, to penetrate the existential depths of a person's being.[33] The fact of being ill is a direct attack on some of the qualities that make people distinctively human;[34] and the obligations of health professionals to help to meet patients' needs are derived from the conditions (physical, psychological, social, and philosophical) imposed by illness.

With recognition that different people exhibit different reactions to the threats posed by illness, an examination of what illness does to the humanity of individuals must be undertaken in order to identify human responses to these threats. One of the first things illness does to people is infringe on human autonomy—people's independence as persons. At the very least, individuals are required to go to another person, to place themselves before that person, to reveal that they have a deficiency or a defect and to ask to have it alleviated. Thus does disease make an independent individual a petitioner—a position that threatens people's views of themselves as self-sufficient and in control. The more personal or the more threatening the disclosure, the more difficult it is for a person to make it.

Ordinarily, when we encounter a threat, we either fight or flee.[35] However, we cannot run away from our bodies or fight what we cannot control within ourselves. This is the threat that, no matter how hard we try, we cannot alleviate without becoming a petitioner. If health professionals are sensitive to this difficulty and to the painful humiliation it imposes, they can take steps to mitigate its effects. Often it seems that health professionals (and nurses are no exception) are so caught up in their own busy-ness, their own knowledge and their own importance that they fail to consider the humiliation of the patient. If nurses remember that they too are vulnerable human beings, they will be more open and more accessible to patients. It is only in doing so that they can assist individuals to overcome this first obstacle and thus begin to address the damage.

The second attack on an individual's humanity involves loss of *freedom of action.* When people are ill, they cannot command their bodies to do what they want them to do; thus, they are damaged in yet another dimension. Human beings use their bodies to express hopes, dreams, ideals and values; that is, they use their bodies to transcend the physical. Nurses must realize that loss of freedom of action (verbal, locomotive, sometimes intellectual) damages the humanity of the patient, sometimes very seriously.

If nurses are sensitive to the needs created by a loss of freedom of action, they can take steps to ameliorate that damage. The state of a patient's vulnerability is exquisite. In some cases, an individual's impairment is in his ability to hear, to see, to grasp, or to understand. In others, it may be just a matter of rate or degree, but nurses often do not take the time to assist patients in the expression of their values. Patients may be disabled, but they do have value systems that nurses tend to ignore. Some nurses even may begin to interpret what is a meaningful or useful purpose for patients' lives. The situation is particularly treacherous when a patient cannot participate consciously in the human exchange called the patient–professional relationship.[36] The deficiencies are at the surface but the value structure is obscure; hence, health professionals have to rely on surrogates, such as families, who are not always advocates. Health professionals must be fully aware of unconscious motivations that affect a decision to be rid of a long-term, vexing problem. In all circumstances, health professionals must be conscious of what it is that the surrogates are saying about the patient; in some circumstances, health professionals may have to assert their own value systems. These are very difficult situations in which patients' rational capacities are damaged and perhaps not even retrievable. These complex problems place onerous burdens on everyone (family, health professionals, and society) and do not lend themselves to easy or unilateral resolutions.

In an extreme form, these situations represent a third dimension in which people may be damaged by injury or disease. Many factors are operant in decision making, chief among which is the ability to make critical distinctions and to weigh facts and values in order to arrive at the best possible solution. Disease interferes with a person's *ability*—not his *right*—to make choices. Pain, disability, shock, and drugs impair one's ability to make choices as does the trauma imposed by loss of one's wholeness and of one's ability to act.

Human beings, including professionals, are inclined to consider that decisions that agree with their own are rational. Nevertheless, in all circumstances, the right to consent rests with the individual. Under certain circumstances, one could presume that the patient would consent;[37] in others one could obtain authorization to act,[38] but the right to consent always remains with the individual. Nurses who are sensitive to this problem are likely to try to discover and act on the patient's value system rather than on their own or on the family's. The potential for conflicting values in such situations has been magnified greatly by the increasing technological powers and the moral pluralism that characterize contemporary society. Therefore, the responsibility to discover and respect the patient's value system has assumed vastly increased significance.[39]

The magnitude of power exercised over patients is another attack on their humanity. For example, it has been recognized widely that consent obtained under duress is not legally binding.[40] Few things in life are as coercive as is the threat of suffering and death (in this case, imposed by illness); however, no legal advocate and no laws of state can protect people from these threats. Thus, people who are perceived as capable of relieving these threats can and do exercise enormous power over individuals. Patients generally lack the knowledge to define the threat and they do not have the ability to reduce the threat; hence, they must depend on health professionals for both. Whether health professionals want it or not, whether they like it or not, they have power over those whom they serve. How is this power used? Refusing to admit that this power exists creates a situation in which health professionals use power as they wish. Only if they recognize this power will they take steps to share it with patients and their families and thus relieve, to some extent, the threat it imposes. Individuals who have been damaged by injury or disease and who have been placed in the power of others, to a large extent have lost their freedom to define for themselves their own image of what it is that they should be. This sounds very esoteric, so perhaps an example would help.

Some years ago, a nurse was involved in the care of a twenty-two-year-old male who was diagnosed as having primary cancer of the testes. There was no evidence of metastasis. He was a jockey by trade, married and the father of two young sons. He was told of his diagnosis. He was told that he needed an orchiectomy and he was told of the physical effect this would have on his relationship with his wife. He and his wife discussed the matter and, considering the alternative, decided on surgery. However, what he was not told was at least as significant as what he was told. He was not told that he would lose his facial hair and develop breasts and a feminine speaking voice. How much did the health professionals impinge on his identity? What image did he present to himself, to his sons, to his wife? What kind of comments did he have to endure from his co-workers at the race track? This is not known; however, what is known is that he committed suicide nine months after surgery.

If a person's values are ignored or replaced with the values of others, the person ceases to exist as a singular human being. People are defined by their value choices. They will lose a sense of meaning or purpose for their existence[41] if others ignore, usurp, or attempt to destroy their value system. At the very least, the individual will die as the person he was. Not only did the health professionals fail to realize what could happen to the jockey, but they actually intensified his existential crisis by deliberately withholding vital information. As the philosopher Nietzsche put it, "He who has the why to live can bear with almost any how."[42] Although nurses deal with *how* a patient shall live, they must learn to recognize that the *why* is much more important.

If nurses accept their own humanity and the humanity of patients, certain actions, attitudes, and obligations will flow naturally. Sensitivity to a patient's humanity and vulnerability will help nurses to look beneath the surface for the human responses to actual or potential health problems.

A TWO-SIDED EQUATION

Health professionals are human beings too and as such they have rights, values, and principles. They are not merely automatons programmed to carry out the wishes of others. They are moral agents who are accountable for their own actions. They are accountable to themselves, to patients and their families, to the institution that employs them, to society at large, and to the profession.

As human beings, health professionals must act in accordance with their convictions, that is, they must act to preserve their own integrity. Because patients and their families are so vulnerable, they do need protection. It is sad to note that they may need protection even from those who should be serving them. However, attempts to coerce professionals into acts that are contrary to their consciences are just as much a violation of human rights as those on the other side of the equation.[43]

Conscience has been defined as "that faculty by which we feel rational approval or disapproval of actions or agents."[44] Although conscience is "far from an infallible source of right and wrong,"[45] in the last analysis, a moral agent must act to preserve his or her own integrity.

In 1919, the famous American jurist, Harlan Fiske Stone, wrote: "All our history gives confirmation to the view that liberty of conscience has a moral and social value which makes it worthy of preservation at the hands of the state. So deep is its significance and [so] vital, indeed, is it to the integrity of man's mortal and spiritual nature that nothing short of the self-preservation of the state should warrant its violation; and it may well be questioned whether the state which preserves its life by a settled policy of violation of the conscience of the individual will not, in fact, lose it by the same process."[46] This passage has been cited in many court cases regarding freedom of conscience, particularly in cases involving conscientious objections to military service (*U.S. v. Seeger,* 380, U.S. 163, 170, 1965).

Thus, although the primary focus of ethical concern in any clinical decision ought to be the welfare of the individual and, although the patient has an integral if not central role in such decision making, the patient has no more right to coerce the professional than the professional has to coerce the patient. If the differences between the patient and the professional are irreconcilable, the professional must withdraw from the care of the patient and refer him or her to someone whose value system is in accord with the patient's. If no such professional can be found, the patient may have to reconsider his or her decision or withdraw from care. In most instances, some form of negotiation is possible.

Another factor to be considered is the difference between patient needs and patient wants. Health professionals, by virtue of the role they have chosen to fill in society, have assumed the duty *in personum* to meet the genuine health care needs of people. Failure to fulfill this duty can be justified only by the gravest of reasons. However, health professionals have no special obligation to try to fill all (or any) of the health care wants of individuals. They may do so, but they have no particular moral obligation to do so.

Moreover, health care professionals have no obligation to meet patient needs that fall outside their area of expertise. In fact, they have an obligation to refrain from acting in areas in which they lack competence. Therefore, a nurse who has worked for many years in labor and delivery, for example, is justified in refusing to work in an intensive care unit because she is not competent to care for the desperately ill patients in that unit. In a truly human relationship, decisions are made jointly and joint decisions should reflect a respect for the values of both parties.

THE PROFESSION OF NURSING

Whether nursing is or is not a profession is a matter of debate among sociologists,[47] possibly because they persist in their attempts to define nursing according to specific care functions.[48] Essentially, sociological definitions of professions have little value because the attributes sociologists assign to professions may or may not be congruent with the characteristics of persons identified by the public as professionals.[49]

It may be more realistic to recognize professionals in terms of the philosophy that embodies the principles and values that define, limit, and direct their activities. The most distinctive characteristic of a professional is full-time commitment to a calling that almost always involves matters that " . . . are among the greatest personal concerns that human beings have; physical health, psychic well-being, liberty and the like."[50] Because of the specialized knowledge and skill required to practice a profession and because of its importance to the welfare of the public, a professional should possess a service orientation, the principles of which are embodied in a code of ethics, that is, the professional views the "occupation and all of its requirements as an enduring set of normative and behavioral expectations."[51] Moreover, as professionals have a body of knowledge and skill that those outside the profession do not have, both the individual professional and the profession itself must exercise self-discipline. The profession as a whole must establish standards of practice and take steps to ensure adherence, while the individual practitioner must be committed to practice according to these standards. Consequently, organizations of professional practitioners have as their primary concerns the protection of the public and the advancement of the profession.

Although autonomy is put forth as the distinguishing characteristic of a profession, the validity of this is questionable. No individual and no group in our contemporary society is truly autonomous. A professional's autonomy not only is restrained by his or her responsibilities, but the professional also is held accountable to various individuals, groups, institutions and statutory bodies. Although a high degree of discretionary judgment in the application of the professional's knowledge and skills is not only desirable but necessary, true autonomy is not possible and probably is not desirable.

Finally, "the professions almost always involve at their core a significant interpersonal relationship between the professional on one hand, and the person who is thought to require the professional's services: the patient or the client."[52]

The philosophy of a profession embodies a set of ideals. Individual practitioners of that profession may exemplify these characteristics to a greater or lesser degree according to their capacities and to the degree of their commitment. However, they may not reject the philosophy totally without rejecting the profession.

Nursing is a true profession, distinguished by its philosophy of care, its full-time commitment to human well-being, its particular blend of knowledge and skill and its valuable service to the community. To the extent that nursing succeeds in regulating its practice and in meeting the health care needs of society, it will remain a profession. Individual practitioners will be viewed as professionals to the extent that they exemplify the characteristics that distinguish the profession of nursing.

DISCUSSION

The view of nursing as a moral art, the purpose of which is "the diagnosis and treatment of human responses to actual or potential health problems," entails knowledge of the individual patient. In other words, knowing the patient as a singular human being is not merely a nicety, it is an epistemological necessity. At the same time, it requires a revolutionary view of the nurse–patient relationship. Knowledge of an individual patient almost always is inadequate. The imbalance of power between the professional and the patient increases the possibility of unjustified, patronizing behavior. These factors suggest that tragic errors may occur unless patients are permitted—indeed, assisted—to become full partners in the development, design, and implementation of their own care. To achieve the potential of this relationship, nurses must provide information readily, share power equitably, encourage individuals to assume responsibility for their own health status, and work diligently to maintain their own integrity and the integrity of patients or clients.

One of the presuppositions of a profession is that there is a special and privileged relationship between the professional and the patient or client. In the past, this relationship entailed role-differentiated behavior that generally took the form of a parent–child relationship. That is, the professional was seen as the parent who defined the "good" for the child (patient) and assured compliance through various subtle and not so subtle means of coercion. The sole justification and safeguard for the patient was the guiding rule that health professionals always must prefer the patient's interests above those of all others.[53] "This is significant because it is the nature of role-differentiated behavior that it often makes it both appropriate and desirable for the person in a particular role to put to one side considerations . . . that would otherwise be relevant if not decisive."[54]

Nursing's task, as it moves to meet the demands of a more sophisticated consumer in a society characterized by moral pluralism, is to adjust roles such that professionals and patients will work together to promote the well-being of individuals. No longer can health care professionals afford to set aside such significant moral considerations as an individual's rights to self-determination and bodily integrity. Indeed, the demands of the adult relationships between nurses and patients are great, but the results, in terms of human integrity, personal responsibility, and professional accountability, are worth the effort.

NOTES

1. Wasserstrom, Richard. "Lawyers as Professionals: Some Moral Issues," *Human Rights,* Vol. 5 (1975) p. 2.
2. *Ibid.*

3. Amundsen, Darrel W. "Medical Ethics, History of Ancient Greece and Rome" in Warren T. Reich, ed. *The Encyclopedia of Bioethics* (The Free Press, New York, 1978) pp. 930–937.

4. Unschild, Paul. "Medical Ethics, History of Pre-Republican China," in Warren T. Reich, ed. *The Encyclopedia of Bioethics* (The Free Press, New York, 1978) pp. 906–916.

5. Jaggi, O. P., "Medical Ethics, The History of India," in Warren T. Reich, ed. *The Encyclopedia of Bioethics* (The Free Press, New York, 1978) pp. 906–910.

6. Moore, Thomas V. *Principles of Ethics,* 4th ed. (J. B. Lippincott, Philadelphia, 1935).

7. Crowder, Eleanor, "Manners, Morals and Nurses: An Historical Overview of Nursing Ethics," *Texas Reports on Biology and Medicine,* Vol. 32 (1974) pp. 173–180.

8. Ramsey, Paul. *The Patient as Person* (Yale University Press, New Haven, 1970).

9. *Ibid.*

10. London, Perry. "The Ethics of Behavior Control," in Richard Wertz, ed. *Readings on Ethical and Social Issues in Biomedicine* (Prentice-Hall, Englewood Cliffs, New Jersey, 1973) pp. 159–161.

11. *Ibid.*

12. Wertz, Richard W., ed. *Readings on Ethical and Social Issues in Biomedicine* (Prentice-Hall, Englewood Cliffs, New Jersey, 1973) pp. 1–5.

13. Hauerwas, Stanley. "Medicine as a Tragic Profession," in David Smith, ed. *No Rush to Judgment* (Indiana University Foundation, Bloomington, Indiana, 1978) p. 69.

14. Fuchs, Victor R. *Who Shall Live? Health, Economics and Social Choice* (Basic Books, New York, 1974) p. 52.

15. Hauerwas, *op. cit.,* pp. 71–72.

16. Ramsey, Paul. "The Nature of Medical Ethics," in Robert Veatch and Willard Gaylin, eds. *The Teaching of Medical Ethics* (A Hastings Center Publication, Hastings-on-Hudson, New York, 1973) pp. 14–27.

17. MacIntyre, Alistair. "How Virtues Become Vices: Values, Medicine and Social Context," in H. Tristam Englehardt and Stuart Spicker, eds. *Evaluation and Explanation in the Biomedical Sciences* (D. Reidel Publishing Company, Dordrecht, 1975) p. 108.

18. Illich, Ivan. *Medical Nemesis* (Pantheon Books, New York, 1976).

19. Hunt, Robert and John Arras. *Ethical Issues in Modern Medicine* (Mayfield Publishing Company, Palo Alto, California, 1977) p. 3.

20. Michaelson, Michael G. "The Coming Medical War," in *The New York Review of Books* (New York Review, Inc., New York, 1971).

21. Curtin, Leah L. "Optimal Care vs. Maximal Treatment," *Supervisor Nurse,* Vol. 10, No. 8 (1979) p. 16.

22. Hauerwas, *op. cit.,* p. 68.

23. Moore, *op. cit.,* Chapter 13.

24. McAllister, J. B. *Ethics With Special Application to the Medical and Nursing Professions,* 2nd ed. (Saunders and Company, Philadelphia, 1955).

25. Langham, Paul. "Open Forum: On Teaching Ethics to Nurses," *Nursing Forum,* Vol. XVI, Nos. 3 and 4 (1977) p. 225.

26. Gustafson, James. "Mongolism, Parental Desires and the Right to Life," *Perspectives in Biology and Medicine,* Vol. 16 (Summer 1973) p. 555.

27. American Nurses' Association. *Code for Nurses with Interpretive Statements* (American Nurses' Association, Kansas City, Missouri, 1976) p. 1.

28. Ladd, John. "Are Science and Ethics Compatible?" in H. Tristam Englehardt and

Daniel Callahan, eds. *Science, Ethics and Medicine* (A Hastings Center Publication, Hastings-on-Hudson, New York, 1976) p. 57.

29. *Ibid.,* p. 55.

30. Gadow, Sally. "Existential Advocacy: Philosophical Foundation for Nursing." A paper presented to the Four State Consortium on Nursing and the Humanities at its Phase I Conference, *Nursing and the Humanities: A Public Dialogue* (Farmingham, Connecticut, November 11, 1977).

31. The claim has been made that medicine is a moral art. For example, see "The Concept of Health and Disease," in H. Tristam Englehardt and Stuart Spicker, eds., *Evaluation and Explanation of the Biomedical Sciences* (D. Reidel Publishing Company, Dordrecht, 1975) and Eric Cassell, "Moral Thought in Clinical Practice," in H. Tristam Englehardt and Daniel Callahan, eds. *Science, Ethics and Medicine* (A Hastings Center Publication, Hastings-on-Hudson, New York, 1976). However, I think this claim can be made as validly (if not more so) for nursing.

32. Kelly, Lucie Young, "Nurse Practice Acts," *American Journal of Nursing,* Vol. 74, No. 7 (1974).

33. Gadow, *op. cit.*

34. Dubois, Rene. *So Human An Animal* (Chas. Scribner and Sons, New York, 1968) p. 121.

35. Gardiner, W. Lambert. *Psychology: A Story of a Search* (Brooks/Cole Publishing Company, Belmont, California, 1970) p. 94.

36. Gustafson, *op. cit.,* p. 529.

37. Treatment that is lifesaving may be rendered without consent if the individual is unconscious or otherwise unable to give consent and if there is no qualified person to authorize treatment.

38. When an individual cannot give consent for himself, for reasons of age, unconsciousness, or mental disability, a legal guardian may authorize treatment.

39. Maguire, Daniel. "The Freedom to Die," in Thomas Shannon, ed. *Bioethics* (Paulist Press, New York, 1976) pp. 171–180.

40. Jonas, Hans. "Ethical Aspects of Experimentation with Human Subjects," *Daedalus,* Journal of the American Academy of Arts and Sciences, Boston (Spring 1969) pp. 219–247.

41. Frankl, Viktor. *Man's Search for Meaning: An Introduction to Logotherapy.* Translated by Isle Lasch (Pocket Books, New York, 1963) pp. 160–163.

42. Nietzsche, Friedrich. *The Birth of Tragedy and the Geneology of Morals.* Translated by Francis Golffing (Doubleday/Anchor Books, New York, 1956) p. 298.

43. Ramsey, Paul. *Ethics at the Edges of Life* (Yale University Press, New Haven, 1978) pp. 43–93.

44. Wellman, Carl. *Morals and Ethics* (Scott-Foresman, Glenview, Illinois, 1975) p. 143.

45. *Ibid.,* p. 14.

46. Stone, Harlan Fiske. "The Conscientious Objector," *Columbia University Quarterly,* Vol. 21 (1919) p. 269.

47. Katz, Fred. "Nurses," in Amitai Etzioni, ed. *The Semi-Professions and Their Organization* (The Free Press, New York, 1970) pp. 82–104.

48. Shulman, Sam. "Basic Functional Roles in Nursing: Mother, Surrogate and Healer," in E. Jaco, ed. *Patients, Physicians and Illness* (The Free Press, New York, 1958) pp. 528–537.

49. Moore, Wilbert. *The Professions: Roles and Rules* (The Russell Sage Foundation, New York, 1970) pp. 5–6.

50. Wasserstrom, *op. cit.,* p. 2.

51. Wilbert Moore, *op. cit.,* p. 5.

52. Wasserstrom, *op. cit.,* p. 2.

53. Hauerwas, *op. cit.,* p. 113.

54. Wasserstrom, *op. cit.,* p.3.

9

The Commitment of Nursing

Leah Curtin

"It has given my heart a change of mood
And saved some part of the day I rued."

Adapted from Robert Frost's *Dust of Snow*

The claim that nursing is a moral art emphasizes nurses' commitment to care for as well as to give care to other human beings. It involves a particularly intense form of the general moral imperative to care for one another. Understanding the content of this commitment is important because it constitutes the scope and depth of ethical concern in nursing and lays a foundation for an approach to any one ethical quandary. Moreover, an understanding of nursing as a moral art challenges the notion that considerations of ethics in nursing are limited to or even solely focused on the discrete ethical quandaries faced by nurses.

THE CONTENT OF COMMITMENT

Commitment in the profession of nursing raises at least two questions: What does being a professional nurse involve? Even more puzzling, what does it mean to be a practitioner of a moral art? Such questions entail an explication of the role, character, and behavior of individual practitioners.

The question of how the nurse is committed to the patient or client necessarily involves what it means to be a professional. The word profession has as its root the Latin word, *profitere,* which literally means "to declare publicly." It was applied to certain occupations because the practitioners of those occupations declared publicly, that is, promised publicly that they would meet certain standards and dedicate themselves to serve people through the fulfillment of certain needs.

The philosopher J. L. Austin developed the now famous distinction between two different kinds of statements: descriptive and performative.[1] Descriptive statements transmit a given fact in the world. For example, "The tree outside my window is 40 feet high." or "You have cancer of the lung." or "Your child was born with a condition called meningomyelocele." However, performative statements alter a reality in the world by introducing a new ingredient—something that would not be there *apart from the declaration.* For example, "I, Leah, take thee, Peter, to be my wedded spouse. . ." or "I will help you." or "I will not abandon you."

Because a promise is a link between what is and what will be, to make or to break a promise is a very serious thing to do. If we want to understand the nature of nurses' commitment to patients or clients, we must examine the performative declarations of the nursing profession. To what have nurses committed themselves? What promises are entailed in the practice of this profession? Briefly, nurses have promised to help those who are ill to regain their health, those who are healthy to maintain their health, those who cannot be cured to maximize their potentials and those who are dying to live as fully as possible until their deaths. The making of such promises entails an honest commitment to their fulfillment because their fulfillment significantly affects people's lives.

By and large, the question of honesty of health professionals has been limited to discussion of whether to tell the patient the truth (or part of it) or, more saliently, who should tell the patient the truth. To be sure, truth-telling in the context of health care is quite important because it involves the imparting of highly significant and risk-laden knowledge.[2] The squabble about who should impart such knowledge to patients is an interdisciplinary conflict that involves the qualifications and roles of various practitioners. However, the performative declarations of a professional expand the demands of honesty in a professional's life. The moral question for the professional (in this case, the nurse) is not simply a matter of telling the truth, but also of *being true* to the promises of the profession.[3] That is, honesty among professionals not only entails truthfulness, but also fidelity.

For professionals to practice effectively, they must have the public's trust. There is no such thing as an automatic right to be trusted; it is a privilege that one earns. To trust a professional, a patient or client must believe that this individual has the knowledge necessary to help him, and that this person will act in his best interests. The first involves knowledge: What special expertise does the professional have that enables her to address a specific problem? The second involves commitment: the promises the profession and the professional both make and imply—and whether the promises are kept.

Because the degree of trust granted by the public to a profession rests squarely on the shoulders of individual practitioners, the consequences of the presence or absence of fidelity in individual nurses are enormous. The total situation for patients includes not only the disease or disability they have, but also whether someone will care for them or abandon them through the course of the disease or through their dying. Taken as a whole, the performative declarations of the nursing profession commit nurses to work to improve the quality of living of those who seek or who receive their services.

While the fidelity of the nurse to these promises may not eliminate disease or prevent dying, it will affect the context in which the patient lives, that is, his or her quality of life. This is precisely why nurses are so concerned about preventing disease, promoting health, engaging in patient teaching and health counseling, maintaining health, and caring for the dying. If they are to fulfill the promises of the profession, they must become equally concerned with developing innovative ways of caring for persons who are chronically ill, handicapped, retarded, or aged. For nursing to be valued fully by the public, nurses must take the lead in developing innovative approaches to elevating the quality of life for those who cannot be cured.

The patient, specifically the institutionalized patient, is surrounded by nursing personnel twenty-four hours a day. Nurses create the atmosphere in which patients live or die. While it is true that some facts cannot be changed (the fact that a person is irreversibly dying; the fact that a child is born with a severely handicapping condition; the fact that a person is quadriplegic as a result of trauma or disease), the conditions under which people live out these facts can be changed. It is nursing's responsibility to create the opportunities and the atmosphere in which patients or clients can actualize their potentials and live their lives as fully as possible. Nursing assessments revolve around identification of an individual's quality of life to enable nurses to improve that quality of life. This is the moral imperative of nursing practice. Indeed, it describes how the nurse is committed to the patient. To the degree to which nurses are faithful to this commitment, they will alter the reality of the lives of patients or clients and their families.

PROFESSIONAL STANDARDS

Unfortunately, professions develop unevenly because the professionals who comprise them are in diverse states of awareness, intellectual attainment, and commitment. Practitioners' perceptions of their roles and their character traits affect the problems they see, the personal presence they bring to them, the manner in which they address them, and the reservoir of personal resources they can call upon to serve another day. At the same time, their moral commitments (or lack of them), as repeated in thousands of their colleagues, will create or destroy the profession.

The license to practice does not include a permission to practice poorly; it presupposes an obligation to practice well. The power to license that society grants to the professions exists prior to the granting of licenses to practice. If the license to practice entails an obligation to practice well, the power to license must include the obligation to judge and to monitor well the practice of individual practitioners.⁴ As individual members of a profession, we share the obligation of assuring that established standards of practice are followed by all members of the profession. Practicing a profession involves internalizing a philosophy, perceiving what is congruent with reality and developing a discretion that enables one to recognize what is "fitting" or appropriate within this role. Among other things, it raises the questions of professional standards, self-regulation and self-discipline. The problem of maintaining professional standards goes to the heart of a profession's obligations to society. Professionals tend to avoid this problem because it involves questions of the virtue, style and character of the individual practitioner.

THE IMPLICATIONS OF NURSING'S COMMITMENT

In general, reflections on ethics in the nursing context have focused on the discrete quandaries faced by individual practitioners. The most obvious reason for this is that nurses naturally desire help in resolving the moral problems they face in every day practice. A less obvious reason may be that quandary ethics tends to ignore problems of professional discipline because it concentrates on particular problems of usually anonymous practitioners. As a result, professional ethics tend to concentrate only on exploring the moral principles that are applicable to concrete cases—what one might call abstract ethics for decision makers. In other words, analytic faculties are focused on how to reach a particular decision and generally fail to address how the decision should or can be implemented. Such an approach tends to obscure the fundamental philosophy that defines the profession and the degree of commitment the individual professional has to this philosophy.

Moreover, while professionals concentrate comfortably on procedural questions of appropriate decision making, larger questions about the social and economic structures within which the profession operates are left to others—political scientists, social engineers, health planners, economists, and administrators. For example, this proclivity tends to obscure nurses' obligations not just to share information with patients, but actually to teach patients and other lay persons about disease and health and to involve them actively in maintaining their own health. In the process of teaching, one does not just give words to people; one helps to interpret what is happening and why it is happening. Teaching has a therapeutic value that extends beyond the explanation of a disease; it can and should enable a person to understand his problem or potential problem, to ask critical questions about it, and to help make whole (or to heal) the individual and thus place him in a position of control over what happens to him. Health professionals really have committed relatively few of their professional resources to developing innovative systems for delivering preventive care and health knowledge to the public.

Concentration on only specific, individual problems may lead to neglect of the demands of social justice. Because the practice of a profession requires knowledge and skill that are essential to the public welfare, the principles of distributive justice require the delivery of such essential services to the whole community. In return, society accords the profession certain powers, status and privileges to the extent that its members help meet the needs of the public.

Clearly, no one professional or profession at large can meet all the needs of the public. In fact, a profession cannot even fulfill its own circumscribed mission without widespread communal support and assistance. However, professionals do have at least four obligations under the principles of distributive justice: (1) to do what they reasonably can do to meet the need for their services; (2) to do what they know how to do competently, whether or not the patient can pay for their services; (3) to help design methods for dealing with the health as well as the illness needs of the populace; and (4) to testify to the community about a social system that fails to meet the fundamental health needs of its citizenry. These obligations obtain not only because of one's role as a professional but also because a professional is in a position to know the injustices that result from the inequitable distribution of health resources. With this knowledge comes both the power and the responsibility to effect change.

In addition, health professionals have been lax in developing adequately systems for the care of long-term, chronic, and disabled individuals. While society has fostered elaborate specialization to handle problems in acute medicine, it has devoted a woefully small amount of its resources to the nursing care needs of large segments of the population. Thus, although medicine has been remarkably successful at prolonging life, nursing has yet to tackle effectively the problem of improving the quality of the lives so prolonged.

These problems of professional ethics require systemic, structural, and institutional reform. They do not fit easily (if they fit at all) into the conventional pattern of case-oriented ethics. The commitment of nursing demands that nurses develop an approach to ethics that is proactive rather than reactive; that nurses concentrate on the deeper aspects of preventive, chronic, and maintenance care rather than on the dramatic problems of acute care; and that nurses direct attention to the milieu in which they must make decisions, that is, environmental and personal factors that inhibit or advance the ability of individual providers to implement decisions.

For example, case-oriented ethics may lead nurses to the decision that it is not ethically defensible to kill an infant who is retarded, but they no longer can afford to ignore what this decision entails: it must address *how* the child shall live. That is, it logically entails a commitment to do what is possible to improve the quality of the child's life. To ignore this logical entailment is to abrogate the commitment of our profession: the commitment to improve the quality of living.

It has been said that knowledge and skill are the foundations of professionalism; this is not the case. Although knowledge and skill are integral to the practice of a profession, the foundation of a profession consists of the performative declarations professed by its practitioners and the fidelity of the practitioner to these promises. The fidelity of the practitioner is at the very root of the relationship between the individual and the professional and between society and the profession. Without fidelity there is no trust, and without trust the nurse cannot practice.

NOTES

1. May, William F. "Normative Inquiry and Medical Ethics in Our Colleges and Universities," in David Smith and Linda M. Bernstein, eds. *No Rush to Judgment: Essays on Medical Ethics* (The Indiana University Foundation, Bloomington, Indiana, 1978) p. 356.
2. Fletcher, John. "The Parent–Child Bond," *Theological Studies* 33 (September 1972) p. 458.
3. May, *op. cit.*, p. 357.
4. May, *op. cit.*, p. 360.

BIBLIOGRAPHY

Bandman, Bertram, "The Human Rights of Patients, Nurses and Other Health Professionals," in Elsie Bandman and Bertram Bandman (eds.). *Bioethics and Human Rights.* Little, Brown, Boston, 1978, pp. 321–330.

Bandman, Elsie L., "The Rights of Nurses and Patients: A Case for Advocacy," in Elsie Bandman and Bertram Bandman (eds.). *Bioethics and Human Rights.* Little, Brown, Boston, 1978, pp. 332–337.

Bok, Sissela. *Lying.* Pantheon Books, New York, 1978, pp. 220–248.

Fried, Charles. *An Anatomy of Values: Problems of Personal and Social Choice.* Harvard University Press, Cambridge, Massachusetts, 1970, p. 217.

Fried, Charles, "Rights and Health Care—Beyond Equity and Efficiency," *The New England Journal of Medicine,* Vol. 293, No. 5, July 13, 1975, pp. 241–245.

Fuchs, Victor. *Who Shall Live? Health Economics and Social Choice.* Basic Books, New York, 1974, pp. 52–58.

Gadow, Sally, "Nursing and the Humanities: An Approach to Humanistic Issues in Health Care," in Elsie Bandman and Bertram Bandman (eds.). *Bioethics and Human Rights.* Little, Brown, Boston, 1978, pp. 305–312.

Hiatt, Howard, "Protecting the Medical Commons: Who is Responsible?" *The New England Journal of Medicine,* Vol. 293, No. 5, July 31, 1975, pp. 235–241.

Kass, Leon, "Regarding the End of Medicine and the Pursuit of Health," *The Public Interest,* No. 40, Summer 1975, p. 39.

Murphy, Catherine P., "The Moral Situation in Nursing," in Elsie Bandman and Bertram Bandman (eds.). *Bioethics and Human Rights.* Little, Brown, Boston, 1978, pp. 313–319.

Pincoffs, Edmund, "Quandary Ethics," *Mind,* Vol. 80, 1971, p. 552.

Ramsey, Paul. *The Patient as Person.* Yale University Press, New Haven, 1970, pp. 252–275.

Urmson, J. O., "Saints and Heros," in A. I. Milden (ed.). *Essays in Moral Philosophy.* University of Washington Press, Seattle, 1958, p. 198.

10

The Nurse–Family Relationship

Jeanne Quint Benoliel

"The essence of man is the experience of his relation to other human beings, and to the cosmos."

Rene Dubos, *So Human an Animal*

A nurse's primary responsibility is to the individual (patient) regardless of whether the purpose of the transaction is to prevent disease, restore health, promote well-being, rehabilitate the person, or relieve suffering.[1] In other words, the nurse–family relationship is subordinate to the nurse's primary responsibility to diagnose and treat the human responses of individuals to actual or potential health problems. According to Logan,[2] the nursing literature typically depicts the family as a support system or resource for an individual member defined as "ill" and in need of assistance. However, across fields of specialization within nursing, the family often is diagnosed as abnormal or dysfunctional in some way and a mode of intervention is prescribed to correct a problem.

The work that nurses do brings them into frequent contact with human situations in which the values, beliefs, and practices of families can be at variance with the values, beliefs, or practices in the health delivery system. These differences can lead to withdrawal from treatment, conflicts among providers, difficult choices and decisions, and problems in communication among all concerned. That is, the nurse's ability to offer sound care or to encourage the patient to engage in health-promoting activities is affected by the attitudes and behaviors of members of his family. If the needs of a family go unheeded, the patient's humanity very often suffers another blow.

VALUES IN HEALTH CARE DELIVERY

Several features of the health care system contribute to this state of affairs. Health services are delivered by many different specialists who may or may not communicate effectively with each other about the people being served. The goals and programs of the health care system are dominated by the ideology of the biomedical model of disease that separates mind and body and considers disease in human beings to be a scientific phenomenon to be studied. According to Engel,[3] the biomedical model of disease has become a cultural imperative (the dominant folk model of disease). Thus, all members of society today are influenced to a greater or lesser extent by a belief system that defines *disease* primarily as biomedical and physical deviations from established norms and *treatment* as activity to destroy the diseased part. Based on principles and methods drawn from the physical sciences, the model does not include behavioral and psychosocial data and it fails to take account of an individual's personal experience of illness. All providers (including nurses) in Western systems of health care delivery have been socialized to this belief system and perform roles in keeping with the biomedical model.

The combined influence of science and of its successes also led to the notion that death is an enemy to be conquered and to the emergence of the physician as an active intervenor between death and the individual.[4] In the twentieth century, the attempt to keep death under control has been industrialized—a state of affairs fostered by social legislation that has made medical care available to most people. Rapid expansion of medical technology and biomedical research in the 1950s contributed to the development of the hospital as a highly technical life-saving establishment and changed the character of human birth and human death. The decade between 1960 and 1970 saw the establishment of a variety of critical care settings, all with heavy emphasis on life-saving medical activity.[5] Increasingly, nurses found their work dominated by the demands and pressures of medical techniques and procedures and by the high value attached to life-saving activity.[6]

Nurses' ideas about their rights and responsibilities as well as about the rights, responsibilities, and obligations of patients and families are influenced strongly by the biomedical model of disease. In addition, the majority of nurses are introduced to practice in settings that support and affirm the primacy of critical care work. The power of the biomedical model is reinforced by educational programs in nursing that emphasize the importance attached to disease processes and medical treatments. Moreover, the primacy of the biomedical model is reflected in the policies and mechanisms whereby funds are made available to agencies providing nursing services to people. Given the power of these beliefs, it is not surprising that many nurses define their responsibilities to patients and families in terms of the primary goals of medical practice. The historical dominance of medical thought over health care delivery and nursing practice also has affected beliefs about the proper behaviors of patients and families. In short, health care delivery in the United States and Canada is designed around the belief that scientific treatment of disease is more important than the care of human beings.

According to Levine,[7] the attitudes and behaviors of nurses toward patients and families also are influenced by a white, middle-class perspective, heavily weighted by a Protestant ethic, that fosters an image of the patient as a dependent child who does not know what is good for him. Such a bias carries an expectation that the patient will behave in certain acceptable ways and, above all, will do as the nurse has told him to do. It also limits understanding of the structure of families and the differing belief systems that influence the adaptations of families to illness, diversity and stressful life experiences. Patients and their families are expected to be "good"; their human rights as well as their cultural differences often are neglected.

DIFFERENCES IN BELIEF SYSTEMS

The people served by nurses and other health care providers come from a variety of cultural backgrounds. Their culturally derived belief systems foster particular definitions of health and illness and prescribe the behaviors expected of individuals and families in response to important life events such as birth, death, and serious illness. Although such events are shared across human groups, individual and familial behaviors, rooted in differing primary values and beliefs, can vary widely.

Some of the misunderstandings between families and health providers have their origins in these differences. For example, in the United States the individual historically has been considered more important and more sacred than the social group. To this day, individualism continues to be a primary value in society and in the field of nursing.[8] However, in many societies the value of the social group is superior to that of an individual. People in cultures that emphasize the importance of the family or tribe learn from infancy that the group is central to their lives. Commonly, when illness appears, members of the extended family gather around the patient to offer assistance. The support offered by the extended family plays an important part in the patient's recovery.[9] However, the appearance of large extended families in the hospital can be prevented by nurses who believe that the patient's recovery is aided by limitation of the number of visitors. For some patients, isolation from kin who function as a support system interferes with their ability to cope with their illnesses.

Differences in cultural beliefs about the proper treatment of serious illness may result in a family's failure to follow the regimen prescribed by a physician. For example, a public health nurse providing home care services to a Navajo woman with terminal cancer found that the family offered exquisite physical care but did not give the medications as directed.[10] The Navajo aide who assisted the nurse thought that the family withheld the prescribed medicine because they feared that more of the drugs would make her worse. The family arranged for visits from the medicine man because they believed that his ceremonies, known as "sings," would help the woman to regain a balanced state. The Navajos believe that illness occurs when an individual has fallen out of a delicate balance with the environment and that restoration of health is achieved through the acts of a knowledgeable religious specialist. Like a number of other cultural groups, the Navajo people do not distinguish between health and religious practices. For them, treatment of illness involves the total environment, including the supernatural.

Families that do not follow the prescribed medical plan of treatment often are labelled "noncompliant"; they have failed to follow the "right" approach to treatment. In this instance, the nurse chose to support the family's choices and to help them provide for the patient's physical comfort through the period of dying. The nurse respected the family's values and behaviors even though she occasionally was uncomfortable with their practices.[11]

Each patient's humanity is linked closely to the values that have shaped his life; his expression of basic human needs is affected by a cultural belief system that prescribes proper behavior in response to many aspects of living. Cultural values and beliefs determine food preferences and eating styles, religious beliefs and rituals, sex-role relationships, verbal and nonverbal communication patterns and obligations to other members of society. The people of the world, through their varied ethnic and subcultural groups, have devised many different ways of responding to basic needs. They also have a tendency to categorize and stereotype groups whose behaviors differ from their own. Ethnocentricism, that is, seeing one's own culture as "better than" another's culture, has the unfortunate consequence of labelling other people as inferior and therefore unworthy of equal consideration.

Vocal minorities in the United States claim that the health care system does not respond to their cultural differences or to their special needs. Leininger[12] supports this view by noting that Western health providers often know very little about the cultures of the ethnic subgroups they serve and believe that their own health ideas are the desirable ones. Such an attitude ignores the special needs of individual members of a cultural subgroup. However, to label all members of a minority group and to expect them to respond in the same manner ignores the special needs of the person. For example, a nurse who has read Zborowski's[13] study of pain responses in Jewish, Italian, Irish, and older American patients now may approach all Jewish and Italian patients with an expectation that they will respond emotionally to pain. An appropriate attitude toward people of different ethnic persuasions is fostered by respect for individual differences based on the knowledge that what may be generally applicable to a particular group may not apply to some persons in that group. In other words, the variations in human behavior within any subcultural group are extensive—and most people thrive on respect for their individualities.

Differences in the belief systems of nurses and other health care workers and family expectations about roles and role relationships also can lead to ethical problems of various kinds. In part, these problems arise because of differences in interpretation of right and wrong behaviors.

ETHICAL VALUES AND CULTURAL VALUES

All human societies provide for the sustenance and survival of their members. The achievement of these broad goals requires a social organization through which necessary resources are provided, the group is protected and children learn their proper roles in society. Across cultures, the kinship system has been the primary social mechanism by means of which individuals have learned their rights and responsibilities as members of society. In a general sense, families have been responsible for socializing new members into society and for teaching them concepts of "right" and "wrong" that they are expected to accept without question.

The problem is that moral practices based on cultural values and beliefs are not always congruent with ethical definitions of human rights and obligations. More than that, unreflected prescriptions about right and wrong conduct infer action without choice in contrast to the ethical premise that choice of "right action" follows a mental process of rational problem solving. Some examples may help to clarify these differences.

Families in all societies carry special obligations to children who are not yet capable of taking care of themselves. In addition, families have special responsibilities to train these new members for their roles as adults and to assist them in learning behaviors deemed appropriate by the group. Although child training is a universal human activity, the general techniques of socialization used by persons responsible for child-rearing may depend on the values, beliefs, and practices of the group.[14] In traditional Japanese society, child-rearing practices during the first five years of life were extremely permissive by Western standards and discipline was exerted primarily through the use of ridicule.[15] In contrast, European societies traditionally emphasized corporal punishment as the principal means for establishment of compliance with authority.[16] Although today many parents still believe that they have the right to discipline their children by means of physical force, ethical concerns about the human rights of children, particularly their right to bodily integrity, has led to a change in law: physical violence has come to be classified as child abuse. Established cultural beliefs about parents' use of corporal punishment have given way to new societal beliefs about the welfare of children and about their rights as human beings.[17] In professional practice, however, nurses still encounter situations in which these values are in conflict and choices must be made about what to do if child abuse is suspected.

Culturally determined beliefs also have had a powerful influence on expectations about and attitudes toward women. The patriarchal system that dominated the Greco-Roman, Semitic, Indian, Chinese, and Japanese civilizations and, in turn, our own society, defined women as subordinate to men and incapable of making decisions outside the home.[18] As a result, women have been treated unequally in many areas of life—economic, educational, civic, and legal. The patriarchal system also contributed to the belief that women are "frail creatures" who must be protected from bad news and guided in their choices by the men in their family. Consequently, there are many women whose husbands or fathers decide that they are not to be given complete information about a diagnosis and prognosis. It is clear that such decisions interfere with the human rights to bodily integrity and self-determination.

Children also are subject to patriarchal control and often are prevented from having direct access to knowledge about their states of health. As minors, children are vulnerable on yet another score—parents' beliefs about disease and treatment may conflict with scientifically grounded medical therapies and can interfere with the application of life-saving treatments. In cases involving the use of blood transfusions, the courts have held that parental control can be limited when the safety and welfare of children or others unable to care for themselves are clearly at stake.[19] However, reliance on court orders may exacerbate differences between a family and the medical care system.[20]

Families share common obligations to provide support for their members, but they may define these duties *in personum* differently. Therefore, while all families may accept the responsibility to care for a sick member, some may not want the patient fully informed and others may think that the patient alone should make all decisions about treatment. Cultural definitions of human rights and privileges are based on beliefs about positions in the family system rather than on beliefs about individual human needs. These definitions determine who has decision-making power over whom and under what sets of circumstances decisions are made. In addition, communication patterns within families are subject to intergenerational differences in values and beliefs and intergenerational differences in personal and familial priorities.[21] Recognition of these powerful influences on the behaviors of patients, families and nurses can help one gain perspective on the complexity of professional relationships with people whose expressions of human needs and social concerns take very different forms.[22]

FOUNDATIONS OF NURSE–FAMILY RELATIONSHIPS

The impact of kinship and friendship networks on the human experience makes attention to families and other living groups a necessary ingredient in the planning and implementing of humane nursing care. There are at least two reasons that attention to families is important: (1) As extensions of individuals, families are influential contributors to the ongoing life experience of their members. (2) Some health care problems can lead to social crises of serious dimensions that interfere with a family's capacity to function or with the human needs of some of the family members.

FAMILIES AS RESOURCES

If one assumes that the unique needs of patients are the central focus of ethical concern in nursing, it follows that families are important resources. They can offer singular contributions to the situation—as sources of information, support, and direct assistance. They also may help make judgments about the capacity of an individual to make decisions. Family members, through choices and actions, may facilitate or limit the patient's opportunities for self-determination and his search for personal meaning. For example, they may think that their loved one should not be told that he is dying, even though the person has asked to be given such information. Although family members usually request that this information be withheld because they fear that it will lead to depression, such practices support deception of the person who is dying and may interfere with opportunities to bring closure to life.

Nursing's commitment to helping the dying person find meaning in dying cannot be fulfilled ethically through disregard of the family's claim. In such a situation, nurses' efforts should be directed to support of the family's concerns, to provide help for them in clarification of their values concerning the loss of someone important and, perhaps, to provide help for them in understanding that lying to a person who is dying can lead to loss of trust in the good intentions of other people.[23] This is not to say that such support is superior to the imperatives of the nurse–patient relationship. One is not substituting concern about the family for concern about the patient. Rather, it is an essential nursing service in support of the patient's life situation.

Families' contributions to a situation can be important, most commonly because families provide information that has bearing on the nurse–patient relationship. Siegler,[24] commenting on the factors that influence a physician's decision to discontinue heroic life-saving activity, observed that a family can be helpful in interpreting whether or not a patient's behavior (for example, a request for no resuscitation) is typical or highly unusual. The family would not make the choice for the patient, but could help the physician to determine the validity of the patient's personal wish in the matter. Although probably useful in a context of critical illness or in an emergency setting, generally speaking, family members' opinions about a patient's values should be viewed with caution, particularly when the situation involves prolonged chronic disease, loss of consciousness or mental illness. In other words, health crises that put prolonged or extreme pressure on the values and needs of family members may color their perceptions of the patient's wishes and needs. In general, the validity of a family member's opinion about a patient's "usual behavior" is enhanced if it is supported by more than one family member. However, family members' interpretations of the patient's values and behaviors should not replace the patient's stated values in the context of the nurse–patient relationship itself. Although often helpful and insightful, family members' observations alone should not determine the course of action.

Families are valuable resources; they can provide information about factors that influence the patient's situation. Families also are the custodians of many resources—fiscal, psychological and social—that have a direct bearing on a patient's recovery or adaptation to a particular health crisis. However, families often need help in recognizing and mobilizing the resources at their disposal in ways that maximize the well-being of all concerned, particularly when the health problems are complex. Young parents with a first-born child, for instance, generally are not prepared for parenthood—the changes in responsibility, routine and lifestyle that result from the introduction of an infant to their home. Support from nurses in the form of information, direct assistance and active listening can make a difference in the way that many new parents meet the human needs of these vulnerable babies. In a general sense, nurses have many opportunities to help families in transition to organize themselves and their resources to meet the human needs of their members in responsible and responsive ways.

The nurse's role in helping a family mobilize its resources does not mean that the nurse assumes responsibility for obligations that properly belong to the patient or family. Rather, it implies a willingness on the part of patient, family, and nurse to exchange information that can assist in problem solving and to collaborate in the achievement of mutually agreed upon goals. The nurse should be sensitive to the private nature of the information shared by the patient and ordinarily should let the patient determine whether that information will be exchanged with family members or other health care providers. Exceptions to this rule may be necessary if the information the patient shares with the nurse contains indications of a threat to the lives of the patient or others. However, a decision to violate patient confidentiality should not be made hastily; it should occur only for proportionately serious reasons. The nurse must realize fully that the patient's right to privacy is being violated and should take account of all factors that are relevant to disclosure.

Effective mobilization of helpful resources also depends on a family's willingness to collaborate with the nurse; that is, the nurse's right to offer nursing care implies an obligation on the part of family members to participate in ways that promote or, at least, do not interfere with the welfare of the patient. A nurse should not be expected to perform treatments that she believes bring harm to the patient, but she has an obligation to explain her position to family members and to tell them why she will not help with a particular course of action. However, nurses cannot expect the family to help the patient at the expense of their own health or well-being. The establishment of collaborative arrangements with family members requires respectful attitudes on the part of both nurse and family and a willingness to negotiate reasonable contractual agreements.

Ideally, these agreements should take place through the open sharing of power by patient, family, and nurses as they work together toward mutually acceptable goals. Communication among participants should be in keeping with the guidelines that Dworkin[25] outlines for the preservation of individual autonomy through attention to authenticity and procedural independence. The methods of influence chosen by the nurse should "support the self-respect and dignity of those who are being influenced." Methods of influence that interfere with the ability of an individual to think rationally about his own interests, make use of deception, are physically intrusive, and show basic disregard for the personal identities of individuals should be avoided.[26] Generally, the autonomy of all participants is enhanced by active involvement—both cognitive and affective—in all the ways and means used to bring about change. Collaboration with families may be difficult to achieve when their adaptive capacity is limited in scope or when the health problem creates other difficulties within the family.

FAMILIES IN CRISIS

Some health problems make unusual demands on a family's coping resources. Catastrophic events, such as the sudden and unexpected death of the principal wage-earner, can magnify the human needs of all survivors in a family, especially those who are particularly vulnerable to the actions of others. The needs of children for sustenance and support are very great following the sudden death of a mother or father. However, caught up in his own needs and preoccupations, the surviving parent easily can overlook the needs of children for information, security, and participation in mourning.[27] The sudden loss of a significant human relationship creates wounds of many kinds. It often leads to social disorganization and problems in communication, psychological distress, and personal disruption. People often experience a need to find meaning in the event and to search for ways of coming to terms with its reality. Just as the dying person searches to find meaning in his death, so the survivors try to find meaning in the event and its circumstances.[28]

In the aftermath of catastrophic events, family members are vulnerable people. The special needs of dependent members may not be met if the responsible adults are caught up in their own human responses without access to caring relationships that support them in their efforts to cope with the full impact and range of change produced by the experience. In such circumstances a family may not be able to mobilize its personal and social resources effectively without the assistance of outside sources of help and guidance.

Another health problem that makes unusual demands on a family's coping resources is one that creates chronic stress—often over a prolonged period of time. The extended illness or disability of one member of the family can create difficulties for other family members as they try to meet their obligations to one another. For example, the terminal illness of a mother in a family with young children can prevent her from functioning in her established role. However, the introduction of another family member as temporary housekeeper, who is likely to use different child-rearing practices, may be disruptive for the children. If these practices are not oriented toward the human needs of the children who already are vulnerable because of the forthcoming loss of a significant relationship, conflict may result.

In similar fashion, the progressive deterioration of an aged parent can lead to stressful living conditions for the adult child who assumes the care-taking functions. According to Robinson and Thurnher,[29] the stress associated with care-taking increases over time as the demands of the role impinge more and more on the child's life and life-style. The stress for the adult child comes from two sources: coping with changes in the mental functioning of the parent and coping with feelings of ambivalence and antagonism toward the parent. The sense of confinement associated with care-taking functions also contributes to stress, especially when the need to be available interferes with the child's established pattern of living or personal need for fulfillment through other kinds of activity. Robinson and Thurnher found that an adult child's decision to relocate a parent—either at home or in a nursing home—was not made precipitously but generally was reached after a lengthy period of physical and mental deterioration of the parent.[30] These transitions imposed severe psychic stress and taxed the child's ability to cope with the situation. From an ethical perspective, the problems associated with late-life parent–child relationships are difficult because they involve conflicting rights and obligations that are not resolved easily. Such situations are tragic because there is no easy solution to the problems presented in a relationship that has few rewards for one of the participants.

Any long-term health problem that makes heavy demands on a family's care-giving resources may disrupt the interpersonal relationships of the whole family. For example, caring for a physically handicapped or mentally retarded child in the home places great strain on parental relationships and inevitably affects the care that parents are able to provide to the other children. As time goes by, such situations tax the human resources and coping abilities of all persons living in the household. By their very nature, such situations shift the rhythm and balance in established patterns of human relationship, just as terminal illness can disrupt the basis for intimacy.[31] Situations of chronic care-giving easily may interfere with the quality of living of some if not all of the members of a family.

Sometimes a health problem experienced by one member of a family leads to a crisis for someone else. For a school girl, an unexpected pregnancy creates an emotional crisis: she must tell her parents and she does not know how they will react to the news. In her study of early pregnancies, LaBarre[32] found that most of the girls were surprised and relieved that their parents took the news reasonably well. She also observed that the mothers identified with their daughters in what is clearly a profound feminine experience. However, LaBarre's findings indicated that the support provided by the parents did not come without moments of distress and periods of soul-searching for them. All of these girls carried their pregnancies to term and the majority of the parents supported them throughout the experience. Of course, there also can be a situation in which a teenager wants to have an abortion but her mother, already upset by the pregnancy, is even more upset because she opposes the practice of abortion. In such a family, a double crisis now exists.

Even though a recent U.S. Supreme Court decision protected a minor female's legal right to opt for abortion without parental consent,[33] conflict between parents and child about the morality of abortion can lead to distressing problems in family relationships. Consideration of abortion can have a dramatic impact on the child–parent relationship and can provoke deep parental concern about decision-making powers within the family. In particular, such a situation can exacerbate conflicts in values and differences of opinion concerning the rights of children and parents and the obligations of both. The point is that recourse to legal power to resolve the problem for the teenager may do little to assist the family to come to terms in positive ways with the human complexities of their situation. The process through which the girl and her parents reach a resolution to the problem may be growth-producing or growth-restricting, and the resources available to aid them in reaching their decisions could make the difference.

Another particularly difficult situation faced by families is that in which one member is faced with making a choice or decision about the life or well-being of an ill member of the family. In such situations, paternalistic decision making is common and many people are unaware that human rights are violated. However, these situations become morally problematic and highly stressful when a life or death decision must be made. Given the use of high technology in medical care today, these decisions often involve choice between continuation and discontinuation of active medical therapies. These are difficult situations, not only because of the personal losses involved, but also because they present ethical quandaries: the decision maker must base his choice on the presumed consent of the person whose life is at stake or, in the case of infants, on the potential quality of their lives.[34]

Moreover, these decision-making situations assume added complexity when the wishes of the family are in conflict with the beliefs of the medical staff. One major difficulty is that families may be deprived of full information because the information they receive is guided by the specific frames of reference of the various professional groups involved.[35] Many families are unable to countermand the powerful influence of the health care establishment and are left with unhappy memories of an unfinished experience. Others may take their case to the courts and make their claim for the patient through appeal to the right of privacy—an avenue that was taken by the parents of Karen Ann

Quinlan in discontinuing the use of a respirator.[36] Such action is costly and many families do not have the resources to choose it. Patients and families need a mechanism that will enable them to have access to full information about the complexities of their lot and to participate fully in the decisions that affect their present and future lives. Because nurses are concerned with the whole human being, they should be involved in the creation and implementation of these important social mechanisms.

HUMAN NEEDS AND FAMILY NEEDS

It has been established that the distinctive needs of patients are the central focus of ethical concern in nursing. It follows that patients' families are also of ethical concern whenever the human rights of patients are jeopardized by the family or whenever the health problem with which they are struggling threatens the humanity of family members as well. The nurse–patient relationship is embedded in a matrix of other interpersonal relationships that greatly influence what happens to the humanity of the patient. In a number of health situations, attention to the family's needs is an essential concomitant to the nurse–patient relationship. In such situations, the structure of the nurse–patient relationship will be determined not solely by the patient's human needs and the nurse's responses to them but also by the family's values, norms and modes of conduct.

The purpose of the nurse–family relationship is to provide support that assists families in at least three ways: 1) in meeting the human needs of their dependent members in ways that show respect for the individual's rights to autonomy and freedom of action, 2) in making decisions that are based on all relevant information, and 3) in creating a context that allows distressing life situations to be used by families and nurses to promote compassion and human concern in their relationships with one another. Nurses' actions may not always avert tragic outcomes, but nurses' choices and decisions may serve to humanize the atmosphere in which families live through their own particular tragedies.

FORM OF THE NURSE–FAMILY RELATIONSHIP

The nurse–family relationship is more complex than the nurse–patient relationship because it requires human-to-human relationships with at least two members of a family and sometimes with many more. The form of the nurse–family relationship will depend on a combination of factors—the nature of the health problem, the context in which the nurse–family relationship occurs and other circumstances that structure its characteristics and duration.

NATURE OF THE HEALTH PROBLEM

When patients are hospitalized for acute illnesses of short duration, the nurse–family relationship often is tangential to the nurse–patient relationship. In other words, the depersonalizing aspects of short term, clearly reversible health problems can be counteracted much of the time by a nurse–patient relationship centered on the human needs of the person who happens to be the patient. However, even in this situation, the creation of an effective nurse–family relationship may be necessary to assist a key member of the patient's family to support the patient's right to self-determination through access to information or opportunity to participate in decisions.

The nurse–family relationship assumes increasing importance when the health problem is long-term in nature, irreversible in its effects, requires difficult decisions about one of the members, or interferes with the quality of people's lives. Unlike delimited illness that requires a temporary adjustment, these problems create the need for major adaptations in living and often test a family's basic value system. For instance, a family faced with a decision to continue or to discontinue active treatment in one who is comatose may find itself caught in value conflicts regarding who among them should make the decision, which course of action should be taken and who should be responsible for long-term care. Because of the tensions they generate, prolonged deteriorating illness and its related problems affect the human capacity to be human and, not uncommonly, may cause family members to behave in a dehumanizing manner toward each other. In a word, any health problem that interferes with a family's established way of life makes heavy demands on the human resources of its members and increases the tendency of the family to use paternalistic practices in reaching decisions. Like the patient whose experience of illness creates new human needs, the family as a human group is vulnerable to the depersonalizing influences of many serious health care problems. The nurse–family relationship may provide one avenue of assistance to family members who must cope with the human problems and the serious decisions associated with major health crises.

CONTEXT OF THE NURSE–FAMILY RELATIONSHIP

Although the nature of a health problem influences the form of a nurse–family relationship, the setting in which interactions take place is important also. The hospital, for example, is a setting that accords high value to life-saving activity and that is governed by the norms and rules of the health care establishment. Judgments about proper behavior for patients and members of families are determined by health care personnel who maintain control over many facets of hospital living. In contrast, the patient's home reflects the values, norms, and rules of living deemed appropriate by the family, and determinations about proper behavior in this setting are subject to the family's control. Usually, the nurse is more at ease in the hospital than is the patient or family, whereas the latter are more comfortable at home than is the nurse who comes for a visit. The point is that the content and focus of discussion in any interaction between a nurse and a member of the family will be affected by the setting in which they meet and the comfort they experience in the exchanged information and ideas.

Types of contacts between nurse and family are determined by the nature of the human problems faced by the patient and family (as judged by the nurse), the setting in which the patient is located and the length of time involved in the finding of a resolution. Moreover, the setting is an important determinant of the number of family members who will participate in the nurse–family relationship. If all contacts between nurse and family occur in the hospital, it is possible that the nurse–family relationship will be limited to interactions with only one or two members of the family. If transactions take place primarily in the family's home, chances are increased that many people will be involved, depending on the size and complexity of the patient's network of human relationships. The actual number of active participants, however, will be determined in great measure by the characteristics of the health problem and the contributions of various members to the decision-making process. The characteristics of the health problem also influence a nurse's decisions about the temporal features of the nurse–family relationship, that is, the frequency and duration of contact with members of the family. The length of the nurse–patient relationship may range from days to years and will depend on two interacting factors: the nurse's position in the system *vis-a-vis* the offering of services to the family and mutual agreement among nurse, patient and family to maintain the relationship.

The form of the nurse–family relationship will be affected also by the family's ability to fulfill its obligations to its members, whether they consist of supporting the human rights of its members or making its resources available to meet the human needs of its dependent members. The establishment of a viable nurse–family relationship will be complicated whenever families are unwilling or unable to fulfill these human-to-human obligations because of conflicts in values among the members, power struggles concerning the allocation of family resources and decisions that strike at the heart of their fundamental beliefs. In a general sense, the more complicated is the problem, the greater is the need for sensitivity and flexibility on the part of the nurse.

The nurse–family relationship will be affected also by the quality of interdisciplinary working relationships among the various providers offering services. One particularly important influence is the manner in which physicians and nurses work together in the delivery of patient care. A spirit of collaboration facilitates the flow of information to patient and family; lack of cooperation creates confusion and obstructs the primary goals of care. Problems in collaboration may rest, in part, in the inequality of power between medicine and nursing in decision-making processes pertaining to patient and family services. They are fostered also by the unwillingness of many nurses to move into active negotiation with physicians on behalf of the human needs of those to whom they offer care. The delivery of personalized services requires more than collaboration between physicians and nurses; it requires nurses to collaborate with each other in working toward the best interests of those being served. The need for nurse–nurse collaboration is doubly important in hospitals that are oriented to new clinical treatments and to the application of technology to the solution of many health care problems. As Adams[37] has noted, settings in which the findings of science and technology are applied to clinical problems create hazards for social workers (and for nurses) because they find themselves caught between the demands of those who control these new treatments and their inclination to advocate for the self-determination of patients and families. The problem with many of these settings is that they do not provide safeguards for the protection of human rights.

OTHER INFLUENCING CIRCUMSTANCES

The form of the nurse–family relationship also will be affected by the numbers and types of human concerns and needs presented by a single family. Clearly, a family with many problems is a greater challenge than is a family with only a few. In fact, there can be families whose needs are so great that more than one nurse may be needed to establish effective communication among the individuals concerned. For example, in the provision of home care to dying children and their families, the same nurse often cannot be the central person in the nurse–patient relationship and in the nurse–family relationship. Services in these situations are improved when two nurses work together in a team relationship with clearly established responsibilities for care and a mutually agreed on working arrangement.

It is clear also that the structure of the nurse–family relationship is determined by the nature of the agreement or contract that the nurse and family have established. According to May,[38] the notion of a contract between doctor (in this case, nurse) and patient includes the following understandings: 1) information will be exchanged on the basis of which agreement is reached and a subsequent exchange of goods takes place—usually money for services; 2) the contract will be enforced by law to protect both parties; and 3) the basis of the contract will be the self-interest of both parties. May also points out that the commercial nature of contracts, as they have evolved in the modern world, makes them insufficient to the needs of either patients or the health professionals who serve them during times of illness and tragedy. At the very least, the needs cannot be spelled out in detail in advance. In May's view, agreements between health professionals and patients are both contracts and covenants: "Contracts are external; covenants are internal to the parties involved. Contracts are signed to be expediently discharged. Covenants have a gratuitous, growing edge to them that nourishes rather than limits relationships."[39]

A contract spells out for both parties their common understanding of the nurse's contribution, such as, how available she will be to the patients, the limits of her accessibility, and what contributions the family will make to the arrangement. On the other hand, covenant refers directly to subjective interpretations of the meaning of the contract and the nurse's commitment to it. Covenant deals primarily with matters of promise and fidelity in the relationship. A nurse's definition of trust and fidelity will influence the manner in which she implements the agreement. It probably is fair to say that the quality of a nurse–family relationship will depend on the trust she earns. Thus, the nurse's recognition of the importance of fidelity to promises is a matter of major importance.

Agreements between nurses and families are affected also by the type of nursing assistance needed at a given time, for example, direct physical care, instruction on matters of health and self-care, or guidance in the use of available community resources. The focus and emphasis of any given nurse–family agreement will be strongly directed by the nurse's definition of the nursing role and her judgments about the primary goals to be achieved. If the nurse adheres strictly to a biomedical model and sees "cure" as the major goal for nursing, her decisions about priorities will be guided by the high value attached to life-saving activity. At the other extreme, a nurse who defines her obligations to patients and families primarily in terms of care will be oriented toward the welfare and well-being of the people involved, the importance of informed decision making by the recipients of services and transactions that emphasize reciprocity and exchange.[40] Of course, in the real world of practice, nurses' attitudes toward the services they offer are a composite of ideals about care and cure; rarely do nurses hold an extreme position that excludes one or the other. Attitudes are powerful forces in the creation of nurse–family relationships because they are predispositions to action. In other words, they guide nurses in their choices and decisions about patients, families, and themselves.

The significance of professional choice is not limited to actions taken within the context of a given nurse–family relationship (although this emphasis permeates the nursing literature). The actual existence of such a relationship depends on some nurse's decision about a family's need for assistance. Not only do nurses make choices and decisions about single cases, they also make judgments about the priorities of needs for help among the patients and families with whom they are working. That is, nurses make many decisions that have something to do with the just distribution of the services they have to offer. Whether aware of it or not, nurses frequently decide that some human responses of patients and families deserve attention whereas others do not— or can wait until another time. Unfortunately, the power attached to the nurse's position is not recognized or appreciated by many practicing nurses.

PROFESSIONAL NURSING AND FAMILIES

The nurse–family relationship comes into being when a nurse recognizes a family's need for support in coping with a serious health care problem. Usually the human needs of one member provide the impetus for its development and the nurse–family relationship functions in a manner that is complementary to a nurse's relationship with the patient. However, serious or tragic problems may impinge on the human needs of other members of the family or on the family as a whole. In these situations, the structure of the nurse–family relationship can be intricate, involve a number of people and be complicated by the kinds of decisions to be made and the length of time needed for resolution of them.

No matter how complex is the nurse–family relationship, its form will depend greatly on a nurse's decisions about the nature of the family's situation, the kinds of assistance needed and the location of decision-making powers among family members. The ability to share power with patient and family will be affected strongly by a nurse's beliefs about the human rights of patients and families and by her willingness to assist them in obtaining knowledge for informed decision making. Willingness to share power with consumers also implies that the nurse knows which clinical decisions are properly hers to make and which decisions properly belong to the patient and his family. In her progression to this point, her commitment to nursing has been flavored undoubtedly by her own personal values and probably by the opportunity (or lack of it) to develop respectful attitudes toward others' values and beliefs.

Decisions about relationships with families are notably difficult when a family's beliefs differ from those of the health providers. When a family wants to use laetrile therapy for a child with cancer, for instance, nurses often find themselves in the center of conflicting opinions about what should be done–with different perspectives advanced by the hospital, by physicians, by the family, and by other nurses. Nurses faced with such a problem in one hospital sought guidance in ethical analysis of the situation and identified four possible alternatives for action: 1) abandon the child and family for their failure to comply with the hospital's protocol; 2) take the physician's position and discourage use of laetrile and encourage use of chemotherapy; 3) support the family's position on laetrile to promote their psychological well-being; and 4) refuse to take any position and stay neutral.[41] The analysis helped them to gain perspective on their situation and the nurses moved from being reactive to rational in their approach to reaching a decision. They found that consultation with professional providers not directly involved in offering services to this family provided them with support in their collection of all necessary information, in determination of all possible courses of action and in the weighing of outcomes associated with each alternative.

Support that assists others—whether nurses or families—in decisions about ethical dilemmas or problems requires more than provision of access to important information. It requires the creation of a climate in which the participants can come to grips with the reality of their choices and with the reality of their situation. In such a climate, one does not try to minimize the suffering of the participants by making decisions for them. The proper climate helps people to understand the full meaning of the problem and encourages their independence in and responsibility for the choices they make. Writing about the special difficulties of decision making when a newborn has many defects, Pauli noted: "Perhaps well-considered choice requires experiential nurturing and a special kind of caring."[42]

Nurses have a long-standing interest in the creation of supporting environments for patients and families. Nursing interventions based on the perceived psychosocial needs of patients and families emphasize the verbalization of feelings and facilitation of communication among the members of a family. Such interventions may suppress temporarily or ameliorate the immediate anguish of distressing feelings or anxieties associated with a serious problem. Yet, in a humanistic sense, such support may interfere with the efforts of family members to deal with the existential meaning of the experience. Commenting on humanistic interventions in nursing, Zbilut observed: ". . . the goal is not to lessen the patient's anxieties, nor to provide emotional support. Rather, the goal is the enhancement of holistic understanding of the self, an understanding that indeed temporarily may increase anxiety and feelings of abandonment."[43] Zbilut then goes on to say: "Strange as it may seem, a nursing intervention that seems inappropriate to fulfill psychosocial needs, may be most appropriate to fulfill humanistic needs of patients and their families."[44]

The point for nurses is that different forms of interpersonal support may result in different outcomes for patients and families in highly diverse states of intellectual and psychological awareness. One set of interventions is not always better than another. Nurses have many options in their choices about which intervention to use with vulnerable people and they make their selections based on personal definitions of what is needed at the time. Sometimes people need emotional support and sometimes they need to deal with ultimate concerns. Knowledge about interpersonal strategies that consider the existential needs of patients and families adds an important dimension to professional nursing practice.

DISCUSSION

The view of nursing as a moral art the purpose of which is "the diagnosis and treatment of human responses to actual or potential health problems"[45] necessarily requires knowledge of the family as well as of the patient. This is particularly true when patient and/or family are caught in the intricacies of a health problem that taxes their human relationships and coping capacities. Diagnosis and treatment of the human responses of patients and families require more of nurses than technical competence and specialized knowledge (although these are essential ingredients of the services that are offered). They demand commitment to the rights of individuals, to the sharing of power, to responsibility for one's own decisions and to recognition of and respect for the decisions that belong to others. A nurse–family relationship that promotes partnership as the central means for seeking solutions and finding resolutions is an essential component of the delivery of nursing care in such a manner that the integrity of each person is preserved.

Partnerships with families require an openness to the possibility that there are many different ways of sharing power within groups. The ability to share power with families demands that nurses learn how to work together with people who may or may not share the same values. The establishment of viable nurse–family partnerships requires a willingness to examine conflicting points of view and to continue communication despite differences in expectations. It demands that nurses function in a respectful manner and protect information shared in confidence by one member of the family. It means using support in the broadest sense of the word to help families in distress to cope responsibly with the human problems imposed on them by illness, injuries, and profoundly difficult decisions. Nurse–family relationships initiated and developed to meet the special needs and circumstances of singular patient–family situations require nurses who are flexible in approach and who can shift roles easily to accommodate to changing needs and conditions. The demands of such relationships are great but their potential rewards—in the human development of patients, families, and nurses—are even greater.

NOTES

1. American Nurses' Association. *Code for Nurses with Interpretive Statements* (American Nurses' Association, Kansas City, Missouri, 1976) p. 1.
2. Logan, Barbara Bryan. "The Nurse and the Family: Dominant Themes and Perspectives in the Literature," in Kathleen Astin Knafl and Helen K. Grace, eds. *Families Across the Life Cycle: Studies for Nursing* (Little, Brown, Boston, 1978) p. 5.
3. Engle, George. "The Need for a New Medical Model: A Challenge for Biomedicine," *Science,* Vol. 196 (April 1977) pp. 129–136.
4. Benoliel, Jeanne Quint. "The Changing Social Context for Life and Death Decision," *Essence,* Vol. 2, No. 2 (1978) pp. 5–14.
5. Hilberman, Mark. "The Evolution of Intensive Care Units," *Critical Care Medicine,* Vol. 3 (1975) pp. 159–165.
6. Benoliel, Jeanne Quint. "Nurses and the Human Experience of Dying," in Herman Feifel, ed. *New Meanings of Death* (McGraw-Hill, New York, 1977) pp. 123–142.

7. Levine, Myra E. "Nursing Ethics and the Ethical Nurse," *American Journal of Nursing,* Vol. 77 (May 1977) pp. 846–847.

8. Leininger, Madeleine. "The Significance of Cultural Concepts in Nursing," in Madeleine Leininger, ed. *Transcultural Nursing: Concepts, Theories and Practices* (John Wiley and Sons, New York, 1978) p. 130.

9. Clausen, Joy Princeton. "Cancer Diagnoses in Children: Cultural Factors Influencing Parent/Child Reactions," *Cancer Nursing,* Vol. 1 (October 1978) p. 398.

10. French, Jean and Doris R. Schwartz. "Terminal Care at Home in Two Cultures," *American Journal of Nursing,* Vol. 73 (1973) pp. 502–505.

11. *Ibid.*

12. Leininger, Madeleine. "Towards Conceptualization of Transcultural Health Care Systems: Concepts and a Model," in Madeleine Leininger, ed. *Transcultural Nursing: Concepts, Theories and Practices* (John Wiley and Sons, New York, 1978) p. 57.

13. Zborowski, Mark. "Cultural Components in Response to Pain," *Journal of Social Issues,* Vol. 8 (1952) pp. 16–20.

14. Whiting, John W. M., *et al. Field Guide for a Study of Socialization* (John Wiley and Sons, New York, 1966) pp. 39–64.

15. Kiefer, Christie W. *Changing Cultures, Changing Lives* (Jossey-Bass, San Francisco, 1974) p. 177.

16. Aries, Philippe. *Centuries of Childhood* (Alfred A. Knopf, New York, 1962) p. 261.

17. Hofmann, Adele D. "The Right to Consent and Confidentiality in Adolescent Health Care: An Evolutionary Dilemma," in Elsie L. Bandman and Bertram Bandman, eds. *Bioethics and Human Rights* (Little, Brown, Boston, 1978) pp. 183–188.

18. Sullerot, Evelyne. *Woman, Society and Change* (McGraw-Hill, New York, 1971) pp. 19–42.

19. Flowers, Ronald B. "Freedom of Religion Versus Civil Authority in Matters of Health," *Annals of the American Academy of Political and Social Science,* Vol. 446 (November 1979) p. 157.

20. Steinman, M. "A Child's Fight for Life: Parents vs. Doctors," *New York Times Magazine,* December 1978. The parents of Chad Green differed with the physician about the use of laetrile to treat his cancer. Court intervention led to the parents "kidnapping" their child and seeking refuge in Mexico—hardly a desirable outcome.

21. Skerrett, Karen. "The Family Across Generations," in Kathleen Astin Knafl and Helen K. Grace, ed. *Families Across the Life Cycle: Studies for Nursing* (Little, Brown, Boston, 1978) pp. 315–326.

22. Leininger, Madeleine. "Culturological Assessment Domains for Nursing Practice," in Madeleine Leininger, ed. *Transcultural Nursing: Concepts, Theories and Practices* (John Wiley and Sons, New York, 1978) pp. 85–106.

23. Bok, Sissela. "Lying to Children," *The Hastings Center Report,* Vol. 8 (June 1978) pp. 10–13.

24. Siegler, Mark. "Critical Illness: The Limits of Autonomy," *The Hastings Center Report,* Vol. 7 (October 1977) p. 13.

25. Dworkin, Gerald. "Autonomy and Behavior Control," *The Hastings Center Report,* Vol. 6 (February 1976) pp. 23-28.

26. *Ibid.*, pp. 27–28.

27. Furman, Erna. *A Child's Parent Dies* (Yale University Press, New Haven, 1974) pp. 57–58.

28. Gadow, Sally. "Caring for the Dying: Advocacy or Paternalism," *Death Education,* Vol. 3 (Winter 1980) p. 398.

29. Robinson, Betsy and Majda Thurnher. "Taking Care of Aged Parents: A Family Cycle Transition," *The Gerontologist,* Vol. 19 (1979) p. 592.

30. *Ibid.*

31. May, William. "The Metaphysical Plight of the Family," *The Hastings Center Studies,* Vol. 2 (May 1974) p. 27.

32. LaBarre, Maurine. "Emotional Crises of School-Age Girls During Pregnancy and Early Motherhood," *Journal of the American Academy of Child Psychiatry,* Vol. 11 (July 1972) pp. 537–557.

33. *Danforth v. Planned Parenthood of Central Missouri.* 44 U. S. L.W. 5197 (1976).

34. Roberts, Carolyn Sara. "Ethical Issues in the Treatment of Neonates with Severe Anomalies," *Nursing Forum,* Vol. XVIII, No. 4 (1979) pp. 355–358.

35. *Ibid.*, p. 361.

36. Kohl, Marvin. "Karen Quinlan: Human Rights and Wrongful Killing," in Elsie L. Bandman and Bertram Bandman, eds. *Bioethics and Human Rights* (Little, Brown, Boston, 1978) p. 121.

37. Adams, Margaret. "Science, Technology, and Some Dilemmas of Advocacy," *Science,* Vol. 180 (May 25, 1973) p. 841.

38. May, William F. "Code, Covenant, Contract, or Philanthropy," *The Hastings Center Report,* Vol. 5 (December 1975) p. 33.

39. *Ibid.*, p. 34.

40. Benoliel, 1977, *op. cit.*, p. 135.

41. Moser, Dorothy and Jean Marie Cox. "Perspectives: Resolving an Ethical Dilemma," *Nursing 80,* Vol. 10 (May 1980) p. 40.

42. Pauli, Richard M. "Commentary–Case Studies in Bioethics: Nurturing a Defective Newborn," *The Hastings Center Report,* Vol. 8 (February 1978) p. 13.

43. Zbilut, Joseph P. "Holistic Nursing: The Transcendental Factor," *Nursing Forum,* Vol. XIX, No. 1 (1980) p. 48.

44. *Ibid.*

45. Kelly, Lucie Young. "Nursing Practice Acts," *American Journal of Nursing,* Vol. 74 (July 1974) p. 1315.

11

The Nurse–Nurse Relationship

Leah Curtin
M. Josephine Flaherty

"The greatest trust between men is the trust of giving counsel."

Francis Bacon

Among the basic commitments for nurses who practice according to generally accepted standards is that they participate as members of the health care team. This involves collaboration with other health professionals, including other nurses. Hence, it is essential for nurses to understand fully how they are embedded personally in the body of their profession. Each nurse is an active and intimate part of nursing—a profession that every nurse both practices and helps to create.

The ethics of a profession not only delimit the role and scope of its activities and prescribe the nature of the relationship that should exist between its members and the lay public, but also establish the duties that professionals owe to one another and to the profession. That the ancients recognized the unique nature of the professional relationship is demonstrated in the Hippocratic Oath: "I swear . . . to hold him who has taught me this art as equal to my parents and to live my life in partnership with him. . . ".[1] Codes of professional ethics usually included a pledge to exert one's best efforts to maintain the honor of the profession, to uphold its public standing and to extend the bounds of its usefulness.[2] Nurses, then, as they assume their professional identities, are pledged to: (1) the work of understanding, interpreting, and expanding the body of the profession's knowledge; (2) the equally disciplined work of criticism and self-regulation; and (3) the work of developing and cultivating in themselves and in their colleagues the character traits on which personal and professional excellence depend. The deep-seated relationship between a profession and its individual members and the relationships among the professionals cannot be forced into conformity with a model; rather, they should be described in terms of the practitioners' actual experiences of the profession.

The moral commitments of nurses to their profession and to one another form a foundation for professional life. The practitioners' perceptions of and fidelity to these moral commitments will affect and, to a large extent, will create the structure of their intraprofessional relationships.

To the extent that nurses recognize their commitment to common goals, the similarity of their knowledge base and their indebtedness to the nurses who went before them, to their teachers and to their peers, they will devote themselves to the advancement of the profession and to the growth of their colleagues. Hence, nursing as a caring profession involves not only care for and of patients but also care for and of fellow nurses. It is on this base that the significance of the nurse–nurse relationship rests. In the fulfillment of nurses' contracts with society, with patients and families and with employing institutions, their relationships with their fellow nurses are crucial.

The importance of intraprofessional relationships in nursing may not be appreciated fully by nurses if they focus their ethical concern solely on the well-being of patients and their families. Mature recognition of their own limits and capabilities leads nurses to rely on and incorporate the knowledge, the experience and the research of other professionals in their own practice. Clearly, the structure of work in most facilities requires nurses to function interdependently, that is, to trust in the professional expertise of colleagues, both in and outside of nursing, as each member of the health care team strives to achieve personal and professional goals. That nurses work collaboratively with members of other professions is obvious. What may be overlooked is the fact that nurses' professional interdependence demands special—even fraternal—relationships *among nurses.* Reflection on these relationships reveals interesting and challenging dimensions.

THE PROFESSIONAL RELATIONSHIP: AN ETHICAL IMPERATIVE

The ethical principles that underlie the formulation of professional relationships derive from several sources.[3] The first source is comprised of the universally applicable concepts of human rights and the duties attached to those rights. Nurses are human beings and they deserve to be treated as such by all persons, including other nurses. As is the case with all other human relationships, nurses' mutual humanity forms the fundamental framework for relationships among the people who belong to the same profession. Therefore, the relationships that obtain among nurses should be characterized first and foremost by respect for one another's human rights. Nurses should guard against behaving in ways that could threaten those rights. Such attention will help nurses to avoid demonstrating a lack of consideration for other nurses as both strive to fulfill professional duties and responsibilities.

A second source of the ethical principles that underlie professional relationships is in nurses' obligations to promote the public's welfare. Because nurses are professionals, they are responsible to the public for the services rendered by all members of the profession. As professionals, nurses assume a duty to practice in accord with established standards and to improve standards as knowledge increases.[4] One of the most effective ways to promote excellence in nursing practice and to disseminate new information is for nurses to offer support, guidance, criticism, and direction to one another. To fail or to refuse to offer this kind of assistance actually constitutes a breach of faith—not just with colleagues, but also with the public because it will affect negatively the quality of nursing service offered. It could result in nurses, in their professional care of patients, displaying a lack of knowledge, skill or judgment, or a disregard for the welfare of a patient. In some statutes, such behavior constitutes professional incompetence.[5] Hence, ethical nurses cannot ignore the practice of colleagues but must assume some responsibility for the promotion of excellence in the practice of fellow nurses. Because all nurses share this corporate responsibility for the work of the profession as a whole, as it fulfills its contracts with society, with patients, and with other individuals and groups, they must look beyond their own specific patient assignments in order to fulfill their duties as members of the nursing discipline.

While human rights and concern for the public welfare form a basic framework for the special nature of intraprofessional relationships, a third source of the underlying ethical principles breathes life into them. When nurses enter the profession, they figuratively "adopt" their colleagues as brothers or sisters.[6] The ethical obligations flowing from this source derive from the professional bond rather than from blood ties or mutual liking. Typically, the duties ascribed to the "fraternal" aspects of the professional relationship are formalized in rules regarding the handling of incompetent colleagues, canons of loyalty and professional courtesies. These superficial manifestations of the professional bond only begin to approach the realities of the human experience that is the professional relationship. It is incumbent on nurses to examine how the professional bond affects the behavior in their professional lives and to decide whether what they see is acceptable.

Professional relationships enable one to be a professional (specifically a nursing professional) through identification with others and through recognition of the dilemmas of others within oneself. Such relationships do not tell one how to act as much as how to be. The discovery and understanding of oneself as a professional stems from one's perception and knowledge of other professionals. This means that each nurse discovers the outline of herself/himself in the human totality of nursing colleagues: each recognizes himself or herself in others and sees the characteristics of others in herself. More precisely and powerfully, between their first experience of the professional relationship and their last, professionals actually exchange characters. The exchange of characters between self and others creates what one is as a nurse and, at the same time, the ideal of what one should be as a nurse—in general and in particular.

In terms of the sociology of the profession, the function of the professional bond may be described as that of role modeling and role internalization. The latter occurs when individuals begin to identify with their role models and to adopt their behavior patterns, both consciously and unconsciously. It has been said that nurses of today may have difficulty with such identification and that role models in nursing practice, in all types of venues, may be conspicuous by their absence. This creates a void for practicing nurses who need competence figures. "Ironically, the deficits in role inculcation probably relate to the educational model adopted by the nursing discipline. In misguided attempts to improve the educational status of nursing, students often have been 'protected' from interaction with practicing nurses, with the rationalization that such interaction smacks of apprenticeship."[7] However, all experts were apprentices or beginners at one time who were taught and guided by master craftsmen. If nursing students remain apart from the mainstream of the work world of nurses, they will be like spectators who sample the practice field but never really feel that they are significant parts of it. As a result, the professional bond in nursing is weak for nursing students; it may remain this way for registered nurses because their professional identity does not develop, either during student experience or after their entry to professional practice following graduation.

The lack of professional identity is evidenced by the large number of nurses who leave the field and by those who practice at subprofessional levels (regardless of what degrees or credentials they earn).[8] Such nurses do not see that their concern, commitment, and genuine involvement in the profession and its development are what makes the profession viable. They do not appreciate the true interdependence of all members of a profession.

Only as nurses discover and create their own practices and identities as nurses, and only as they understand the roles that these play in the viability of nursing will they discover, add to, and create their profession. In the end, the sources of the ethical principles underlying intraprofessional relationships—human rights, commitment to the public welfare, and the professional bond—give structure and life to the practitioner's experience of the profession. This, in turn, revitalizes the profession itself. It follows that where positive professional relationships are weak or absent, both the profession and the professionals suffer. It is incumbent on nurse educators and nurse leaders to ensure that professional relationships are fostered and maintained. This is a challenge that forms an essential part of the daily professional life of a nurse.

PROFESSIONAL PREROGATIVES

When one becomes a professional, one assumes a number of obligations and earned rights. Earned rights, as distinct from human rights, encompass those prerogatives that are necessary to the fulfillment of professional obligations. They are not privileges in the sense of mere courtesies (although the importance of true courtesy never should be underestimated) because they are essential to the practice of the profession. They are not rights in the sense of something that automatically is owed to all persons; rather, they are enabling qualities that one merits through effort, education and experience, that is, they are earned. If one proves unworthy of them, one no longer has them: they can be removed formally by a statutory body, by an institution or by the profession, and informally by fellow professionals or by patients or clients and their families.

Earned rights are not extras, pleasantries, or even behavioral expectations of other professionals and members of the public, because they are necessary—indeed, integral—to the practice of a profession. Among the earned rights of nurses are:

1. The right to practice nursing in accord with professionally defined standards
2. The right to participate in and to promote the growth and direction of the profession
3. The right to be trusted by members of the public
4. The right to intervene when necessary to protect patients, clients or the public
5. The right to testify authoritatively to the community about the health care needs of people
6. The right to be believed when one is speaking in the area of his/her expertise
7. The right to be respected by those inside and outside the profession for one's knowledge, abilities, experience and contributions
8. The right to be trusted by colleagues
9. The right to give to and to receive from colleagues support, guidance and correction
10. The right to be compensated fairly for services rendered.

These earned *rights* are, in fact, accurate reflections of the *duties* of nurses, all of whom have the duty to:

1. Practice nursing in accord with the standards of the profession
2. Participate in and promote the direction and growth of the profession
3. Fulfill the promises the profession has made to the public
4. Intervene to protect patients or clients from the unethical or illegal actions of any person
5. Testify to the public regarding the health care needs of people
6. Speak out accurately and honestly in one's area of expertise

7. Strive constantly to increase one's knowledge and experience

8. Give to and to receive from one's colleagues guidance, support and correction

9. Render adequate and safe nursing services within professionally defined standards and institutional or agency policies.

Failure by nurses to fulfill these duties cancels the rights that are attached to them. However, failure by both nurses and others to recognize that rights are attached to these duties leaves nurses powerless in the face of awesome responsibilities. Germane to the nurse–nurse relationship are nurses' rights: (1) to be trusted by their colleagues; (2) to give to and to receive from their colleagues support, guidance, and correction; and (3) to be respected for their knowledge, experience, and contributions to the profession. These earned rights of nurses translate into guidelines—actually, behavioral imperatives that are well grounded in ethical principles—for their professional relationships. Nurses should be treated and should treat one another in congruence with these professional imperatives.

These rights and responsibilities of nurses make it incumbent on nurses at all levels to ensure not only that nurses *do* fulfill their duties and responsibilities but also that conditions in the work situation are such that nurses *can* fulfill them. Failure of nurses and others—including employers, fellow professionals, and society—to provide conditions that make it possible for nurses to fulfill their duties constitutes infringement of the human and professional rights of nurses and it is unethical behavior. Hence, the rights and duties of nurses are inseparable and are essential to each other.

PROFESSIONAL CHARACTER TRAITS

Contemporary nurses appear to have been far less interested than were their predecessors in the identification and cultivation of the character traits that are necessary to the life of a profession. This may be due in part to a reaction to the almost monastic life that used to be required of nurses and in part to the fact that this area may seem to be subjective and elusive. Whatever the reason, the result is that too little thought has been given to the question of the virtues that are appropriate to the development of professional character.

For a person to enter fully into professional relationships with peers requires:

1. Fidelity to the promises of the profession: a shared commitment to the profession's goals provides identity for the group and forms a solid foundation for cooperative effort. Nurses must decide what are the basic beliefs and values of the profession and adhere to them so that practice can be sufficiently predictable and consistent that both nurses and the public can be confident that the behavior of members of the profession will fulfill nursing's contracts with society, patients, colleagues *et al.*

2. Respect for the human and earned rights of oneself and of one's colleagues: self-respect enables one to stand up for one's beliefs; respect for

others infers openness to discussion and debate in order to clarify differences of opinion, fact, and intent; both are essential to healthy relationships. Nurses must be prepared to articulate their beliefs and values and to submit them to the scrutiny of their peers. Failure to appreciate that colleagues have opinions and values and to give consideration to them connotes lack of respect that will hinder the development of effective professional relationships.

3. Honesty and intellectual integrity: these virtues are at the very heart of a "community of scholars"; they are essential to sound relationships within the profession and between the profession and the public; they infer a willingness to share knowledge and to work with others toward mutually defined goals. Shakespeare has noted that one who is true to himself cannot be false to others, and so it is with nurses in their professional relationships with one another.

If these character traits are appropriate to professional life, the virtues that nurses must seek and nurture in themselves and in others are benevolence, honesty, respect, fidelity, and integrity. Without these virtues, the moral fiber of the profession will be weakened and the activities of the profession itself will be reduced to commercial transactions at best. The dictum, *caveat emptor* (let the buyer beware) certainly is not an appropriate motto for the nursing profession. If matters of professional virtue—and the presence or absence of it in each nurse—are not addressed, the vast resources of the profession will be for sale to the highest bidder.

THE GROWTH OF THE PROFESSION AND THE PROFESSIONAL

If nursing is to become and is to continue to be a justifiable and viable profession, three developments must take place. All are possible because all exist today, although in muted form.

First, the profession must regain and must nurture a sense of commitment—of vocation—in its members. The knowledge that nurses possess and the skills that they acquire are more a public trust than a private acquisition to be prized and sold on the open market. Nurses' current concern with their economic status can be salutary but, if it becomes a preoccupation, nursing will be placed in an extraordinarily vulnerable position because money is far too narcissistic a focus for a profession. Opportunities for financial gain and personal advancement within a profession flourish only in the context of the valuable services that the profession provides to the public; the utility and the advancement of a profession depend on individual members who have some sense of professional identity, commitment, and responsibility. When the professional bond is weak and each practitioner thinks of himself or herself as an entrepreneur—alone, unencumbered by a public and professional trust—the profession is wounded, perhaps mortally. By virtue of its traditions and its contract with society, nursing can ill afford to deny its public function, the interdependence of its practitioners, or its inherently altruistic goals. However, to engage in critical inquiry into the tension between adequate remuneration and altruistic service is, itself, a social act that infers accountability and responsibility for judgments and decisions and that assumes that these actions can be evaluated by others. "Critical inquiry is part of the public life of the mind, an indispensable ingredient to a professional life that has more to offer than the technical services for personal gain."[9] Such inquiry necessarily includes a weighing and weighting of the values, obligations and goals of the practitioner and of the profession. The sense of commitment to the profession and to the public trust is embodied in professional and ethical codes for nurses[10,11] and in standards of nursing practice,[12,13,14] in both Canada and the United States, some of which are covered by statute.[15,16]

The second development is that members of the nursing profession must become far more aware of their responsibilities to one another. Nurses must recognize, more fully than they have done to date, their duty to nurture, support, guide, and correct one another.[17] Cooperation and mutual growth must be recognized widely as norms in professional relationships—instead of competition or acquisition of power. Practically speaking, one's own success depends largely on the knowledge and skill of one's colleagues as well as on their willingness to share information and insights and to engage in the constructive criticism that is part of collaboration, cooperation and peer review. The nurse–nurse relationship is one vital factor that is notorious for being inexplicably weak. However, without a strong intraprofessional relationship, nurses will be unable to fulfill their commitments to the public and to achieve their personal and professional goals. Hence, nurses must take action to improve their relationships with one another.

The third development that must take place is that nursing must address the systems, institutions and structures that shape the environment in which nurses practice. Indeed, the ethical spirit of the profession today has been shaped largely by institutions—both schools and work places. In the eighties, perhaps more than ever before, health care professionals, including nurses, must go beyond direct patient care to consider and act on factors associated with the nature and shape of the health care system and the practice of members of the health care team.[18] Nurses are required by ethics and by law to question directions, including direct orders of other health professionals such as physicians and supervisory and management nurses, as well as policies and practices of institutions, about which they have concern.[19]

Therefore, it is appropriate and necessary for nurses to examine health-related institutions and systems and to strive to improve them. Such examination includes scrutiny of the customs and taboos of the situations in which they find themselves, including their own behavior and that of their colleagues, to identify whether what they see is consonant with the standards of practice for which they stand accountable.[20] Efforts to improve health care situations include the making of suggestions about and the testing of new methods and patterns of practice and of organization and willingness to be open to the ideas of other participants in the health care enterprise, including fellow nurses.

Do schools of nursing prepare students to engage in critical inquiry into the values that shape society and the profession? Do they provide opportunities for students to become skilled at such inquiry? Are they developing the kind of professional who can function effectively to meet the needs of the public and to advance the profession? Do nurses' workplaces provide environments that are conducive to excellence in nursing practice? Does the socialization process in both schools and workplaces promote the development of the professional bond? The answer to all of these questions is no—or at least not to the degree necessary to advance the profession.[21]

Nursing's institutions of higher learning, reflecting the general trend in higher education after World War II,[22] have concentrated chiefly on the development of operational and technical intelligence. "For example, in adopting the behavioral objective many nursing programs have eliminated all attempts to inculcate values, attitudes, thought processes, that defy a simplistic behavioral translation."[23] Although, in contrast, the counter-culture movement of the late sixties and early seventies stressed the affective component to learning,[24] both of these approaches reflect a far too narrow concept of intelligence. The result is a constellation of nurses who define themselves in terms of the technical tasks that they perform and who discuss values, goals, and ethics in terms of how they feel rather than what they think.

Development of operational intelligence helps the learner to determine how to get from here to there. It deals with means but it does not criticize ends. On the other hand, critical intelligence involves the making of judgments about the worth and value of the ends and the means that are appropriate for achievement of the ends. The word critical has its roots in the Greek verb, *kritikos,* that means "to judge, to discern, to separate, to distinguish."[25] The intellectual activity that is demanded in professional life includes the task of normative as well as descriptive inquiry—the use of critical as well as operational intelligence. If nursing's institutions of higher learning are to develop fully the intelligence of their students, nurses must take seriously the proposition that they constitute a community of scholars, learn how to behave in a scholarly fashion and then do so. Nursing educators in particular must demonstrate scholarly behavior and demand that students question and challenge nursing's propositions, methods, and goals. Thus, reasoned discourse and debate can take place and discriminating judgments can be made about ends and values. This will create the atmosphere of open and critical inquiry that is essential to the task of giving to and receiving from one's colleagues criticism, support, direction, and guidance. Such discussion and debate should be an ongoing part of nursing practice at all levels, from the daily nursing care conference to the highest level nursing boards and councils in the profession. This type of activity will provide the opportunity and the basis for critical inquiry into the development and utility of the profession's goals and activities. If nurses are to be the change agents that their profession mandates them to be, they must define goals clearly and judge critically the value of those goals. It is the responsibility of nursing leaders and managers to create environments in which such activity can and will take place.

Sociologists and economists may offer valuable services to the nursing profession by describing the systems within which nurses work,[26] but they cannot offer nursing the conceptual tools that are necessary for critical analysis of the values and goals either of the systems or of the profession. The value or disvalue of hierarchical structures, interprofessional relationships, dependent versus interdependent and independent practice, social attitudes toward women, remuneration for nursing services, specialization and diversification among nurses and the like must be addressed by the profession as a whole—and this will be achieved only if nurses recognize and cherish their professional bond and work together within it. By and large, the institutions and systems in which nurses work were designed to serve laudable utilitarian ends and have functioned to provide services to the community. Their destruction is unlikely to serve the public's interests. Hence, nursing must weigh the social impact of its strivings for change if its struggles to reform "the system" are to serve the health needs of the populace as well as the aspirations of the profession. The enhancement of the profession and the strengthening of the professional bond among nurses must never become more important to nurses than their commitment to public well-being. Rather, these two elements of nurses' professionalism must be directed specifically toward fulfillment of nursing's commitment to society. Otherwise the profession will degenerate into a self-serving occupation and the professional bond will become an excuse for protection of professionals rather than a relationship that enhances practice.

In short, a profession that derives its authority and its influence from the fact that people need its services can become exploitative unless its members possess a high degree of altruism and work together to promote and foster high ideals in themselves and in their colleagues. People need to trust nurses, and to maintain this trust, nurses need to trust and to rely on one another. In fact, the very nature of nursing supports the claim that to be a nurse is to be a part of creative, constructive, professional relationships that involve being a partner in the development of a profession, the primary goal of which is to serve the needs of others. The extent to which each nurse demonstrates a caring quality in nurse–nurse relationships is proof of the extent to which the claim "to be a nurse" is being realized by the profession through the behavior of its members.

NOTES

1. "Appendix: Codes of the Health Care Professions," in Warren T. Reich, ed. *Encyclopedia of Bioethics* (The Free Press, New York, 1978) p. 1731.

2. *Ibid.,* pp.1732–1815.

3. Veatch, Robert. "The Ethics of Professional Relations," in Warren T. Reich, ed. *Encyclopedia of Bioethics* (The Free Press, New York, 1978) pp. 178–179.

4. American Nurses' Association. *Code for Nurses with Interpretative Statements* (American Nurses' Association, Kansas City, Missouri, 1976) Statement No. 8.

5. Ontario. *The Health Disciplines Act, 1974, Part IV, Nursing.* 1974 c. 47, s. 84(4), as amended by 1975, c. 63 (Toronto, 1975).

6. Veatch, *op. cit.,* p. 178.

7. Stevens, Barbara J. *Research in Nursing Education: Perspectives for the Future* (Teacher's College, Columbia University, New York, 1979) pp. 12–13.

8. *Ibid.,* p. 12.

9. May, William F. "Normative Inquiry and Medical Ethics in Our Colleges and Universities," in David Smith and Linda Bernstein, eds. *No Rush to Judgment* (Indiana University Foundation, Bloomington, Indiana, 1978) p. 334.

10. American Nurses' Association, 1973, *op. cit.*

11. College of Nurses of Ontario. *Guidelines for Ethical Behaviour in Nursing* (College of Nurses of Ontario, Toronto, 1980).

12. American Nurses' Association. *Standards of Nursing Practice* (American Nurses' Association, Kansas City, Missouri, 1973).

13. College of Nurses of Ontario. *Standards of Nursing Practice: for Registered Nurses and Registered Nursing Assistants.* Revised, May 1979 (College of Nurses of Ontario, Toronto, 1979).

14. Canadian Nurses Association. *A Definition of Nursing Practice. Standards for Nursing Practice* (Canadian Nurses Association, Ottawa, 1980).

15. College of Nurses of Ontario, 1979, *op. cit.*

16. Ontario. *Regulation made under The Health Disciplines Act, 1974, Part IV, Nursing. Ontario Regulation 578/75,* s. 24 (Queen's Printer, Toronto, 1975).

17. *Ibid.,* s. 21, i.j.

18. Flaherty, M. Josephine, "Accountability in Health Care Practice: Ethical Implications for Nurses." Chapter 23, in Davis, John W., *et. al.,* eds. *Contemporary Issues in Biomedical Ethics* (The Humana Press, Clifton, New Jersey, 1979) p. 273.

19. *Ibid.,* p. 271.

20. *Ibid.,* p. 276.

21. Many sources could be cited here. For example, see Fromm, Linda, "The Problem in Nursing, Nurses!" *Supervisor Nurse,* Vol. 8, No. 10 (October 1977) p. 15.

22. May, *op. cit.,* p. 338.

23. Stevens, *op. cit.,* p. 12.

24. Alinsky, Saul D. *Rules for Radicals* (Vintage Books, New York, 1971) pp. i–xxvi.

25. *Webster's New World Dictionary.* Unabridged, Second Edition (World Publishing Company, New York, 1968).

26. For example, see Dachelet, Christy Z. "Nursing's Bid for Increased Status," *Nursing Forum,* Vol. XVII, No. 1 (1978) pp. 19–45.

12

The Nurse–Physician Relationship

M. Josephine Fluherty

*". . . the trained nurse has become one of the great blessings of
humanity, taking a place beside the physician and the priest and
not inferior to either in her mission."*[1]

Sir William Osler

Of all the relationships of the nurse, perhaps the best known and least
understood is that with physicians. Members of the public tend to see nurses
and physicians working together as the main functionaries of the health care
system. The nurse, however, is the ever-present or constant element, with
whom patients and families have the greatest amount of direct contact and
with whom patients and families often communicate most fully and most
frankly. In spite of this, nurses may be regarded—by patients and families, by
other health care workers such as physicians, and even by some nurses—as
somehow inferior, subservient, and unequal to physicians, rather than as
partners on the health care team. The basis for such perceptions lies in the
historical foundations of physicians' and nurses' roles and functions.

HISTORICAL ROOTS AND PATTERNS OF DEVELOPMENT

Sir William Osler, that great man of medicine in Canada and in the United
States at the turn of the century, who saw the nurse as "taking a place beside
the physician and priest and not inferior to either in her mission,"[2] also noted
that "In the gradual division of labour, by which civilization has emerged
from barbarism, the doctor and the nurse have been evolved, as useful
accessories in the incessant warfare in which man is engaged."[3] It should be
noted, however, that these two workers have inherited rather different basic
images from history. An understanding by nurses and physicians of each

other's historical roots and patterns of development may assist them to develop and maintain effective inter-professional relationships.

Nursing's earliest image, from primitive times, is the folk image of the nurse as a simple, mothering care-giver. This is in contraposition to the early image of the physician as medicine man—a person who was set apart from others by the length and difficulty of his training and who was in possession of special knowledge and ability to influence gods and evil spirits. For this, he was honored and rewarded. The third member of Osler's trinity of "useful accessories" was the priest who, like the physician, was thought to be able to do something other than simply accept the "will of the gods." The authority of each of these three workers was derived from a different source.

The authority of the priest was based on the *summum bonum*; he helped to direct people towards the greatest good. The physician, by contrast, derived his authority from the *summum malum* because of the fact that he helped to protect people from evil. Failure to be effective in the battle with the *summum malum* was perceived by many physicians, and still is today, as a threat to their authority. This may account in significant part for the concentration of the medical profession on "success." The authority of the nurse, who was "of the people" rather than set apart, rested in her nurturing skills, which were instinctive or were learned by chance or were common knowledge. This view of nursing knowledge has persisted in the minds of many people for a long time. Even Florence Nightingale, although she regarded nursing as an important field of work and said that she would like to "open a career, highly paid,"[4] noted that "Every woman, or at least almost every woman, in England has, at one time or another of her life, charge of the personal health of somebody, whether child or invalid—in other words, every woman is a nurse."[5]

Although both medicine and nursing have developed through several stages since these early times, there is still considerable lack of appreciation and understanding by both groups for the other's roles and responsibilities. The evolution of roles and functions of physicians has been reflected in codes and position statements related to the medical profession.

Ethical Policy for Medicine

Ethical standards have been formulated for physicians in their professional duties, for persons conducting medical experiments involving human beings and for various other health professions. Ethical codes are the expression of standards but there are also principles and professional rules of conduct in prayers, oaths, creeds, and institutional directives and statements of professional organizations.[6]

Ethical policy for the health care professions is fashioned by two principal methods: 1) formal and relatively public professional positions that become codes of ethics, policy statements, oaths, pledges, creeds, vows, and by-laws;

and 2) less formal and less palpable practices that foster the development of influential oral traditions that may supplement or even supplant what has been included in codes and statements that were issued earlier. Ethical issues are grouped in two categories: (1) broad moral imperatives that resemble the Ten Commandments or the Golden Rule and (2) detailed statements regarding the technical and commercial aspects of professional practice. Many of the earliest codes and statements were weighted more heavily in the first group than in the second, partly because it was believed that an honorable and worthy person could not help but do the right and proper thing and that being a gentle person, in the broad social as well as immediate behavioral sense, was desirable. Even today, it is considered a compliment to be labelled "a real gentleman" or "a real lady."

In the medical profession, the ancient "prayers" outlined the personal commitment of the physician to a professional duty. The oaths were public pledges of new physicians to uphold the recognized responsibilities of members of the profession. The codes were comprehensive statements of standards to guide the practicing physician. Each form of ethical statement, most of which were developed by physicians, contained a moral imperative that was either to be accepted by a physician personally or enforced by a medical organization or its members. In ancient times, the physician allied himself, in the treatment of disease, with the deity, who was beseeched to inspire physicians to fulfill their moral obligations, to reward those who honored their sacred trust, and to punish those who violated it.[7]

The well known Hippocratic Oath consists of: a contractual agreement between pupil and teacher that pledges the novice physician to become an adopted member of and to assume some responsibility for his teacher's family, thus forming a basis for the strong medical professional bond that is fraternal in nature; and an ethical code that delimits to some extent the techniques of the physician and points to his relationships with his patients' families.[8] For some time, this oath was not accepted by a number of physicians. With the rise of Christianity, it was modified to put it in harmony with Christian ideology and it continued to be the model for succeeding medical oaths including the *Declaration of Geneva* of 1948.[9] This is a secular oath that, by pledging physicians to uphold the honor and traditions of the medical profession, offers a basis for professional pride and solidarity.[10]

History reveals that modern physicians have inherited a tradition of elaborate professional codes beginning in China in the sixth century. The first and best known Western statement, the treatise of Thomas Percival of 1803, influenced subsequent codes of medical ethics such as the *Code of Ethics, 1847* of the American Medical Association.[11] At that time, physicians in the United States were experiencing a crisis in public confidence and it was hoped that the *Code* would establish standards for medical practice and help to prevent the worst abuses of the doctor–patient relationship and re-establish public respect for the medical profession.[12] Twentieth century codes echo the

Percival tradition and include attention to modern problems and issues such as concern for public as well as individual well-being. By the middle of this century, physicians were focusing more on patient treatment and less on formal intraprofessional and physician–patient relationships than had been the case earlier. The year 1949 saw the adoption of the *International Code of Medical Ethics*[13] and in 1957, the American Medical Association adopted the *Principles of Medical Ethics (1957).*[14] These dealt with issues related to practice, the supremacy of the patient's well-being, professional association with nonscientific practitioners, and the use of discretion regarding professional confidence.[15] Subsequently, the American Medical Association issued additional sets of guidelines for special areas such as *Organ Transplantation (1968),*[16] *The Physician and the Dying Patient (1973)*[17] and *Human Artificial Insemination(1974).*[18] Recently, codes of medical ethics have been prepared by groups other than physicians—such as religious bodies—that focus on moral rectitude, civil governments and consumer groups that demand rights for patients to participate in decision making about their own welfare. As a result, physicians are facing competing ethical authorities with conflicting standards and the responsibility for the development of ethical guidelines. The medical profession has run the gamut—from directives to preserve human life, to be gentlemen and good citizens, to strive for professional excellence, to expose unethical colleagues even though the professional bond often directed them to demonstrate solidarity to the nonprofessional world, to promote comfort, dignity, and autonomy of patients, and to provide service to all who needed it, regardless of their status in society and ability to pay—to recent moves by some groups in the United States and in Canada to challenge fellow professionals, both inside and outside medicine, to resist third-party payment for medical services, to opt out of health care insurance plans in some provinces in Canada, and to resist strongly suggestions for changes in the health care system. For example, members of the Canadian Medical Association reacted negatively and publicly to recommendations made by the Honourable Emmett M. Hall in his study of *Canada's National-Provincial Health Program for the 1980's.*[19] Members of organized medical associations in the United States have protested strongly about proposals made by some legislators for health insurance schemes for the country.

   Major developments, such as the changing role and structure of hospitals, unprecedented advances in knowledge and technology, the predominance of empirical science as opposed to the humanitarian principles that reigned supreme at one time and the development of specialization in most fields with resultant proliferation of types and groups of workers, have changed the face of the health care system. Today, "it rivals the industrial complex in the production and delivery of services to the people. But it has grown worse as it has grown better—it is now available to all, but in a more impersonal way."[20] This new phenomenon, that has been referred to as "megamedicine," has yielded both new benefits and new risks. Physicians could become sufficiently dependent on test results and on their computer printouts that they would pass over clinical judgment, that is based on direct experience with their patients,[21] in favor of technology that yields mechanically generated data to which impersonal or mechanical responses are possible.[22]

Ethical Policy for Nursing

Similar trends have been observed in nursing, but many are not of as long standing as those in medicine and the more recently observed ones may not be recognized as involving risks. Ethical considerations have been significant in nursing education and nursing practice, with distinct ethical principles forming an important element, along with the major emphasis that has been placed on the character, etiquette, and subservient obligations of the nurse. During the nineteenth century, Florence Nightingale wrote extensively about nursing and how nurses should conduct themselves.[23] The first formal statement that was thought of as a well known statement or pledge of ethics was the Florence Nightingale Pledge for nurses, which was prepared by a special committee at the Farrand Training School of Harper Hospital in Detroit in 1893. This pledge was named after Florence Nightingale because "it represents the highest type of nurse and an ideal";[24] it was part of the graduation ceremonies in many schools of nursing for a long time.

In 1903, Isabel Hampton Robb, a Canadian nurse who became a nursing leader in the United States, wrote on "nursing ethics for hospital and private use." In the *American Journal of Nursing,* at the turn of the century, there was discussion of nurses' ethical concerns. These early expressions focused on manners, obedience to physicians, adherence to institutional norms and policies and nursing's contract with the patient to ensure that no harm came to him—an early indication of the advocacy role of the nurse as well as of nursing's commitment to the quality of care.

It was not until 1950 that the *Code for Nurses* was adopted by the American Nurses' Association. The *Code,* which has been revised periodically, has served to inform the nurse and society of the profession's expectations and requirements in ethical matters. The *Code* and the "Interpretive Statements" that accompany it provide a framework for the nurse to make ethical decisions and to discharge responsibilities to the public, to other members of the health team, and to the profession.[25]

The Code for Nurses and the *Interpretive Statements,* which were revised in 1976, are directed toward present-day practice. Previous *Codes* were more prescriptive and pointed to desirable standards for both personal and professional behavior. They described appropriate relationships with physicians and other health professionals and identified certain responsibilities of the nurse as a citizen, an employee, and a person. The 1976 *Code,* while it is still prescriptive, depends more on the nurse's accountability to the client and in that sense, represents a change of focus in an ethical code.[26]

The *Code*'s requirements may exceed but are never less than the law's requirements. Violations of the law may result in civil or criminal liability for nurses. Violations of the *Code for Nurses* may result in reprimands, censure, suspension, or expulsion of nurse members from the American Nurses' Association, as well as the sanctions, which are serious for the nurse, of loss of the respect of society and of colleagues. Each nurse has both a personal obligation to uphold and to adhere to the *Code* and a corporate responsibility to ensure that nursing colleagues do likewise.[27] The ultimate impact of the *Code for Nurses* depends on the extent to which nurses are familiar with it and prepared to implement its precepts in their professional lives, and on the extent to which they are able and willing to enforce it.

In 1973, *The ICN Code for Nurses—Ethical Concepts Applied to Nursing*[28] replaced the International Council of Nurses' earlier *International Code of Nursing Ethics* that was developed in 1953 and revised in 1965.[29] The new *Code,* which outlines the fundamental responsibility of the nurse and the nature of the need for nursing and nurses' responsibilities to people, to practice, to society, to co-workers, and to the profession, was endorsed for all their members by a number of nursing organizations, such as the College of Nurses of Ontario,[30] the statutory body that is responsible for the registration, regulation, and disciplining of the nursing profession in the Province of Ontario.[31]

In 1980, the College adopted its own code of ethics when it approved the *Guidelines for Ethical Behaviour in Nursing,*[32] a set of eleven statements accompanied by an interpretation of each statement. These decisions about ethical codes represent statutory action to fulfill the College's mandate to develop standards of practice and of ethical behavior to be used as a reference point in the development and assessment of the ethical component of any nurse's professional practice. The *Guidelines* focus on the role of the nurse, competence, expanding knowledge, quality of care, accountability, truth, consent, confidentiality, the health team, professional goals, and the nurse as a citizen.

It should be noted that the *Guidelines* constitute the second Canadian code of ethics for nurses that has become part of provincial nursing statutes. The first was the Code of Ethics[33] for nurses in Quebec that was approved by the Government of that province and by the Order of Nurses of Quebec in 1976, and to which, by statute, nurses in Quebec are bound to adhere. It embraces nurses' duties and obligations to the public and those to clients or patients— integrity, availability and diligence, liability, independence and disinterest, professional secrecy, accessibility of records, determination and payment of fees, nurses' duties and obligations to the profession, their relationships with the Order of Nurses of Quebec (the statutory or registering body), and their contribution to the advancement of the profession. In 1980, the Canadian Nurses Association published the first draft (which is being revised) of its *Code of Ethics*[34] which, like the ANA *Code,* is permissive rather than statutory in nature; however, it is the official statement of the national nurses' association for Canada. Themes and sessions related to ethics are seen frequently in nursing meetings and conferences. Consideration of the ethical components of professional nursing practice has prompted nurses to press for clarification and modification of conditions under which and situations in which nurses exercise their roles. These developments have important implications for the physician–nurse relationship and for the nature and shape of the health care system.

Sources of Conflict

Because nurses are prepared in a variety of types and levels of programs, it is difficult for some members of the public and for some health professionals to have a consistent view of what nursing is and what nurses can and will do. Even members of the nursing profession are still discussing roles, functions, relationships and levels of education that are appropriate for entry to nursing practice. Both the American Nurses' Association and the Canadian Nurses Association had lively discussions of the latter issue at their 1980 conventions. There is agreement that sound preparation, at every level, is necessary for nurses and that the public should be able to expect nurses to demonstrate specified standards of practice. Peer review is considered by most nurses to be essential, although relatively few members of the profession are implementing it fully. Physicians, health care administrators and other health workers have been evaluating nurses for a long time, without necessarily having the expertise to do so, and with at least tacit acceptance of this state of affairs by many nurses. This has led to tensions between physicians and nurses and has hindered effective communication. Physicians are thought to belong to a more homogeneous profession than do nurses, because of physicians' university level of preparation—the only route to entry to the profession. However, this apparent homogeneity is probably more illusion than fact.

Many nurses and other persons perceive that the nursing profession's failure to agree on a definitive definition of the discipline leads to confusion and lack of focus. This, too, may be more illusion than reality, for there are few, if any, completely clear and all-embracing definitions of medicine or of some of the other major helping professions. The focus of nursing appears to be unclear because of institutional bureacracy—in specific health care agencies and in the health care system as a whole—that helps to suggest that nurses simply follow physicians' orders. This is a result of the failure of physicians and other health care workers, including some nurses, to recognize the independent, dependent and interdependent functions of nurses. Although both Canada and the United States claim to have health care systems, in many ways, these are episodic illness care systems, the entry to which is possible only through physicians, the health care professionals who usually are responsible for transfer and/or discharge of patients from health care agencies and from the system. In 1980, the Canadian Nurses Association took a strong and public stand that there should be multiple entry points to the Canadian health care system,[35] a position that was not received with an excess of enthusiasm by very many groups, and certainly not by the organized medical profession. However, it was recommended in a major study of health care that the nurses' brief be studied carefully by governments at all levels.[36]

Another aspect of the institutional bureaucracy that contributes to problems with the nurse–physician relationship is that most nurses are employees of health care institutions, while physicians, nurses' apparent "co-workers" on the health care team, are "guest practitioners" in the same agencies, who wield a great deal of power over most aspects of the organization. Nurses, in spite of the fact that they are the largest group of health care professionals, have relatively few opportunities to make significant contributions to decision making and even to exercise the control over their own practice for which they are accountable by statute and by professional standards of practice and of ethics. This tradition of self-employed "guest practitioners" in health care institutions having so much power over the large groups of "full-time employees" of the institutions defies explanation, but it is a fact of life in health care.

Collaboration and Cooperation

With the increasing depersonalization of health care services and the diminution of direct contact with patients by some health professionals in the face of a rise in the amount of mechanically generated data, more than ever before there is a need for checks on the quality and relevance of information that enters diagnostic and decision-making processes in health care. It has been suggested that in medical practice, the family physician will play a central role in this responsibility.[37] However, unless the human resources of nurses, who are with patients in hospitals, for example, on a twenty-four-hour basis, and on a long-term basis in many other situations, are used in a collaborative and cooperative manner in the assessment and application of clinical information, including, but not restricted to, that generated solely by nurses, to the diagnostic, prescriptive, implementation, and evaluative aspects of health service to patients in all venues, there is grave danger that inhumane, depersonalized, unsafe, careless, fragmented, and inappropriate care will be given. Thus will both physicians and nurses fail to provide the ethical and professional standards of care for which they are accountable to society and the human rights of citizens to health care will be violated.

Many physicians believe that they alone are ethically and legally responsible for the totality of the health and illness care provided to patients; they fail to recognize that the health care team includes patients and their families, nurses and other health professionals, and health care administrators, all of whom have significant roles to play in the health care enterprise. When nurses attempt to exercise their broad ethical and legal responsibilities to and for patients, in situations in which they have limited authority, they feel powerless, excluded and dependent if there is a lack of nurse–physician collaboration and cooperation. Frequently, nurses are accused of being defensive when they insist that nurses be responsible for nursing, even though nurses' responsibility for their own behavior and for the regulation of their own profession is explicit in many nursing statutes. By law, medicine is not accountable for nursing; hence, nurses believe that medicine cannot be responsible for nursing and that nursing must assume that task.

The nurse of the eighties is responsible for professional judgment at two levels: (1) at that of a professional who influences and promotes change in health care policies in national, provincial, state, and local domains and who has input to policy decisions and to the establishment of standards in the profession at large and in the employing institution, and (2) at the level of an individual practitioner—who may be a clinician, an administrator, a teacher, or a researcher—who is responsible for the quality of care provided for individuals, families, or groups. Nurses' attempts to exert leadership in these areas for which they are accountable are met often with opposition from physicians, some of whom perceive nurses to be encroaching on their "professional territory," and some of whom reject and may even try to block the attempts of nurses to move beyond the "care taker" role, that is directed toward the well-being of another person in whatever setting and manner in which it needs to be fulfilled and that has evolved into the nursing and female role, and to enter the traditionally male-oriented, "healer role," that has been directed more specifically toward the tasks that are necessary to restore an individual to a functional status; this role, that is carried out usually in a specialized health setting, has evolved into the traditionally masculine and medical role.[38]

MODERN CONCEPTS OF NURSING AND OF THE ROLES OF WOMEN

The existence of these differences of opinion about the roles of the two major health professions has done little to modify nursing's poor and somewhat limited self-image; it is in serious conflict with major modern concepts of the nature of nursing, such as that it is a nurse–patient interaction that stems from the assessment of a patient's needs and levels of functioning and that it is designed to optimize the patient's adaptability through modification and/or reinforcement of the environment, modification and/or reinforcement of behavior and biological care and maintenance. This process is accomplished through the use of nursing care strategies in appropriate measure.[39] This and comparable other definitions include the notion that nursing is aimed toward the restoration and maintenance of functional competence, an idea that is similar to the goal of the traditional "healer." Hence, it is logical for nurses to perceive themselves as being very involved, in both their independent and interdependent roles, in the healing process.

It should be noted that even in the medical profession, there has been evidence of the perception that women ought to function in the "care taking" aspects of health care and leave most of the "technical" aspects to men. Female physicians, who because of home and family responsibilities have practiced on a part-time basis more than male physicians have done, have been more conspicuous in patient care roles than in administrative and academic roles, which seemed to be reserved for men.[40] Nurses in hospitals, who are predominantly women and who constitute the largest group of health workers, often are conspicuous by their absence from decision-making committees at high levels, even though the scope and extent of their responsibility are wide and far-reaching.

In general, women who remain in traditional roles do not threaten existing patterns or the status of other workers. History suggests that women in many fields, especially in some of the senior professions, have been considered less important, and their contributions less substantive or critical, in terms of national pride and prestige than are men. While major changes in these patterns and advances for women have been seen in times of war and of major cultural reorganizations, such as those in China and in the Union of Soviet Socialist Republics (USSR), these changes have not been as persistent or far-reaching as one might have predicted would be the case.[41]

These trends do not augur well for the nursing profession, which is part of a complex, hierarchical, and traditional health care system, the structure of which has encouraged a sense of limited expectations by and for persons at the lower levels of the hierarchy. As a result, there is a wide range of talents and abilities in health providers that may not be recognized and utilized by decision makers at many levels. Less than a decade ago, a Michigan court, in a malpractice liability related to nurses, noted that "A nurse, although obviously skilled and well-trained, is not in the same category as a physician who is required to exercise his independent judgment on matters which may mean the difference between life and death. Her prime function is to observe and record the symptoms and reactions of patients. A nurse is not permitted to exercise judgment in diagnosing or treating any symptoms which develop. Her duty is to report them to the physician. . . . A nurse by the very nature of her occupation is prohibited from exercising an independent judgment . . . ."[42]

This statement of the Michigan court is regressive, but it demonstrates the current ambiguity in nurse–physician roles and responsibilities. Some blurring of roles and overlapping of responsibilities and areas of function can be expected in situations where two professions such as medicine and nursing have the same clients and the same type of interests in those clients—the promotion of the well-being of individuals, families and communities. The practice entailed in such promotion necessarily involves intervention in the lives of others. Hence, it has an ethical component, whether the practice is direct patient care, the teaching of those who will enter the profession or who will increase their competence in it and/or the advancement of the theoretical aspects of the profession through research involving individuals or groups. Ethical decisions, which are based on values, are made by these health care professionals. Their ability to fulfill their ethical responsibilities depends on the professional context in which nurses and physicians work: appropriate professional preparation, suitable conditions for the exercise of professional practice, social respect for the professional as a decision maker and social recognition of professional expertise.[43]

NURSES, PHYSICIANS, AND PATIENTS

The ethical judgments made by nurses and physicians flow from personal conscience and include a weighing of alternatives—what *could* be done—and the making of decisions—what *should* be done. As alternatives are weighed, past experience, possible consequences, and personal strengths and weaknesses come into play. Once the decision is made, personal inventiveness and strength of will are important in the implementation of the action that flows from the decision.[44] Nurses and physicians pride themselves on their sensitivity to cultural and family factors that influence the patient's problems;[45] continuing recognition of and consideration for the values of other persons should be helpful to these health professionals as they search for the solutions to ethical problems.[46] At the same time, when the patient's wishes and values are in sharp conflict with those of the health professionals, whose values should take priority? If health professionals believe that their values are more significant because compromise of them could represent failure by professionals to be true to their personal and professional ethics, how would this affect the patient–professional relationship? On the other hand, if the patient's values take precedence, how would this affect the professionals' responsibilities to practice their profession and to care for the patient in the way that they believe is best for the patient?[47] How can health professionals make decisions that may be advantageous to their patients but a burden or a strain on society as a whole? Should continuing and complex health care be provided for patients whose conditions are self-induced? Should beds in a special care unit be provided on an equal basis to people whose major injuries are the result of their being drunken drivers or the victims of self-administered drug overdoses or of self-induced obesity?[48]

Both nurses and physicians are committed to recognize and to take action on their responsibilities to look beyond day-to-day patient care issues such as these and, in so doing, they will be examining issues that affect society as a whole.[49,50,51] However, they must guard against the temptation to focus on global issues at the expense of the principal focus of their professional practice—their patients, and their relationships with them. Although it is stylish for health care professionals to talk about working with patients as partners in the health care enterprise, patients have reported that they do not feel they are part of such an arrangement. Instead, they feel like numbers "being shuttled around" in the absence of psychological preparation for certain experiences, such as intensive care units, where the prevalence of electronic monitoring equipment is in sharp contrast to the lack of human warmth and compassion. Some patients have felt like "intruders" and they have experienced, from health professionals, little or no inspiration to make the special effort that is necessary to get well.[52]

It is obvious that nurses and physicians share the "commitment not just to individual life but to the institution of life."[53] If their professional associations are concerned solely with professional and territorial questions, the professions and their members could become and remain insulated from this control role, with the result that they would "trail happily after illness while ignoring . . . [their] obligation to help humanize society and to make it safe and fit for human beings."[54] This requires not only expertise in professional practice, but also knowledge about ethics or understanding of ethical systems or moral reasoning and "good moral reflexes."[55] These can be refined through the help in the clarification of ethical values and issues that is available from colleagues who understand the situations involved. Physicians and nurses who demonstrate what they profess, that is, participatory membership on a health care team, practice as colleagues—with respect for each other's expertise and contributions, consideration of each other's points of view in their decision making and genuine collaboration in the common goal of the promotion of functional competence in the recipients of health care. Such practitioners feel no obligation to shoulder the burden of blind obedience to prescribed procedures and the maintenance of traditional values. Like Socrates, they believe that the "unexamined life is not worth living"; hence, they assert themselves and challenge existing beliefs and practices.

The result will be that no longer will nurses silently reinforce the image that a few physicians have of themselves as gods. No longer will physicians view and treat professional nurses as servants. Rather, the kind of cooperative nurse–physician participation that takes place in emergency situations—in which whoever is closest to the item or action that is needed and whoever is better prepared to do something in the particular situation does it—will become the rule in nurse–physician relationships rather than the exception.[56] Until this is a universal phenomenon in health care, what can nurses do about the nurse–physician relationship?

CONCLUSIONS

McGuire has suggested that decency and courtesy are essential components that must be used by nurses who will start today—not next year, not tomorrow—to: (1) speak up: a keen mind cannot be discovered unless its owner learns to open up; (2) keep a sense of humor and perspective and remember that only a minority of physicians have no appreciation of nursing's contribution to health care; (3) enhance academic preparation through taking responsibility for their own education; (4) document what was done and observed and be prepared to subject it to the scrutiny of peers who include physicians; (5) exercise the patient advocacy role that has been made explicit in formal position statements of some professional associations,[57] by speaking for patients and intervening if necessary; (6) keep an open mind and a short memory by never holding a grudge about incidents that take place in the heat of difficult moments; and (7) ensure that diplomacy prevails in accordance with the diplomatic craftsmanship that is a hallmark of nursing skills. McGuire believes that when nurses learn to use these resources that are available, problems with the nurse–physician relationship will be solved.[58]

NOTES

1. Osler, Sir William. "Nurse and Patient," Address at Johns Hopkins Hospital, 1897, in *Aequanimitas (with other Addresses to Medical Students, Nurses and Practitioners of Medicine)*, by Sir William Osler (H. K. Lewis and Co. Ltd., London, 1920) pp. 153–166.
2. *Ibid.*
3. Osler, Sir William. "Doctor and Nurse," Address at Johns Hopkins Hospital, 1891, in *Aequanimitas, op. cit.*, p. 17.
4. Woodham-Smith, Cecil. *Florence Nightingale 1820–1910* (Collins (Fontana Books), London, 1951) p. 361.
5. Nightingale, Florence. *Notes on Nursing: What It Is and What It Is Not* (Dover Publications, New York, 1969) p. 3.
6. Konold, Donald. "Codes of Medical Ethics: History," in Warren T. Reich, ed., *Encyclopedia of Bioethics* (The Free Press, New York, 1978) pp. 162–171.
7. *Ibid.*
8. Oath of Hippocrates, in "General Codes for the Practice of Medicine," in Warren T. Reich, ed. *Encyclopedia of Bioethics* (The Free Press, New York, 1978) p. 1731.
9. World Medical Association. "Declaration of Geneva, 1948 and amended 1968," in Warren T. Reich, ed. *Encyclopedia of Bioethics* (The Free Press, New York, 1978) p. 1749.
10. Konold, *op. cit.*
11. American Medical Association. "Code of Ethics, 1847," in Warren T. Reich, ed., *Encyclopedia of Bioethics* (The Free Press, New York, 1978) pp. 1738–1746.
12. Konold, *op. cit.*
13. World Medical Association. "International Code of Medical Ethics, 1949," in Warren T. Reich, ed. *Encyclopedia of Bioethics* (The Free Press, New York, 1978) pp. 1749–1750.
14. American Medical Association. "Principles of Medical Ethics (1957)," in Warren T. Reich, ed. *Encyclopedia of Bioethics* (The Free Press, New York, 1978) pp. 1750–1751.
15. Konold, *op. cit.*
16. American Medical Association. "Guidelines for Organ Transplantation (1968)," in Warren T. Reich, *op. cit.*, p.1752.
17. _____. "Report on the Physician and the Dying Patient (1973)," in Warren T. Reich, *op. cit.*, pp. 1752–1753.

18. _____. "Report on Human Artificial Insemination (1974)," in Warren T. Reich, *op. cit.*, pp. 1753–1754.

19. Hall, The Honourable Emmett M. *A Commitment for Renewal: Canada's National-Provincial Health Program for the 1980's* (Health and Welfare Canada, Ottawa, 1980).

20. Tiberius, Richard G. "Medical Ethics in the Next 25 Years," *Canadian Family Physician*, Vol. 25 (January 1979) pp. 73–78.

21. Allentuck, Andres. "Megamedicine: It brings new benefits—and new risks," *The Canadian* (Nov. 11, 1978) pp. 5–7.

22. Tiberius, *op. cit.*

23. Nightingale, *op. cit.*

24. "Editorial Comment: *American Journal of Nursing* 11(10):777," cited in Barbara Tate (project director). *The Nurse's Dilemma: Ethical Considerations in Nursing Practice* (International Council of Nurses, Geneva, 1977) p. 72.

25. American Nurses' Association. *Code for Nurses with Interpretive Statements* (Kansas City, Mo., American Nurses' Association, 1976) p. 1.

26. *Ibid.*

27. *Ibid.*

28. International Council of Nurses. *ICN Code for Nurses—Ethical Concepts Applied to Nursing* (Geneva, International Council of Nurses, 1973).

29. Lamb, Marianne. *Nursing Ethics in Canada: Two Decades.* Unpublished Master's thesis, University of Alberta, Edmonton, Alberta, 1981, p. 41.

30. College of Nurses of Ontario. *Standards of Nursing Practice: for Registered Nurses and Registered Nursing Assistants. Revised May 1979* (College of Nurses of Ontario, Toronto, 1979) p. 2.

31. *The Health Disciplines Act, 1974, Part IV, Nursing.* Statutes of Ontario, 1974, Chapter 37, as amended by 1975, Chapter 63 (Queen's Printer, Toronto, 1975).

32. College of Nurses of Ontario. *Guidelines for Ethical Behaviour in Nursing* (College of Nurses of Ontario, Toronto, 1980).

33. *Code of Ethics. Regulation respecting the code of ethics (Nursing). Professional Code* (1973, c. 43, 5.85) (Quebec Official Gazette, Quebec, P.Q., September 22, 1976).

34. Canadian Nurses Association. *CNA Code of Ethics: An Ethical Basis for Nursing in Canada* (Canadian Nurses Association, Ottawa, 1980).

35. Canadian Nurses Association. *Putting "Health" into Health Care.* Submission to Health Services Review '79 (Canadian Nurses Association, Ottawa, 1980).

36. Hall, *op. cit.*, pp. 78–79.

37. Tiberius, *op. cit.*, p. 74.

38. Nadelson, Carol C. and Malkah T. Notman. "Women as Health Professionals," in Warren T. Reich, ed. *Encyclopedia of Bioethics* (The Free Press, New York, 1978) pp. 1713–1720.

39. Adaptation of definition after personal communication with Dr. Marian McGee (University of Western Ontario, London, Ontario, 1975).

40. Nadelson, *op. cit.*

41. *Ibid.*

42. Kambas v. St. Joseph's Mercy Hospital, 205 N.W. 2d 431, 389 Mich. 249 (1973). Cited by Nadelson, *ibid.*

43. College of Nurses of Ontario, 1980, *op. cit.*, p. 4.

44. *Ibid.*

45. Tiberius, *op. cit.,* p. 78.

46. College of Nurses, 1980, *op. cit.,* p. 5.

47. Tiberius, *op. cit.,* p. 76.

48. *Ibid.*, pp. 75–77.

49. College of Nurses, 1980, *op. cit.,* p. 16.

50. American Nurses' Association, 1976, *op. cit.,* p. 3 (#11).

51. Cousins, Norman, "Commentary: Medical Ethics—Is There a Broader View?" *Journal of the American Medical Association,* Vol. 241, No. 25 (June 22, 1979) pp. 2711–2712.

52. *Ibid.*, p. 2712.

53. *Ibid.*

54. *Ibid.*

55. Tiberius, *op. cit.,* p.77.

56. McGuire, Margaret A., "Nurse–Physician Interactions: Silence Isn't Golden," *Supervisor Nurse,* Vol. 11, No. 3 (March 1980) pp. 36–39.

57. See, for example: Registered Nurses Association of Ontario. *Statement on Patient Advocacy* (Registered Nurses Association of Ontario, Toronto, 1977).

58. McGuire, *op. cit.*, p. 39.

13

The Nurse–Institution Relationship

M. Josephine Flaherty

*"In Institutions the corroding effect of routine can be withstood
only by maintaining high ideals of work; but these become
the sounding brass and tinkling cymbals without corresponding
sound practice."*[1]

Sir William Osler

Nurses are employed today by many kinds of institutions, the scope and complexity of which vary from the corporate bureaucracy that may be seen in a large multi-service hospital to a two- or three-person community clinic or a physician's office. Between these two extremes are large numbers and types of health-related organizations including community health agencies in large cities, small urban centers, rural areas or outpost locations, elementary and secondary schools, industrial settings, nursing education institutions in hospitals, community colleges or universities, research institutes, supplemental staffing agencies, professional nursing statutory and voluntary organizations, and other types of voluntary health-related associations.

In spite of this variety, the majority of nurses in North America are employed in hospitals of various kinds. It is essential that the nurse employee understand fully the nature, purpose, and obligations of the hospital (or other employing agency) in order to understand the obligations, rights, and responsibilities of the nurse as employee.

The hospital in contemporary society has undergone a transition from a philanthropic institution that was essentially free from public accountability to an institution that is subject to public scrutiny like other social institutions. By definition and description, the hospital of today is a service agency in which a large number and variety of skills and services, offered by members of many

153

disciplines and supported by costly facilities and equipment, are organized and managed in the best interests of patients. The trustees of the hospital or other health care agency are held morally and legally responsible for everything that goes on in the institution, including the activities of all professionals who work in it. This corporate responsibility for the quality of the health care provided means that society can expect hospitals and other health-related agencies that employ health care professionals to require accountability from those professionals, including the nurses. This suggests that the nurse in the health care setting should have two roles. The first and primary role is to apply professional skills to the total care, that includes but is not restricted to nursing care, of sick and/or well people, depending on the setting in which the care takes place. The second role is to be involved appropriately in the management of the agency. For nurses who are identified as nurse managers at various levels, this role is explicit. For others, the role may be implicit, but it is genuine because of the nature of the responsibility and accountability that makes the nurse a professional.

The employment of registered nurses in and by institutions results in the formation of a nurse–institution relationship that involves rights, responsibilities, and expectations for both parties to the relationship.

Within that institutional relationship, the nurse is engaged, of course, in a number of other relationships that involve patients, their families, physicians, other nurses, health professionals in other disciplines, students, and other workers in the agency. All of these relationships are crucial to the day-to-day conduct of the work place.

In the nurse–institution relationship, it is incumbent on both employee and employer to make clear at the beginning the nature and scope of the rights, responsibilities, and expectations of both parties to the relationship and to keep open the lines of communication between the parties. There is a number of steps that should be taken in the development and maintenance of the nurse–institution relationship.

PRE-EMPLOYMENT PROCESS

A prospective employee should prepare a résumé for the prospective employer, that is, a current summary of academic qualifications and professional experience, and should make formal application in writing for a position. One or more interviews or planned meetings, between employer and employee, should be held with the explicit purpose of ensuring that both parties understand clearly the nature of the position and the mutual responsibilities and obligations. Details of the personnel policies and other items of concern should be discussed and understood before an offer of employment is made or a position is accepted. At the end of the interview(s), the applicant should understand the date by which an offer of or a notice of rejection for a position can be expected and the date by which the applicant must accept or reject an offer.

The employer's offer of a position should be in writing and should include a clear statement of the scope and nature of the position, the date of appointment, the salary and benefits, any other relevant conditions and, if applicable, a copy of the negotiated collective agreement. The candidate should accept or reject the offer in writing. A candidate who accepts an offer of employment has professional and ethical obligations to honor the commitment unless he or she is released formally from it after adequate notice of intent.

All aspects of the position that might pose problems or concerns should be discussed during the pre-employment process. For example, nurses should request and receive information about the lines of authority and the decision-making structure of the employing agency. In special care units in some agencies, clinical nurse specialists and nurse clinicians have considerable breadth of decision-making power, whereas in others, this is quite limited. Such specialty nurses may be in either staff or line positions and this should be clarified. Head nurses and other middle management personnel may be within or outside collective bargaining units and are obliged to respect the relevant policies of agencies in which they accept employment.

Prospective employees should be apprised of responsibilities, outside their normal duties, that they may be required to assume. For example, if a nurse assigned to a surgical unit may be required to work on some occasions in a unit where abortions are done, the nurse should be made aware of that possibility prior to employment. A nurse who, for reasons of conscience or personal conviction, will not take part in abortion procedures, is obliged to make that known to the employer prior to accepting employment. This nurse, on accepting employment after being told that the job may include work in the abortion unit, is making a professional and ethical commitment to fulfill an employment contract. What should he or she do on being assigned to assist in an abortion procedure?

Before this question can be answered, one must examine the kind of obligation that the nurse has assumed in this employment situation. The nurse's professional obligation is quite clear: it is to fulfill the employment contract. The nurse also has an ethical obligation to fulfill the employment contract. However, the nurse was not behaving in an ethical manner in the making of a contract for employment that clearly could result in a conflict situation if it called on that nurse to perform procedures that, for reasons of conscience or personal conviction, he or she would not be prepared to perform. A nurse who views abortion as a wrongful destruction of human life in conscience could not take part in the abortion procedure unless refusal to do so would constitute a direct danger to the patient or would constitute abandonment of the patient because there was no other nurse available to assume the responsibility for the particular tasks. Such a circumstance would take precedence over the nurse's personal feelings or convictions and would direct the nurse's action in this work situation.

The nurse who refuses to take part in abortion procedures because of personal convictions might feel perfectly justified in doing so and might believe that the employer should respect that stand. However, it should be noted that in a circumstance such as the one cited above, the particular nurse, who entered the employment situation in full knowledge that this conflict situation might arise, could and should be censured for his or her behavior. Such action toward the nurse would not be taken because of the refusal *per se* to participate in the abortion procedure but rather because of the nurse's dishonesty in the making of a contract in the knowledge that he or she would not or could not fulfill it under certain circumstances.

TERMS OF EMPLOYMENT

The terms of employment of nurses are governed by relevant legislation and by the policies of the agency. These terms should specify conditions of the probationary period, transfer, promotion, and seniority. Hours of work should be specified with indication of how much flexibility of hours and/or of tours of duty is permissible. Salaries, which must be specified, should be equitable with current practice in the jurisdiction involved. Salaries should reflect the professional status of the nurse, including the responsibilities and obligations of the position, the education and experience required for the position and the potential of the individual in the position. Provision should be made for annual increments according to the collective agreement or, in the absence of such an agreement, according to a consumer price index or similar indicator. Promotions to positions of greater responsibility should involve an increase in salary.

Employee benefits should include vacation and paid statutory holidays, premium pay for special circumstances (such as overtime, standby, call back, reporting in, responsibility and shift differentials), and sickness and maternity leave (in some jurisdictions, paternity leave is being considered). Provision should be made for pension, insurance coverage for disability, sickness, medical, hospital, and dental care where available, and for life insurance coverage. Leave of absence should be provided for compassionate reasons, court duty, public office, and educational and professional development. Some agencies may provide for sabbatical leave.

A salary and benefit package similar to that outlined above, although it would represent considerable outlay for the employer, is not unusual for nurses in some jurisdictions where employers are committed to progressive terms of employment. Employees who benefit from such a package have professional and ethical responsibilities to honor the terms of employment and to live up to the responsibilities of their positions. Similarly, employers have ethical responsibilities to honor the agreement.

CONDITIONS OF WORK

It is reasonable to assume that in most employment situations, problems will arise. To promote equitable adjustment of such problems, a well-defined procedure should be established with the steps to be followed known and understood by all concerned. Both employers and employees have obligations to participate in good faith in all steps of employment problem procedures, using honest and forthright documentation and discussion of issues. In nursing, this involves participation of professional nurses on both management's and employees' sides of the questions.

In western society, professionals have been thought to be management oriented because, by virtue of their education, expertise, and desire to control the quality of their "product" (such as the health care provided), they have input to managerial decisions and they often assumed administrative positions. Health care institutions today are bureaucracies, the structure of which has resulted in apparent erosion of professional prerogatives. This has created a schism between salaried professionals, such as nurses, and their employers. Collective bargaining, involving the formation of unions, has been seen as a means of "preventing a further diminution of the role and rights of the professional employee,"[2] while providing for collective action by professionals toward improvement in the quality of professional service delivered and in the economic and general welfare of professionals.[3]

Nurses are divided on the issue of collective bargaining. Some believe that it results in "a loss of professionalism [that] diminishes the nurse's self-image, negatively affects the nurse's image before the public, and ultimately causes a deterioration in the nurse's professional practice."[4] Others see collective bargaining negotiations that focus on practice issues such as practice committees, adequate staff development, appropriate equipment for patient safety and well-being, adoption of specific standards of practice, peer evaluation, and other factors intended to improve the quality of nursing care delivered, as "one of the clearest possible expressions of professionalism."[5] Many nursing practice issues are purported to be able to be solved easily by unions, professional associations, hospital associations and governments. Many unions see the solutions to problems being enshrined in rigid and isolated assertions of what workers and employers will or will not do in narrowly defined, unchangeable (if that is possible in nursing), and isolated sets of circumstances. As a result, issues such as promotions, salary increases that may ignore the question of merit, and job security that may rest solely on seniority rather than on competence, may threaten the quality of nursing service, professional responsibility, and professional stature.[6] Professional nursing associations are engaged in the development and revision of guidelines on which to base resolution of professional problems in work situations. Some hospital associations promote hospital structures that make appropriate use of nursing expertise improbable if not impossible. Governments in some jurisdictions control hospital budgets in such a way that provision of adequate nurse staffing may be difficult and unlikely to occur. That these problems continue to exist suggests that today neither unions nor professional associations, alone or together, appear to be able to stem the erosion of nurses' autonomy, that is, both authority and responsibility for their own practice—individual or collective—and the effect of that on job relationships. Is it any wonder that self-determination, one of the essential criteria for a profession, is one of the most prevalent issues in nursing? It is one of the basic factors that determine the conditions under which nurses practice. Who is responsible for the conditions of work for nurses?

At the international level, several years ago, the International Labour Organization (of which the United States was not a member) approved a convention (agreement) on conditions of life and work for nurses, the first ever to be formulated for a specific professional group. Member countries were asked to ratify it at the national level; such ratification involves agreement by the country to ensure that all provisions in the convention will be implemented. Canada could meet all of the requirements for nurses but many countries were unable to do so.

At national, state, and provincial levels, there are professional, statutory, and government-wide regulations that affect working conditions for nurses. However, it is at the local, institutional, and unit levels that the major responsibility lies for scrutiny, evaluation, and modification, if appropriate, of the conditions under which nurses practice their profession. The parties involved include, individually and collectively, the members of the governing councils or boards of trustees, the non-nurse administrators, the power figures, such as physicians, the nurse administrators and managers, and the staff nurses. Each of these groups has its priorities, biases, skills, abilities, and mechanisms for dealing with modification and/or reinforcement of working conditions. Both leaders and followers have significant roles to play and the success of the enterprise, which has major implications for the efficiency and effectiveness of nursing practice and service, will depend on the extent to which each group plays its part responsibly. With the nurse manager rests the additional challenge to orchestrate the entire performance so that the conditions necessary for provision of quality nursing care will obtain.

It has been recognized that it is the responsibility of the statutory (registering or licensing) body to determine what is the scope of nursing and what are acceptable standards for practice. The professional association attempts to examine, describe, and prescribe the work and role of nurses, not only in specific terms of what nurses do, but also in terms of the place of nursing in society, how nurses can move the social order forward and how professional knowledge can be increased and diffused so that the integrity of the profession will be enhanced. The employer specifies who shall do what in the agency and allocates resources (physical and human) accordingly. Finally, the individual practitioner decides how he or she will carry out the nursing function in response to patients' needs for care. By definition, then, the nursing practice situation presents several loyalties that demand recognition as nurses are confronted by pressures from peers, superiors, subordinates, other health care professionals, non-nurse administrators, and patients.

Recently, the economic pressure of inflation has resulted in nurses' strikes in Canada and in the United States. Conflict between nurses' obligations to the profession and to the employing agency, that is, between professionalism and institutionalism, resulting in pressure for compromise between loyalty to professional standards and loyalty to institutional demands[7] is inevitable in modern health care institutions. The challenge to nurses is to recognize and accept that they and their colleagues have multiple loyalties that, from time to time, will assume different orders of priority and to implement sound, palatable, and above all, *practical* methods of dealing with these.

All responsible nurses must examine the corporate frameworks in which they function, the professional frameworks that guide their own behavior, the extent of their tolerance for other professional frameworks that motivate their peers, subordinates and superiors, to determine whether these are compatible. In so doing, they will ask whether as professionals individual nurses, wherever they practice, are seeing their work in the light of an interplay of ideals from a variety of disciplines and points of view and directing their practice accordingly. Are they truly conscious of the contexts in which their patients and their colleagues see themselves? Do they see hospitals, for example, as social institutions in which it is the collective responsibility of the professionals who provide service to determine the standards of practice in the agency and, hence, the quality of service delivered? Or, are they pursuing individual goals without due consideration of patients and colleagues? Are the health care institutions exercising social initiatives or are they maintaining the *status quo*? Can and do institutions really control their human and physical resources? Can and will they attempt to reorganize themselves in the future to reflect the importance of disease prevention and reduce the public's "addiction to curative medicine"?[8] Are the professional associations blazing new social pathways and having a greater voice in the affairs of society, in major policy decisions within health institutions and in determinations about the nature, distribution, and financing of the health care system? Or, are they simply mending their fences and erecting "No Trespassing" signs within narrow frameworks to preserve their territories? Are the nurses' unions restricting themselves to wage increases (most of which are the result of economic changes in society rather than the result of union activity) and representation in the grievance process in order to secure equitable treatment for members? Or, are they engaging in professional modes of collective action that focus on issues that directly affect the quality of nursing practice? The answers to these questions will be found by nurses—individually and collectively—in assessment of the extent to which the responsibilities and expectations of nurses and institutions are appropriate and are fulfilled. This involves both ability and ethical commitment on the parts of both parties to exert the required effort.

RESPONSIBILITIES AND EXPECTATIONS OF NURSES AND INSTITUTIONS

When persons qualify, apply for, and accept registration as nurses, they accept the commitment to exercise generally accepted standards of nursing practice in all situations in which they agree to function as registered nurses. A clause that outlines such a commitment for registered nurses appears in many nursing acts or statutes and/or in regulations under these statutes. Statutory bodies that are responsible for the registration of nurses either develop standards[9] of practice for the performance of nursing services by their registrants in their jurisdictions or endorse a previously formulated set of standards.[10] This is in line with the responsibility of the statutory bodies to protect the public by ensuring that those persons who are registered as nurses are qualified to be so registered. It is through the establishment, maintenance, and development of standards of nursing practice that the registering bodies are able to evaluate and monitor the practice of their registrants. It is through these functions that the registering authorities for nurses define the scope and nature of nursing practice, regulate the practice of the profession, and discipline or investigate registered nurses about whom there is concern. This includes issues related to initial and continuing registration of nurses and to allegations of professional misconduct, incompetence, and incapacity against registrants.

In many jurisdictions, the title "registered nurse" is protected. This means that no person shall hold himself out as competent to practice as a registered nurse, shall use the title "registered nurse" or the designation "Reg. N." or "R.N.," or other designation representing the title, unless that person is the holder of a current certificate of registration in the state, province, or territory in which he or she seeks employment. In some jurisdictions, such as the Canadian provinces of Quebec and Prince Edward Island, the title "nurse" is protected; hence, no person shall use the title "nurse" or other designation representing the title or hold himself out as competent to practice as a nurse unless he or she is the holder of a current certificate of registration in the particular province.

An institution considering the employment of a person as a registered nurse, or the granting of permission to the person to function in the institution as a registered nurse without being employed by the institution (as in the case, for example, of a post-RN student or a teacher working with students), has the responsibility to require the presentation of documentary evidence of current and appropriate professional registration. On receipt of this, the institution has the right to expect that the registered nurse will meet at least the minimum standards of practice as specified by the registering body. In the statutes and/or regulations under the statutes for the registration of nurses, definitions of professional misconduct, incompetence and incapacity outline ways of behavior that are unacceptable in the nursing performance of registered nurses. Some of these are well known and easy to identify, whereas others may be less familiar even to nurses. For example, in the Province of Ontario, Regulation 21 under the *Health Disciplines Act, 1974, Part IV, Nursing,* defines professional misconduct as including among other items, the following:

> . . . (i) failure to inform the member's [the nurse's] employer of the member's inability to accept specific responsibility in areas where special training is required or where the member does not feel competent to function without supervision; (j) failure to report the incompetence of colleagues whose actions endanger the safety of a patient; . . . (m) conduct or an act relevant to the performance of nursing services that, having regard to all the circumstances, would reasonably be regarded by members as disgraceful, dishonorable or unprofessional.[11]

This gives registered nurses in Ontario the responsibility, by statute, to communicate to their supervisors their inability to accept specific responsibilities, when they do not feel competent to function in those situations. The employer should be able to be confident that nurses will do this and hence should not be surprised if nurses refuse to work in areas with which they are unfamiliar and for which they should have special training and/or supervision. Registered nurses who accept such situations without comment or action are demonstrating professional misconduct and unethical behavior as they knowingly fail to live up to the standards of nursing practice for which they stand accountable. Hospitals and other health care agencies that knowingly place nurses in such situations are guilty of failure to provide the "treatment" (that in Ontario, for example, is defined for hospitals in *The Public Hospitals Act* as "the maintenance, observation, medical care and supervision and skilled nursing care of a patient . . . ")[12] that they contract to supply to patients who are admitted.

An employer of registered nurses can expect those nurses to be competent, that is, to possess and demonstrate, in the professional care of patients or clients, the knowledge, skill, and judgment that are generally expected of registered nurses as well as the regard for the welfare of patients that registered nurses profess to demonstrate according to the standards of nursing practice for the jurisdiction. An employer also can expect that nurses will have the capacity to practice nursing as registered nurses. If they are suffering from physical or mental conditions or disorders of a nature and extent that make it desirable in the interest of the public and in the interest of the nurses that they no longer be permitted to practice or that their practice be restricted, they may be declared by the statutory body to be incapacitated and their registrations may be revoked, restricted, or suspended. Notice of disciplinary action of this sort may be published by the statutory bodies in many jurisdictions, in the interest of protection of the public. Incapacity of an applicant to complete a nursing education program, because of the physical handicap of severe deafness, resulted in the refusal of a community college to admit the applicant.[13] This decision was upheld by a United States District Court, later overturned by a U.S. Circuit Court of Appeals and then reversed again and upheld by the U.S. Supreme Court.[14] Had the candidate been admitted, it is doubtful whether the college could have fulfilled its professional and ethical commitments to the agencies in which students received clinical practice experience, to ensure safe practice by students. Had the candidate graduated and become registered, it is doubtful that she would have been able to practice clinical nursing according to the standards of nursing practice of the jurisdiction.

Since nurses who are employed by health care agencies function within current legislation affecting the practice of nursing as well as that affecting the function of health care agencies, and according to professional standards of practice and codes of ethics, the health care agencies are obliged to provide circumstances and resources that permit nursing and other professional health care to be provided within these dimensions. The authority for nursing and for other professions is based on a social contract under which society grants to the professions authority over their own functions, together with significant autonomy in the conduct of their own affairs. In return, the professions are expected to behave responsibly in accordance with the public trust. Basic to the contract is self-regulation of the profession to assure quality of practice, the hallmark of a mature profession.[15] As a result of such self-regulation, nurse practice acts and legislation and regulations for registration and licensure have been enacted to define legal authority to practice. The legislation was preceded by and derived from the profession's contract with society.

Since public and private health care institutions offer services that are defined both by legislation and by the policies of the institutions, the public has a right to expect that when these services include care rendered by registered nurses, conditions will be provided under which generally accepted standards of nursing practice can be met. Such standards identify criteria for assessment of the practice of registered nurses and include definitions of the functions of registered nurses, at least in general terms.[16,17,18]

Use of the nursing process governs all nursing practice; recognition of this is reflected in the American Nurses' Association *Standards of Nursing Practice,*[19] to which ethical nurses in the United States are committed. In some jurisdictions, nurses also have a legal commitment to the nursing process because the statutes that govern nursing practice require nurses to demonstrate specific behavior. When the standards specify that "The Registered Nurse effectively uses the nursing process,"[20] the nurse must engage in assessment of the health status of the individual patient, identification of his or her health needs, development, evaluation, and modification of a nursing care plan based on the assessed health needs and the prescribed medical regime and implementation of this plan; the employing agency is required to provide the necessary staff and structures to make effective use of this nursing process possible. This includes freedom and resources, including significant appropriate staff, for the nurse to assess needs, plan, implement, and evaluate the effects of nursing care. Where the standards of practice call for the nurse to participate as a member of the health team,[21] provision must be made for collaboration, coordination, and communication by all members of the health care team. Where the standards of practice call for the registered nurse to fulfill his or her responsibilities as a member of the nursing discipline,[22] provision must be made for the nurse to be able: to collaborate, supervise, and be supervised by appropriate others who contribute to the provision of nursing care; to function competently within relevant legislation, appropriate codes of ethics, and the policies and practices of the agency; to maintain competence relative to current practice; and to be accountable for his or her own actions. Where nursing care situations do not provide adequate resources (physical and human) and lines of authority and communication that are appropriate for exercise of nursing practice according to these standards, they are not fulfilling their legal, ethical, and social responsibilities to provide health and/or illness care by nurses and other health professionals.

The phenomena that are within the scope of nurses' responsibility in professional practice are human responses to health needs and problems; these are under constant examination and refinement by the profession. All registered nurses are accountable for professional behavior, exercised either by themselves or by those for whom they have administrative responsibility, as defined by the standards of nursing practice for their jurisdictions; however, the level and sophistication of application of the standards will vary with the education, experience, and skills of the individual nurses involved. Variations in the practice of nursing occur in relation to the collection, assessment, and analysis of data, the breadth and depth of knowledge and the application of theory to the identification of nursing problems and to the implementation of nursing actions to deal with these, the range of nursing techniques (simple to complex) used by the nurse, the nature and extent of assistance and supervision by other nurses, and the evaluation of the outcomes of nursing and other health care activities.

All nurses, according to the extent of their particular expertise, have responsibility for the provision of preventive nursing care that is directed toward the promotion of health; the prevention of disease; the health education of patients and families; the securing of appropriate medical attention for diagnosis and treatment when the presence of disease, or of predisposition to disease, becomes apparent from the nursing assessment; the early recognition and management of complications and other results of disease or treatment; and the informing of the public about actual or potential health problems.

As part of their social and institutional responsibility, nurses can be expected to demonstrate initiative in the development of new patterns of nursing and health care. To do this, nurses must have the appropriate professional authority and self-regulatory power, the ability and the will to work effectively and efficiently with patients and families, with other health professionals, and with appropriate other workers, within the policies and practices of the health care agency, in the effort to meet the health needs of care recipients. Unfortunately, many nurses are locked into a health care system in which they are hampered because entry of patients to the system is possible only through a physician. In a submission[23] to a Special Commission to review the state of health services in Canada, the Canadian Nurses Association made far-reaching recommendations on remuneration of health care workers, including professionals; the nature and shape of the Canadian health care system; points of entry to the health care system for patients; and utilization of human resources in health care, especially nurses. These recommendations were very well received by the Commissioner. In a chapter of the report, which was devoted to the nursing proposals, the Canadian Nurses Association was commended by The Honourable Emmett M. Hall for the excellence of its brief. "Well structured and carefully documented it was affirmative and forward looking."[24] One of the recommendations of the Hall Commission was: "The whole submission of the Canadian Nurses Association demands close study by all Governments, and I recommend that this be done in a serious and objective way."[25] This is simply one more, and very public, example of nurses' exercise of their social responsibility. The Canadian Nurses Association is working actively to keep the content of its proposals before the public and Governments at all levels.

ISSUES THAT THREATEN THE NURSE–INSTITUTION RELATIONSHIP

The reality of today is that in health care agencies there are real differences that lead to conflict. Inflation and fiscal constraints are facts of life today that push nurse managers to promote cost containment in the face of professional desires to maintain high quality of service and of personal needs to protect one's own standard of living.[26] Thus are nurses, at all levels, pulled to serve two masters. As they attempt to choose between them, their orientations to their discipline and/or to their employing institutions are disrupted.[27] Among the other issues is that structures frequently are designed (or allowed to evolve) to conform to the power structure—real or perceived—and to "vested interests rather than according to what will best serve the evolving purposes of the professional organization."[28]

In their one-to-one and group relationships, nurses have expended a good deal of effort in identification of methods of negotiation and bargaining that preserve professional aspirations, fulfillment of what they see as their obligations, and social and economic security. Collective bargaining in good faith, in a variety of patterns, is thought to be able to achieve this, as it involves both staff and management nurses who discuss issues with a view to the achievement of professional and institutional goals. In spite of this theoretical elegance, many nurses have difficulty with both the concept and the practice of dealing with working conditions issues; in implementation of it, they see themselves functioning in adversary positions.

Expert nurse managers have accepted responsibility for the creation and maintenance of an atmosphere of inquiry in their units and for the promotion of critical thought on the scientific base for nursing. It has been suggested that nurse educators, who feel obliged to prepare nurses to be "leaders," may not be paying enough attention to the preparation of "followers."[29] When the collective bargaining function (discussion of issues on which there are differences of opinion becomes a collective bargaining function when it relates to the conditions under which nurses practice) takes place, it seems to involve acceptance by nurses of a false and probably dangerous dichotomy between staff nurses on the one hand and management nurses on the other.[30] If both groups are members of the same profession, with commitment to a common mission concerning "all things that affect nursing participation in health services," there should be no problem with the achievement of a common understanding;[31] acceptance of the dichotomy would be a contradiction.[32] Just as worrisome is the separation of concern for remuneration and conditions under which professional practice is carried out from the professional association's concern for the nature and development of nursing practice. Certainly, both of these are part of the professional ethos that today's nurse inherited from Florence Nightingale who wrote (in the face of the public's conception of the nurse as a "self-immolating sister of charity" instead of the "professional woman, trained, efficient and highly paid" that she was preparing), "I would far rather than establish a religious order, open a career highly paid."[33] Nightingale did not want fanatics who would engage in rebellion and warfare; she believed that the way to improve the conditions and techniques of contemporary nursing was through thoughtful and wise reform of regulations, which she believed were essential to sound organization[34] of an institution.

More than a decade ago, economists were suggesting that unions' noneconomic contributions would be their most important functions and that soon they would take on additional kinds of involvements, such as political activity to promote legislation dealing with employment measures, public expenditures, social change such as environmental pollution control, occupational health and safety and other conditions of work, such as workloads, that impinge on the ability of workers to achieve the standards of work for which they are accountable.

This has happened already in Canada, where the eighties represent an important new era of labor relations in health care institutions. During the summer of 1980, a ten-day strike by nurses in Alberta and a work-to-rule campaign by medical interns and residents in Ontario pointed to the need for hospital management to become more democratic in response to collective bargaining for health care professionals. As an example of a successful demand for a greater voice for nurses in the determination of workloads, the Ontario Nurses' Association (ONA—the largest nurses' union in that province) achieved the inclusion of *professional responsibility clauses* in contracts between ONA members and hospital boards. Such clauses state that when nurses believe their work is being handicapped by an overload of patients, they may lodge a complaint before an assessment committee of three independent registered nurses from outside the hospital involved. Such committees have concluded, for example, that too few nurses had been assigned to hospital intensive care and coronary care units and that such staffing patterns could jeopardize patient safety.

Since registered nurses, by the very nature of their profession, are required to exercise judgment in carrying out their duties, there may be instances in which the institutional goals or directives seem to be at odds with their professional judgment. However, just because a nurse is a professional with the capacity for judgment, he or she does not cease to have certain responsibilities, as an employee, to the employer. In most collective agreements it is recognized explicitly that there are institutional goals, and an employer is not required to shut down his institution during discussion of a difference of opinion. Normally, attempts are made by nurse managers in health care situations to operate the institution in the interest of both parties to the dispute. If this is not achieved, in many instances the worker will *obey now* and *grieve later.* He or she has access to grievance procedures that may culminate in adjudication of the dispute by a neutral arbitrator, who, if the dispute is well-founded, will be able to protect the interest of the deserving party, whether that is the employer or employee.

In a health care agency, however, there is a third set of interests that are paramount to both employers and employees; they are those of the patients or consumers of the health care produced and delivered by the agency and its employees. One might ask how the interests of patients would affect the application of the *obey and grieve* rule.

During the period of employment, neither employer nor employee can change conditions of the contract for employment without renegotiation of conditions and mutual agreement to the new conditions. All too frequently in nursing situations, conditions are changed by one party without consultation with the other party, and conflict results.

Recently, for example, a nurse, a skilled writer and educator, who was employed as a continuing educator in a specialized hospital, had been engaged for about six months in the preparation of an educational program to be taught by her in several institutions and to be copyrighted eventually and published by the specialized hospital. She discovered that her nursing superior had removed the continuing educator's name from that program and from other work she had authored and had replaced it with the nursing superior's own name. The employee discussed this with her superior who retorted that, as head of the department, she had the right to have her name on all work done in the department. When the nurse employee questioned the propriety of this, the superior asserted that the employee had agreed to this condition when she had been engaged. The employee denied having made this agreement; there was no indication of such an agreement either on the letter of appointment or in the job description. When the nurse said that, in conscience, she could not accept such a condition, the superior told her that this was a firm condition of employment and that either she would have to work under it or she would have to resign. When the employee said that she could not work under such a condition, the employer prepared a letter of resignation and instructed the nurse to sign it then and there, to gather her belongings, and to leave the agency immediately. Unfortunately, the nurse, who was inexperienced in situations of this type and upset by the events, followed the instructions and thus terminated her employment in the hospital.

This is an apparent case of questionable practice by the employer and a less than ideal response by the employee. One would question first the propriety of anyone attaching his own "by line" to material written by someone else. Indeed, this is a practice that, although it has been well known, is deplored in academic and literary circles. While the head of a department has ultimate responsibility for the work done in his or her unit, under normal circumstances this should not include claims to authorship of materials that are the work of another person.

A second issue here is the imposition of a condition with which one party to the employee–institution relationship was not acquainted. If this had been such a firm condition of employment, why did it not appear either in the job description or in the letter of appointment? Why did the nurse employer take such a strong and uncompromising stand on the issue? Why did she not produce a more compelling reason for the placing of her name on work than the fact that, as head of the department, she had "the right" to have her name attached to all work? Why was her name the only one to appear on the work?

A third issue relates to the propriety of an employer preparing a letter of resignation for a senior employee and instructing that employee to sign it immediately. Should an employer *ever* write the letter of resignation for an employee? What motivated the employer to demand an immediate resignation?

Did these events represent discussion in good faith of an employment problem? Was such behavior typical of the agency and will it continue? Did the employer's presentation to the employee of the letter of resignation and instruction to sign it and to leave the premises immediately represent harassment and/or oppression of the employee? Was this incident an appropriate separation process?

Another issue is the situation in which the employee found herself. Should she have resigned under such duress? The letter of resignation that she signed (and she realized immediately afterward that she should not have done so) gave no reason for the resignation and did not allow for appropriate time of notification of separation according to applicable legislation, professional standards, and agency policies. The record shows simply that the employee resigned without notice. This is hardly a healthy situation from which the employee can expect to obtain a positive reference for a future employer.

A reality of the eighties that health care is long on opinion and short on fact has grave implications for health care institutions, for those who work in them and for those who are served by them. The paucity of hard facts and of sound, dispassionate advice to help in decision making constitutes a major threat to the health care manager on his or her main battlefield: resource allocation and determination of priorities within allocated financial resources.[35] The experienced health care administrator realizes that a great deal of this work involves the making of value judgments.[36] Most of the decisions cannot be substantiated fully by data as the health care manager tries, for example, to compare the need for surgical equipment with the need for fetal monitoring equipment. There is a pull between the budgeting of funds for staff development and the allocation of funds for an additional technical staff member. The number and scope of conflicting priorities will increase as fiscal restraints are intensified. A decision maker's value system influences his judgments; therefore, a clear set of values will lend consistency to the making of judgments. It follows that health care agencies, which administer many of the life-saving or life-improving technologies, must have a clear value system in order to make sound and consistent decisions about the scope and nature of health services to be offered and about the use to be made of physical, fiscal, and human resources and to provide an identifiable framework within which relationships between the institution and health professionals can be developed.

McGeorge suggests that agencies such as hospitals, through their expert professionals, should be furnishing data for debate on issues such as admission criteria for critical care areas, cost–benefit of various medical–surgical procedures, numbers of acute care beds needed per thousand population, rationales for the scope and nature of services to be offered, optimum utilization of beds, admission practices in clinical teaching units, informed consent for patients and spouse consent.[37] By recognizing and exposing these issues, by debating them and offering leadership in their resolution, the "towers of technology," as hospitals have been called,[38] may shrug off the modern obsession with repair of damaged bodies in favor of creative responses to social pressure in the shaping of laws and policies that will transform modern health care from a "reactive care" system to the "proactive or anticipatory care" system that will contribute to optimization of the functional competence of people.

Health care delivery is a power struggle—a struggle between diverse vested interests with shifting alliances depending on the issue and the disparate interests therein.[39] Recent events in society indicate that in a democracy, most people still identify individual rights and freedom as extremely important, if not inviolable. However, group efforts and participation of many people are seen as useful approaches to the solution of common problems through legislation and/or change of behavior at societal levels. The "new social man of the eighties" sees the need for improvement in the quality of life.[40] Many of the major health problems today are related to individual life styles based on personal decisions and habits and on environmental factors over which individuals have little control. Personal responsibility for one's own health, together with collective action on certain social, occupational, and environmental problems, will be necessary for realization of improvements in the health of individuals in western society. Public accountability can lead to different approaches to policy setting and decision making.[41] Today, more and more people are questioning programs and expenditures as they never did before. They are demanding moral leadership in health care. Industrial democracy is seen as suited to the real needs of human beings.[42] There is a growing recognition in health care that responsible leaders must be sensitive and responsive to the people who provide health care as well as to those who receive it. Health care workers, including professionals, are prepared no longer to have little or no input to the nature and shape of the health care system. They realize that they have knowledge and experience that suggest directions for health care and they insist on being heard. If their advice is sound, it will contribute to optimization of the use of human and physical resources.

"If the health care industry is to fulfill its mandate, the wise manager would be prudent to re-examine, in consort [sic] with his peers and other colleagues, the goals of his institution in the light of present social needs and current fiscal realities, and ensure that the services of his institution have relevance to the needs and aspirations of the citizens in the community. The alternative is organizational obsolescence and, finally, demise."[43]

A growing awareness of the limitations of available resources has stimulated attempts at the development of a "conserver society."[44]

In most developed countries, there is increasing government financing of health care services. That this has resulted in ever increasing health costs has become a major political issue in developed countries.[45]

Government action, in response to social pressure, to reduce expenditures is not part of an organized plan to alter and improve the health care system.

This can be done only by the providers of health services who must work within the resources allocated to them. They also must work cooperatively with the other disciplines and services involved to provide a health care system in general and specific services in particular that are most appropriate for the people to be served in a particular context.

NOTES

1. Osler, Sir William. "Nurse and Patient," Address at Johns Hopkins Hospital, 1897, in *Aequanimitas (with other Addresses to Medical Students, Nurses and Practitioners of Medicine),* by Sir William Osler (H. K. Lewis and Co. Ltd., London, 1920) p. 166.
2. Beletz, Elaine E. "Organized Nurses View Their Collective Bargaining Agent." *Supervisor Nurse,* Vol. 11 (September 1980) p. 41.
3. Jacox, Ada. "Collective Action: The Basis for Professionalism." *Supervisor Nurse,* Vol. 11 (September 1980) p. 22.
4. Rotkovitch, Rachel. "Do Labor Union Activities Decrease Professionalism?" *Supervisor Nurse,* Vol. 11 (September 1980) p. 16.
5. Jacox, *op. cit.,* p. 23.
6. Rotkovitch, *op. cit.,* p. 17.
7. Levenstein, Aaron. "Dual Loyalties," *Supervisor Nurse,* Vol. 11 (April 1980) p. 23.
8. Laver, Ross. "Hospitals Called Ill With Excess," *Globe and Mail* (July 30, 1980) p. 9.
9. College of Nurses of Ontario. *Standards of Nursing Practice: for Registered Nurses and Registered Nursing Assistants, Revised, May, 1979* (College of Nurses of Ontario, Toronto, 1979).
10. American Nurses' Association. *Standards of Nursing Practice* (American Nurses' Association, Kansas City, Mo., 1973).
11. Ontario. *Regulation Made Under the Health Disciplines Act, 1974, Part IV, Nursing,* Ontario Regulation 578/75, s. 21 i, j, m. (Queen's Printer, Toronto, 1975).
12. Ontario. *The Public Hospitals Act,* Toronto, R.S.O. c. 378, Vol. IV.
13. Southeastern Community College v. Davis, 99 S. Ct. 2361 (U.S. Sup. Ct. 1979).
14. Creighton, Helen. "Physical Handicaps," *Supervisor Nurse,* Vol. 11 (March 1980) p. 44.
15. Donabedian, A. "Foreword" in M. Phaneuf. *The Nursing Audit and Self-Regulation in Nursing Practice,* 2nd edition (Appleton-Century-Crofts, New York, 1976).
16. College of Nurses, *op. cit.*
17. American Nurses' Association, *op. cit.*
18. Canadian Nurses Association. *A Definition of Nursing Practice. Standards for Nursing Practice* (Canadian Nurses Association, Ottawa, 1980).
19. American Nurses' Association, *op. cit.*
20. College of Nurses of Ontario, *op. cit.*
21. *Ibid.*
22. *Ibid.*
23. Canadian Nurses Association. *Putting "Health" into Health Care.* Submission to Health Services Review '79 (Canadian Nurses Association, Ottawa, 1980).

24. Hall, The Honourable Emmett M. *A Commitment for Renewal: Canada's National-Provincial Health Program for the 1980's* (Health and Welfare Canada, Ottawa, 1980) p. 71.

25. *Ibid.*, pp. 78–79.

26. Levenstein, Aaron. "The Adversaries," *Supervisor Nurse,* Vol. 11 (May 1980) p. 47.

27. Levenstein, April, 1980, *op. cit.*

28. Gilchrist, Joan. "Profession or Union: Who Will Call the Shots?" *Nursing Papers,* Vol. 1 (November 1969) p. 5.

29. Brown, Billye. "Follow the Leader," *Nursing Outlook,* Vol. 28 (June 1980) p. 357.

30. Gilchrist, *op. cit.*, p. 4.

31. Levenstein, May 1980, *op. cit.*

32. Gilchrist, *op. cit.*, p. 5.

33. Woodham-Smith, Cecil. *Florence Nightingale* (Collins (Fontana Books), London, 1951) p. 361.

34. *Ibid.*, p. 362.

35. McEwan, E. Duncan. "The Realities of Medicare," *Health Management Forum,* Vol. 1, No. 1 (Spring 1980) p. 27.

36. McGeorge, R. Kenneth. "A Call for Moral Leadership in Health Service Administration," *Health Management Forum,* Vol. 1, No. 1 (Spring 1980) p. 27.

37. *Ibid.*, p. 30

38. Laver, *op. cit.*

39. McEwan, *op. cit.*, p. 38.

40. Chenoy, Neville. "Technology and Human Choices in Health Care," *Health Management Forum,* Vol. 1, No. 2 (Summer 1980) p. 47.

41. Williams, K. J., "Beyond Responsibility: Towards Accountability," *Hospital Progress* (January 1972) pp. 44–50.

42. Jenkins, David. *Job Power—Blue and White Collar Democracy* (Penguin Books, New York, 1974).

43. Chenoy, *op. cit.*, p. 54.

44. Science Council of Canada, Report No. 27, *Canada as a Conserver Society* (Ottawa, 1977).

45. Mechanic, David. "Rationing Health Care: Public and the Medical Market Place," *The Hastings Center Report,* Vol. 6, No. 1 (1976) pp. 34–37.

Section IV

Introduction to Case Studies

M. Josephine Flaherty

*"Le problème technique ne peut être qu'un problème
secondaire, car l'existence de l'oeuvre dépend de l'âme qui s'y
trouve et non des moyens techniques mis en oeuvre."*[*][1]

Antoine Pevsner

"Contemporary literature reflects considerable interest in and concern about the ethical dimension of nursing."[2] It suggests that nurses are trying to clarify ethical dimensions that have relevance for nursing when they discuss moral issues and moral concepts, the ethical dimensions of recent changes in nursing practice and the ways and means of promoting moral conduct.[3]

The nursing profession of the eighties has been affected markedly by the unprecedented scientific and technical changes of our age and by changes in the delivery of health care.[4] Nursing has as its goal to promote the adaptation of patients or clients in situations where changes in health status (including but not restricted to illness) place new demands on those patients. Nursing prides itself in being a profession that gathers and analyzes data relative to human beings and their health problems; that plans with clients to deal with the problems—mental, physical, and social—taking into consideration the factors in the environment affecting health status; that implements a plan of care; and that evaluates the effects of that care.[5] As practitioners of their profession, nurses are among the custodians of the public health[6]—a custodial responsibility that pertains to society as a whole. The nurse–patient relation-

---

[*]"A technical problem can be only secondary because the essence of a human action depends on the heart and soul to be found in it and not on the technical means used to accomplish it." (Translation by the author)

175

ship involves caring for a "patient," a person who, in asking for and receiving nursing care, is reaching for and is in need of both physical and emotional support.[7]

On entering the nursing profession, each nurse inherits a measure of the responsibility and trust that has accrued to nursing over the years and the corresponding obligation to adhere to the profession's code of conduct and relationships for professional practice.[8]

Nurses in Canada and the United States have endorsed standards of nursing practice, some of which are permissive[9,10] and some of which are statutory[11] in nature, in that the requirement to practice according to these standards, which are viewed as being achievable by all registered nurses, is part of the expectation of the registering body of the jurisdiction involved for all persons who are registered by that body.[12]

Nurses in Canada and the United States also have endorsed codes of ethics, as has the International Council of Nurses. Like the standards of nursing practice cited above, some of the ethical codes are permissive[13,14,15] and some are statutory[16,17] in nature. The development of a code of ethics is an essential characteristic of a profession; it provides one means for the exercise of professional self-regulation. A code indicates that a profession accepts the responsibility and trust with which it has been invested by society.[18]

Nursing ethics refers to beliefs about the moral values, ideals, virtues, obligations and principles identified by nurses as important ones. These are affected by the context of nursing ethics, that is, the mode of nursing practice, the organized nursing profession, the health care system, and the social conditions in which the nursing takes place.[19] Storch has indicated that changes in these contextual factors have had ethical implications for nursing.[20]

Nurses, physicians and other health care workers are responsible for the provision not only of scientific and technical competence but also of the spiritual nourishment patients need. Nurses, by the nature of their work, then, are concerned not only with professional questions but also with ethical questions. Ethical decisions must be made by nurses in a modern social climate of moral uncertainty and pluralism.[21] Lamb, who suggested that the "newness" of ethical problems, together with changes in the context of nursing, seem to have directed attention away from the past, described and analyzed nursing ethics in Canada over time. She concluded that the nursing ethics of half a century or more ago focused on the service ideal, on duty to the community, and on the "spirit" of nursing. Nursing ethics of the eighties direct attention to person-centered care, patients, rights, and quality of care.

As she compared nursing ethics of the twenties in Canada with those of the seventies in that country, Lamb noted that nurses in both decades believed that there was a moral dimension to nursing and that moral considerations were important in nursing practice.[22] However, in the twenties, Canadian nurses were likely to make judgments of moral value or to practice what Frankena called the "ethics of virtue."[23] The ethical nurse of that time was described, in terms of motives, virtues, or qualities, as unselfish, tactful, devoted, and kind. Moral conduct in nursing was thought to depend largely on character and on the disposition to act in a certain manner.[24]

During the seventies, nursing ethics were described in terms of Frankena's "ethics of duty"[25] that involved judgments of moral obligation. The issues in nursing ethics of the eighties are centered on actions and duties rather than on traits and virtues, that is, on *doing* rather than *being.* The ethical nurse of today informs patients about treatment and care, maintains competence through continuing education and acts as a patient advocate.[26]

The promotion of the well-being of the patient by nurses has been an enduring theme; today, that theme encompasses the physical, psychological, and social aspects of well-being. Nurses have been committed also to promote the welfare of society. A concern for improvement of nursing services generated comments about the accessibility of services in the twenties and has led to statements about the quality of services today.[27] Respect for the human dignity and autonomy of patients is *au courant* in the eighties, along with increasing emphasis on the individual nurse's responsibility to maintain competence.[28]

The emphasis on rights in the early part of the century concerned nurses' rights to shorter hours and patients' rights to nursing services. Recently, the emphasis has been on nondiscriminatory and nonjudgmental care for patients.[29]

Changes in statements about the obligations of nurses during this century often had relevance for nurses' relationships with other workers. In the twenties, for example, the obligation to obey physicians' orders was altered to cooperation with physicians; in the seventies, nurses stopped referring to the carrying out of medical orders as a moral obligation, dropped all specific references to physicians from the *ICN Code* and inserted an obligation to cooperate with all health professionals.[30]

It has been suggested that the scope of ethics for nurses seems to have changed during the last half century. Psychology and sociology were recognized as applicable to nurses' relationships with other people in the twenties. By the seventies, this was supplemented by knowledge of the formal ethical code and nurses began to realize that because the code was an insufficient basis for decision making regarding ethical dilemmas, there was need for a new code of ethics and improvement in the teaching of ethics in schools of nursing.[31]

A change was noted also in the fact that during the early decades of the century, nurses' obligations included exemplary personal conduct that reflected credit on the profession, whereas in recent years, nursing ethics have emphasized nurses' behavior within their professional roles rather than in their personal lives, and have stressed moral duties and obligations rather than virtues. Nurses' obligations changed from being "ethical" to "professional" during the twenties; today, they are referred to usually as "legal, ethical, and professional obligations," and these are seen often as very closely related or even overlapping. Nurses of the twenties rarely discussed uncertainty about their ethical decisions whereas today, nurses often acknowledge ethical conflicts in their practice and less certainty about their decisions.[32] Lamb suggested that this may account for the fact that Canadian nurses ignored a proposal for formulation of a code of ethics for nurses in the twenties,[33] but developed codes at provincial[34,35] and national[36] levels during the last decade.

The contextual factors, or environmental dimensions, of nursing practice have changed during the last half century from an emphasis on continuous, private duty care and the "adaptability of the nurse," to the more recent phenomenon of highly specialized secondary and tertiary care for groups of patients, in which nurses have not felt capable always of providing truly patient-centered nursing care. Nurses throughout this period have been frustrated by limitations on their professional decision-making power.[37] Modern nurses, as they try to influence the organizational context of their practice, meet opposition that provokes inter-professional tensions and gives rise to concerns by nurses about their ability to fulfill their legal and professional as well as ethical responsibilities. Budget constraints in health care agencies have been a source of conflict for nurses who feel responsible for the quality of nursing and health care in general, as well as for the quality of care given by individual nurses.[38]

Ethical issues in the eighties may be more challenging to nurses than ever before, because of the complexity of the issues, the recognition by nurses of their collegial responsibility, with other health professionals and patients, for ethical decision making and the changing roles and beliefs of patients about their own health care.

Technology in health care brings both benefits and risks. The quality and use made of information in health care is being discussed widely. Computerization of medical records is a mixed blessing because, as it brings ready access to information for health care professionals, it also carries the risk of violations of confidentiality.[39] The recommendations of the *Report of the Commission of Inquiry into the Confidentiality of Health Information*[40] in the Province of Ontario have been discussed by government and by the health professions; the implications of the Report for health care in Ontario, and probably in the rest of Canada, are considerable. For example, a recommendation that patients always have access to their own health care records, if implemented, could affect markedly the nature of those records if health professionals decided to change the content of their recording because of the possibility of patients being able to read them. Nurses and organized nursing in Ontario submitted commentaries on the Krever Commission Report to the provincial government.

Questions about mass immunization, personal *versus* societal responsibility for health, whether health care at public expense will be provided for people whose problems are the result of self-induced risks, patients' needs *vis-à-vis* patients' demands, patients' rights as opposed to health care professionals' rights, the kind and amount of health care research that should be done and whether patients' rights and dignity are being preserved when the research is done on human subjects, mass genetic screening and engineering and even more exotic techniques, are future possibilities[41] that may confront nurses and other health professionals and challenge their ethical positions— personal and professional—to an extent that was not thought possible a short time ago.

Nurses regularly confront "concrete, troublesome and often poignant dilemmas in their daily practice. Their ability to face these dilemmas is unlikely to be improved by exposure to the remote and scholarly ethical argumentation practiced by academic 'ethicists.' Exhortations to be good and sermons to avoid evil, . . . are usually too simplistic to touch either the troublesome questions or the questionable practices. Discussions of shocking and bizarre cases usually do little to illuminate the myriad ordinary practical difficulties."[42]

Although each ethical situation will not be unique in every respect, there are aspects of each situation that are different from what the nurse has encountered previously, because each individual who is involved in a nursing interaction has a "human dimension," that is, a unique set of biological, spiritual, psychological, and social characteristics. This is true of the patient, the nurse, other people who care for the patient, family members, and so forth. This "human dimension" commands respect even as it entails rights and responsibilities.[43]

Nurses are attempting to articulate clearly the nature and scope of nursing. Some members of the profession believe that there is a scientifically sound solution for every nursing problem. Some may even believe that codes of ethics for nurses provide the scientific rules to which nurses can turn for expert help in the solution of ethical dilemmas in nursing. It has been suggested that such a notion is "worse than an illusion" and that it represents "a declaration of moral bankruptcy on the part of the profession," that never used to believe that the dilemmas of caring for the ill could be solved neatly.[44] There is danger that ethical guidelines and procedures, the work of ethics committees and the encouragement of statutory regulations in ethics will be used as substitutes for common sense and discernment in the search for the patient's good. Kass has warned that this could represent a search for yet one more technical solution—this time a technical ethical solution—to problems produced by "our already foolish tendency to seek technical medical solutions for the weighty difficulties of a human life."[45] Like physicians, to whom Kass directed his words of caution, nurses who want to be more than "body technicians" must also be "knowers of souls, those of [their] patients and, not least, [their] own."[46]

The discipline of ethics is distinct from a number of other disciplines because it relies on the method of reason. Its "tool" is the human mind; it uses logical argument only. Although it does not rely only on empirical data, as do sociology and psychology which are also "human sciences," the human mind does not deny the existence or usefulness of data from these disciplines.[47]

The purpose of the case study section of this book is to present a series of studies in which actual situations in nursing practice have been examined and analyzed. There is no attempt to provide a single answer to the ethical dilemmas that are described as there is no one answer. Rather, it is hoped that the case studies will be useful for personal reflection by nurses and for group discussion, through which members of the profession will be helped to keep nursing's ethical dimension under constant scrutiny—and to develop and apply it—as part of the profession's constant pursuit of optimal impact.

This is part of the challenge that nurses of the eighties have accepted: to subject their own profession to constructive criticism in order to determine the need to transform the old order into a new and better one. Such action will not provide solutions for all of the ethical problems in nursing practice. However, it can stimulate members of the profession to continue to strive for excellence, to apply appropriate ethical concepts to the situations in which they work and to be sensitive to the need for thoughtful and sound decision making in the face of ethical dilemmas.[48]

NOTES

1. Reflections of the artist Antoine Pevsner on the value of works of art executed by human beings.
2. Lamb, Marianne. *Nursing Ethics in Canada: Two Decades.* Unpublished Master's thesis, University of Alberta, Edmonton, Alberta, 1981, p. 1.
3. *Ibid.*
4. Flaherty, M. Josephine. "Nursing Expertise in Canada," Chapter III in Glennis Zilm, Odile Larose and Shirley Stinson, eds. *Ph.D. (Nursing)* (Canadian Nurses Association, Ottawa, 1979) p. 23.
5. *Ibid.*, p. 24
6. Cousins, Norman. "Medical Ethics—Is There a Broader View?" *Journal of the American Medical Association,* Vol. 241, No. 25 (June 22, 1979), p. 2712.
7. *Ibid.*
8. American Nurses' Association. *Code for Nurses with Interpretive Statements* (American Nurses' Association, Kansas City, Missouri, 1976) p. 1.
9. American Nurses' Association. *Standards of Nursing Practice* (American Nurses' Association, Kansas City, Missouri, 1973).
10. Canadian Nurses Association. *Definition of Nursing Practice and Standards for Nursing Practice* (Canadian Nurses Association, Ottawa, 1980).
11. College of Nurses of Ontario. *Standards of Nursing Practice: for Registered Nurses and Registered Nursing Assistants, Revised, May 1979* (College of Nurses of Ontario, Toronto, 1979).
12. Ontario. *Regulation Made Under the Health Disciplines Act, 1974, Part IV, Nursing,* O. Reg. 578/75, S. 24. Statutes of Ontario (Queen's Printer, Toronto, 1975).

13. American Nurses' Association, 1976, *op. cit.*

14. Canadian Nurses Association. *CNA Code of Ethics: An Ethical Basis for Nursing in Canada* (Canadian Nurses Association, Ottawa, 1980).

15. International Council of Nurses. *ICN Code for Nurses—Ethical Concepts Applied to Nursing* (International Council of Nurses, Geneva, 1973).

16. Quebec. *Code of Ethics. Regulation respecting the code of ethics (Nursing). Professional Code 1973, c. 43, 5.85* (Quebec Official Gazette, Quebec, P.Q., September 22, 1976).

17. College of Nurses of Ontario. *Guidelines for Ethical Behaviour in Nursing* (College of Nurses of Ontario, Toronto, 1980).

18. American Nurses' Association, 1976, *op cit.*

19. Lamb, *op. cit.*, p. 3.

20. Storch, J. L. *Consumer Rights and Nursing.* Master's thesis, University of Alberta, Edmonton, Alberta, 1977.

21. Curtin, Leah. "Human Values in Nursing." *Journal of New York State Nurses Association,* Vol. 8, No. 4 (1977), pp. 31–40.

22. Lamb, *op. cit.*, p. 82.

23. Frankena, W. K. *Ethics,* 2nd ed. (Prentice-Hall, Englewood Cliffs, N.J., 1973).

24. Lamb, *op. cit.*, pp. 82–83.

25. Frankena, *op. cit.*

26. Lamb, *op. cit.*, p. 83.

27. *Ibid.*, p. 84.

28. *Ibid.*, p. 85.

29. *Ibid.*, p. 86.

30. *Ibid.*, p. 87.

31. *Ibid.*, pp. 88–89.

32. *Ibid.*, pp. 89–91.

33. *Ibid.*, p. 91.

34. Quebec, 1976, *op. cit.*

35. College of Nurses of Ontario, 1980, *op. cit.*

36. Canadian Nurses Association, 1980, *op. cit.*

37. Lamb, *op. cit.*, pp. 92–93.

38. *Ibid.*, p. 98.

39. Tiberius, Richard G. "Medical Ethics in the Next 25 Years," *Canadian Family Physician,* Vol. 25 (January 1979), pp. 73–78.

40. Krever, The Honourable Mr. Justice Horace. *Report of the Commission of Inquiry into the Confidentiality of Health Information* (J. C. Thatcher, Queen's Printer for Ontario, Toronto, 1980).

41. Tiberius, *op. cit.*

42. Kass, Leon R. "Ethical Dilemmas in the Care of the Ill, Part I," *Journal of the American Medical Association,* Vol. 244, No. 16 (October 17, 1980), pp. 1811–1816.

43. College of Nurses of Ontario, 1980, *op. cit.*, p. 4.

44. Kass, Leon R. "Ethical Dilemmas in the Care of the Ill, Part II," *Journal of the American Medical Association,* Vol. 244, No. 17 (October 24/31, 1980), pp. 1946–1949.

45. *Ibid.*

46. *Ibid.*

47. Lynch, Abbyann. *Ethics and Nursing.* Nursing Education Media Project, Volume I (The Ontario Educational Communications Authority, Toronto, 1977) p. 4.

48. Flaherty, M. Josephine. "Accountability in Health Care Practice: Ethical Implications for Nurses," Chapter 23 in Davis, John W., *et al.,* eds., *Contemporary Issues in Biomedical Ethics* (The Humana Press, Clifton, N.J., 1979) pp. 267–276.

Case Study I: Conflicting Obligations

Leah Curtin

I first met Brady on a bleak day in January. She was sitting on a bare mattress in an attic room, a torn robe thrown hastily over her shoulders and a tiny baby in her arms. Brady was a thirty-year-old woman who previously had been institutionalized with a diagnosis of schizophrenia. She was also the mother of six children. Brady was unmarried and unemployed, and what little money she had came from welfare. Cockroaches crawled over the ceilings, walls, floors, and furniture. A big grey rat sat under the kitchen table eating the remains of the breakfast cereal that the older children had spilled on the floor.

As a visiting nurse, I was assigned to see Brady because the doctor was concerned about the effects that the added responsibility of another child would have on her mental state. The four oldest children were at school and the three-year-old was toddling about partially dressed. I cleared off a spot on the table, heated some water for coffee, and Brady and I sat down to talk. Brady's baby (she had not yet given him a name) was sleeping in a rickety crib in the corner. We talked for a long time and Brady expressed her feelings of frustration, anger, isolation, and hopelessness. I promised to talk to her social worker about more money and a safer, warmer place to live. It was so cold in that room!

I met with the social worker and asked her to allot more money for Brady or at least to make a home visit so she could see for herself the deplorable conditions. However, she had so many cases and there was no extra money. So I went to every social agency in town. I even went to the churches and talked to the pastors. I spoke to the landlord about increasing the heat to the attic room, but he could not because there were no heat ducts. Nobody had time, everybody had problems, and no one seemed to care.

My second visit to Brady was not a happy experience. I told her what had happened and she was not surprised. No one had cared in the past; why should they care now? Brady's baby was pathetically frail and weak. I bathed his tiny body and bottle fed him while Brady dressed. We talked about Brady's

183

needs, the baby's needs, the needs of the older children and how to fulfill them—or at least strike a feasible balance. It was so cold in that place that I shivered even though I was wearing my winter uniform.

Several days later, I once again was struggling up the steps to Brady's attic room. Even before I saw him, I heard the rattling, gasping sounds of a tiny infant struggling to breathe. When Brady saw me she jumped up, grabbed the baby, and started to spoon milk into his mouth. I tried patiently but urgently to explain to her that the baby was very ill and must be given clear liquids and not milk. I examined the baby: temperature 104°F.; severe congestion; circumoral and fingernail cyanosis; pulse 154 and weak; skin, hot and dry. It took almost an hour to convince Brady to take the child to the hospital, but finally she agreed. It seemed to take years for her to dress herself and Tanya (the three-year-old).

In my opinion, the baby was too ill to be taken to the hospital by bus, Brady had no transportation and the only recourse was the police. Brady was deathly afraid of the police because she thought they would take her children away from her. Therefore, I ignored policy and drove her to the hospital myself. When we finally arrived at the hospital, I had to use a lot of pressure and persuasion to have the baby seen in a reasonable amount of time.

The intern came into the examining room, gave the baby a quick "once-over," diagnosed the condition as a "cold," prescribed clear liquids, ¼ baby aspirin every four hours and a decongestant and sent us home—all in the space of five minutes. Brady was livid; I was flabbergasted. I begged Brady to let me take her to the emergency room of another hospital, but she refused. I called my supervisor who suggested that the only other option open to me was to contact Children's Protective Services and have the baby removed from Brady's care. However, if I was wrong and the physician was right, I was taking the risk of liability—not to mention the effect it might have on Brady.

Brady was very angry because I had frightened her unnecessarily. I probably was trying to prove that she was an "unfit" mother. She thought I was going to have the police come and take her baby away from her. The rage and frustration accumulated over many years surfaced and she beamed them directly at me. I could not take HER baby anywhere, she exclaimed. I was very much concerned that Brady would have another "nervous breakdown" if I persisted, but I was afraid that the baby would die if I did not.

In the end, I returned Brady to her home and left. That night Brady rushed the baby to the emergency room. Despite all efforts, Brady's baby died of pneumonia within an hour. He still didn't have a name.

Even now, fifteen years later, I wonder why Brady's baby had to die. Officially, of course, he died of pneumonia, but that wasn't the real cause of death. He died because no one cared. He died because I made the wrong decision. He died because of poverty, disease, ignorance and cold. Most of all, he died because of the cold: the coldness of a social system that forgets that it is social. No one cared quite enough: not me, not Brady, not the doctors, not the social workers or pastors or charitable institutions. The baby is dead. Brady was readmitted to an institution and the other children were placed in an orphanage.

IDENTIFICATION AND CLARIFICATION

As with most real life situations, this case is not paradigmatic of any one ethical problem but rather involves a complex interrelationship of ethical, legal and social problems. The more complex the situation, the more difficult it is to sort out and clarify the issues and to identify what realistically *can* be done to resolve a particular problem. The pervasive problem underlying this case is one of social justice or, more accurately, the injustice of a social system that fails to meet basic human needs. Although health professionals can agitate for change and should criticize a society that deprives its members of warmth and adequate nutrition,[1] these activities rarely bring relief in individual, immediate crises.

In addition, this depicts the general ethical and social issues involved in both rights of people to at least minimal health services and the rights of people in health care. The right to at least minimal health care services is a function of the social system and generally deals with the problem of access to the health care system. Considerations of human rights in health care presuppose that an individual already has established contact with the system and depend largely on the behavior of individual practitioners and the quality of the relationship established.[2]

The second set of problems for the nurse involves what could be called "civil disobedience" in health care. That is, it involves a nurses' disagreement with a physician about a medical decision regarding medical care. Cases of civil disobedience presuppose that there is legitimate authority.[3] That is, the nurse did not challenge the legitimate authority of physicians to make decisions regarding medical care; rather the nurse challenged the legitimacy of a particular medical decision.

Within the matrix of these general ethical problems, the nurse is faced with a complex ethical quandary. Does she have the right or the authority to override the mother's decision? Is the mother capable of making a decision? Who is the patient—mother or child? Whose needs are paramount? Where do the nurse's professional obligations lie and how can she best fulfill them?

RIGHTS TO HEALTH CARE SERVICES

In general, rights to at least a decent minimum of health care services[4] involve various formulations of the principles of social justice, among which are that health services should be provided to people according to (a) their merit as measured by actual personal achievements or potential achievements, that is, their moral worth; (b) their contribution or potential contribution to the welfare of society; and (c) their need for the services.[5] Moreover, some theorists claim that justice requires that similar situations should be accorded similar treatment.[6]

The first two formulations are rejected for a variety of reasons. For one thing, health care crises often occur for reasons beyond the control of individuals. For another, there is a difference between goods or services that are earned by effort and those that are required by need.[7] Although some health care services certainly could be placed in the "desirable but nonessential" category, others are required by all persons to sustain life. Therefore, while services that are in the former category safely can be placed in the competitive market place, essential services should be made available to each according to his need.[8]

The notion that health care services should be provided according to a person's contributions to society ignores the human rights of individuals. These should not be disregarded for the sake of long range social benefits.[9] Indeed, the development and application of any of the various social criteria for worth are exceedingly problematic.[10] Ramsey takes the position that life is a precondition for all social goods. He notes that "the equal right of every human being to live, and not relative personal or social worth, should be the ruling principle."[11] The rationale for Ramsey's position includes the concept that life is a precondition for all social goods as well as a final skepticism regarding how one really and truly could measure a person's social worth.

Moreover, people's health care needs change significantly during their older years when both income and economic productivity decline.[12] As each person inevitably grows older, all people are threatened by the establishment of a standard of social utility as a criterion for access to health care services. However, to establish a system based on needs, one must distinguish between basic needs and felt needs. Basic needs encompass considerations of survival; felt needs include personal preferences and desires generated by life in an affluent society.[13]

The final principle, that is, similar treatment for similar situations, is based on the needs concept and on considerations of justice. It must be recognized that without the inclusion of a needs-access model, this principle could mean no treatment for anyone. That is, it would be perfectly fair to refuse to treat a child who has pneumonia as long as all children who developed pneumonia were not treated. The principle, similar treatment of similar situations, serves as a guide for actual choices in a manner that is compatible with the goal of equal access.[14] It can serve as a guide for conduct in the disposition of situations irrespective of the wealth or social worth of the patient or client. With specific reference to this case, the child had a need for health care services and deserved to be treated in the same manner as would any other child presenting the same needs. The mother's needs were less specific and could be characterized as needs for psychosocial support—an area of ambiguity for some observers in their consideration of rights to health care services.

HUMAN RIGHTS IN HEALTH CARE

Once a relationship is established between a health professional and a patient or client, it is presumed to be therapeutic. At minimum, such a relationship will require that the professional practice competently, that he or she consider the patient/client's needs paramount, that the professional not harm the patient through acts of commission or omission, and that the professional be faithful to both the patient and the promises of the profession.

The nurse in this case seemed to perceive a conflict between the needs of the mother and the needs of the child. Consequently, she was uncertain about to whom she should be loyal. In fact, this conflict was not a real conflict but rather a perceived conflict, because what helped the mother would have helped the child, and conversely, what helped the child would have helped the mother. Their rights and needs did not conflict, although the particular handling of this situation produced the illusion that they did conflict.

CIVIL DISOBEDIENCE IN HEALTH CARE

In the final analysis, individuals have a qualified right to determine the type and amount of medical or nursing care they receive—they have a right to determine what is or is not done to their own bodies.[15] However, the rights of parents or guardians to authorize care of an incompetent patient are limited by the best interests of the patient and the duties of both individual and institutional providers.[16] The decision-making authority of health professionals is circumscribed by their area of expertise, the degree of their relationship with the patient, the rights and needs of the patient, institutional policies and procedures, and legal restrictions.

In this case, we see a conflict between what the nurse perceives to be the medical needs of the infant and what the physician perceives to be the medical needs of the infant. Although there was no conflict between what the referring physician perceived as the mother's needs and what the nurse perceived as the mother's needs, the point at issue is whether a nurse has the competence to challenge a physician's medical diagnosis under any conditions.

Two matters are clear in this case: (1) the nurse acknowledged the expertise of physicians in general as indicated by her attempts to convince the mother to seek the advice of a second physician; and (2) the nurse definitely thought the physician had not gathered enough data to arrive at a conclusion: "the intern . . . gave the baby a quick once-over, diagnosed the condition as a cold, prescribed . . . and sent us home —all in the space of five minutes." The nurse was not questioning the legitimacy of physician decision making in general; rather she was questioning the legitimacy of this particular decision on the grounds of insufficient data. The question then, is not whether nurses are competent to judge the quality of medical care in general, but is whether a nurse is competent to judge what constitutes a medical examination. Because nurses frequently perform physical assessments and because physicians regularly depend on nurses' findings and observations of patient conditions in their determinations of appropriate medical care, it can be concluded that nurses are competent to judge what it is that constitutes a physical examination.[17]

Although some would question a nurse's authority to challenge a physician's decision, few would question the legitimacy of a nurse or a patient seeking a second medical opinion. In this particular case, the nurse unquestionably was acting within the scope of her expertise in questioning the legitimacy of the physician's decision and within the scope of her professional authority in urging the mother to seek a second opinion.

In summary, the ethical questions raised in this case involve (1) the demands of social justice (with particular application to access to health care services); (2) the demands of personal justice (human rights) in the equal treatment of similar situations; (3) the commitment of health professionals to act in the best interests of patients or clients; and (4) the legitimacy of a nurse questioning a physician's decision. The following analysis will deal with the specific problem the nurse faced within the matrix of these general ethical problems.

AN ANALYSIS OF THE DISCRETE ETHICAL PROBLEM

Background Information

1. Brady was a thirty-year-old unmarried mother of six. Her sole source of income was Welfare.

2. She had been diagnosed as schizophrenic, and institutionalized at some time in the past. There was concern expressed by the referring physician that her present mental condition was unstable.

3. Her youngest child was a newborn who might not have been premature, but who appeared to have been small and somewhat weak.

4. The visiting nurse was assigned primarily to assess conditions and to stabilize the situation by providing psychosocial support for the mother.

5. The physical conditions under which Brady and her family lived were deplorable.

6. The baby became ill and the mother was persuaded by the nurse to seek medical assistance.

7. The nurse and the physician disagreed about the diagnosis and gravity of the baby's condition.

8. The mother refused to seek further medical help. She also exhibited increasing hostility toward the nurse and the entire situation. The mother repeatedly expressed the fear that her children would be taken away from her.

9. The nurse sought consultation and finally decided to leave the scene.

10. Brady's baby died of pneumonia, she (Brady) was readmitted to a mental institution, and the other children were placed in an orphanage.

In sum, the questions are: did the nurse act appropriately? Was there anything more she could or should have done? If so, what and why?

THE INDIVIDUALS INVOLVED IN THE DECISION MAKING

1. Brady

Brady was the mother of the child, and although she had been diagnosed as a schizophrenic, she still had legal custody of her children. Clearly, the responsibility for the children rested on her shoulders. Although Brady demonstrated concern for the infant's welfare (she did permit him to be taken to the hospital), she did so only after considerable persuasion by the nurse.

One might wonder just how free Brady was to act. Although she repeatedly expressed the fear that she would be declared an "unfit" mother and that her children would be taken from her by the authorities, this fear does not appear to be an irrational one. She had been institutionalized previously for her mental condition, and it can be assumed that her children were removed from her care for an unspecified period of time. Her fear may explain her reluctance to take the baby to any institution, even a hospital. Clearly, Brady did not trust those in authority, nor does it appear that there was much reason for her to do so.

A second factor that could have affected Brady's freedom to act was her unstable mental condition. The diagnosis of schizophrenia is ambiguous at best, but if she was affected also by paranoia or delusions of any nature, these definitely would impinge on her ability to make a rational decision. Further, she was faced with an unfortunate dilemma. The physician indicated that her child suffered nothing more serious than a bad cold. The nurse indicated that her child was seriously ill. Which one should she believe?

A third factor that could have affected her ability to make decisions was the force of the emotions she was feeling and expressing. Brady was very angry, but was her anger inappropriate under the circumstances? The nurse reported that in addition to anger, Brady was expressing feelings of frustration, hopelessness, fear, and isolation. Apparently there were few, if any, support systems for Brady. Her isolation may explain, in part, her fear that her children would be taken from her. They were all that she had. It is not known whether Brady was or was not under psychiatric care; it will be presumed that she was, because she was diagnosed as schizophrenic and referred to the visiting nurse.

In sum, although the legal authority to act rested with Brady, her freedom to act may have been limited on several counts that were related to her:

(a) confusion with regard to the baby's actual condition

(b) fear that the authorities would find her an unfit mother

(c) social isolation to a degree that indicated to her that there was no one to whom she could turn in this dilemma

(d) possible mental instability that could interfere with her ability to make a rational choice, and

(e) strong emotions that may have clouded her ability to choose a rational course of action.

2. The Visiting Nurse

The principal reason that the nurse became involved in this situation apparently was to offer psychosocial support to Brady. She attempted to do this by providing emotional support for Brady and her family and by attempting to improve the physical conditions under which the family was living. As the situation progressed, the life and health of Brady's baby became an obvious concern.

The nurse also was angry, although the expression of her anger was not overt. She was very angry with the authorities, the social worker, the physician and, in fact, the entire system. Every avenue that was open to her in the quest to help Brady and her family was blocked. She appeared to be as appalled by the indifference of society to this family's plight as she was by the physical conditions in which the family was living.

When the baby became acutely ill, the nurse took steps to see that the child received medical attention. Although she must have been aware of the effect that an open disagreement with the physician might have on Brady, she did openly disagree with him. Her reason for doing so seems to have been a genuine concern that the infant would die without medical treatment.

When Brady refused to seek further medical consultation, the nurse faced a dilemma. She sought consultation from her supervisor, but that only resulted in a deepening of her dilemma: the only alternative course of action offered to her was that of taking steps to remove the infant from Brady's care—and this was without a supporting medical diagnosis.

If the nurse had taken this course of action and had been successful, she would have confirmed Brady's fear that her children would be taken from her. If the nurse had been incorrect in her assessment of the infant's condition, she would have been open to legal retribution. Further, the possibilities of success (in removal of the infant from Brady's care) without a supporting medical diagnosis were slim if not nonexistent.

In sum, although the nurse felt a responsibility to act, her freedom to act was limited. She also might have believed that further action on her part would have a negative effect on Brady's mental stability and thus threaten the stability of the family unit.

3. The Physician

The concern of a physician should be for the welfare of patients and their families and, in an emergency room situation, specifically for the physical well-being of the presenting patient. His responsibility is to diagnose the patient's condition accurately and to treat the patient. The physician's freedom to act did not appear to be limited in this case. The rationale for his action is not clear, but it must be presumed that he was unaware of the gravity of the infant's condition. Any other presumption leads to another set of motives and actions to be examined. It may have been that he was extremely busy and that the time involved in examination of an infant who appeared to him to have nothing more than a cold may have irritated him. Moreover, the emergency rooms of many general hospitals often are used as if they are a family physician's office and he may have felt that his time was being wasted. It may be presumed also that the nurse's difference of opinion with him increased his irritation.

In sum, although the physician had the authority and responsibility accurately to diagnose and treat the infant, he did not do so for reasons that are unclear.

4. The Nursing Supervisor

The first concern of the nursing supervisor should be for the well-being of those patients/clients referred to the agency; the second should be for the guidance and support of staff members; the third should be for the appropriate functioning of the agency.

The supervisor's freedom to act as a consultant to the staff nurse may have been limited to some extent by the fact that the staff member had violated policy in at least two ways: 1) the staff nurse should not have been in the emergency room with the patient and 2) the staff nurse should not have provided transportation to the hospital in the first place. In addition, the supervisor had not seen the infant and therefore was not in a position to determine the validity of the staff nurse's evaluation of the infant's condition. In view of the fact that the staff nurse already had violated policy, the supervisor also may have been concerned about the liability of the agency.

She did remind the nurse that she could take steps to have the baby removed from Brady's care, but she made it quite clear that if the nurse did so, she would be acting on her own initiative and without the support of the agency. However, the supervisor did not withdraw all support by ordering the nurse to remove herself from the case and to refrain from further violation of policy by transportation of Brady and her children elsewhere (home or another hospital). She did permit the nurse freedom of movement in this regard and had enough confidence in her judgment to leave the disposition of this case in her hands. However, the supervisor made it clear that the responsibility for the course of action chosen would remain the staff nurse's alone.

POSSIBLE COURSES OF ACTION

1. The nurse could have advised Brady simply that her child was ill and that she should seek medical attention and then gone on to her other patients for the day. This course of action is rejected, although it has the attraction of removing the nurse from the situation. To adopt this course of action, particularly in view of the nurse's education and experience and her knowledge of Brady's problems and the severity of the infant's condition,

would be to abrogate her responsibilities. If it took a great deal of persuasion before Brady agreed to take the baby to the hospital, it can be presumed that Brady was unaware of the gravity of the situation. The nurse also was aware of Brady's fears with regard to the "authorities" and may have presumed that she would not seek medical help without support and some assistance with transportation and so forth.

2. The nurse could have decided to initiate action to have the infant removed from Brady's care. This course of action is rejected for several reasons, chief among which is that such action probably would have been unsuccessful because there was no medical diagnosis to support the action. Second, such an action would have been unfair to Brady who was doing the best she could under the circumstances. Third, this course of action would have destroyed any relationship that the nurse had managed to establish with Brady and possibly could undermine further Brady's mental stability.

3. The nurse could have returned Brady and her children home and removed herself from the scene for the time. Although this option was the one actually followed in this case, it is rejected because of the danger to the infant's life and subsequently to Brady's mental health and the stability of the family that is inherent in it.

4. The nurse could have asked immediately for further consultation in the emergency room, before the physician left the examining room. Such a course of action, although likely to be unpleasant in the extreme, might have been the only viable alternative in this situation.

If the nurse had acted immediately, and if she had remained adamant, it is quite likely that further examination of the infant would have taken place. A more thorough examination probably would have resulted in hospitalization and treatment of the infant. This might not have saved the infant's life, but it certainly would have offered him a greater potential for survival. It also would have offered the nurse an opportunity to consult with the social service department of the hospital. The involvement of the social service department of the hospital might have increased the nurse's chances of success in demonstrating to the welfare department the unhealthy conditions under which this family was forced to live and might have resulted in better living conditions for this family.

THE ACTION ITSELF

The nurse's actions were chosen freely and were intentional. They are not wrong in themselves. Her decision to leave the scene (at least at this time) did not represent an irresponsible or unjust action, but perhaps it may be regarded as an ineffective action. It is quite possible that she was so surprised by the physician's diagnosis and treatment that the fourth alternative did not present itself to her until much later. That she remains concerned about her course of action in this situation and that she thinks that her decision was responsible, at least in part, for the baby's death is quite clear. That she also feels responsible, at least to some extent, for the disintegration of this family also is apparent. Obviously she has reflected on this case and this reflection may lead to more definitive action by her in the future.

THE ETHICAL IDEAL

The general approach or ethical spirit is normative, in that any human act (*i.e.*, one that is freely chosen and deliberate) or choice is right as long as it protects and promotes dignity, inviolability, freedom, and respect for each human being. Actions are wrong when they detract from these general ideals. This explains the nurse's anger with the whole "system"—she thinks that the human rights of Brady and her family are being violated. The notion that one may not intentionally violate another's human rights is normative.

The crucial dilemma that the nurse perceived revolved around the choices of her (a) taking a course of action that would recognize and respect Brady's dignity and freedom, enhance her opportunity to exercise an independent judgment, promote her mental health, and subsequently benefit her family or (b) taking a course of action that would protect the life of Brady's baby. That is, the nurse perceived a conflict of interests between mother and child when, in fact, it did not exist. With effective intervention, an apparent conflict between the interests of mother and child would not have emerged. Option 4 offered the best hope for the nurse to maximize the interests of both mother and child; hence, it is seen as the right action in this case. Although this case does not represent a clear cut example of right and wrong, it is a realistic situation in which there are positive and negative results to any course of action taken.

It should be noted that the designation of option 4 as the right course of action in no way represents a judgment that the nurse was bad or evil. It is quite easy to do a *post-facto* analysis of a situation and determine what course of action ought to have been chosen; it is another matter altogether when one is in the midst of the problem. However, such reflection can be quite useful to us in determination of future courses of action and, if shared with others, can be of great assistance to them if or when they are faced with similar circumstances.

Quite specifically, this analysis approached relevant environmental, social, and psychological factors and, in this sense, is relativistic and situational. It is deontological in that the duties and responsibilities of those active in the decision making constitute a major factor in the deliberations. The emotional impact of the situation also is considered, particularly because it may have bearing on the freedom to act of the various participants. In this sense only, it may be considered to be emotive.

The nurse and Brady both appealed to authority for guidance and the nurse seemed to feel instinctively that the course of action decided upon was inadequate. How much of this was professional expertise and how much was instinct is a moot point. This analysis also is teleological in that the results of the various courses of action have direct bearing on the designation of option 4 as the right or acceptable course of action. It is seldom desirable to separate an action completely from the results or consequences it produces.

COMMENTARY: CASE STUDY I

M. Josephine Flaherty

Although some aspects of the scenario described here may appear to be extreme, they are typical of more situations than members of the health professions would like to admit. The ethical problems in the situations have been identified and the actions of the persons involved have been described. It is a sad story but not a unique one.

The *mother* did what she thought was right and probably she was acting at the level of her capacity at the time, given her history, her experience, and the pressures—physical as a result of her environment, emotional in light of the state of her mental health and social because of her fear of "the authorities" who might take her children away from her—that were on her. One cannot help but identify with the mother's feelings of hopelessness; she had good reason to feel negative about life and about the world.

The *nurse* tried. She saw several options for action, weighed each one and chose what she thought would be most effective for the child and least unsettling for the mother. She took specific action to help both mother and infant when she persisted in her visiting, bathed the baby, and talked with the mother. She succeeded in the establishment of enough confidence in the nurse on the part of the mother that the latter agreed to go to the hospital. The nurse approached a number of persons and groups for help but the responses were either absent or ineffective. As she noted, community based authorities seemed "to be too busy" or "not to care."

The *nursing supervisor's* qualified support was not sufficient to make a major difference in the situation, but it was enough to permit the nurse to decide for herself what she would do. It appears that the nursing supervisor was not completely familiar with the situation, even though one could assume that the family was known to the visiting nursing agency. One would wonder whether the role of that supervisor included home visiting with members of the staff, particularly when the family situation was as complex as this one. It can be assumed that the supervisor's ability to act in this case was limited, as has been noted. One would also wonder how well she knew the nurse involved (perhaps she was a fairly new staff member) and hence how secure she could feel about the quality of the staff nurse's judgment. One would wonder also how many other similar calls for help the supervisor had received that day and what was the nature and extent of her workload. It would be interesting to know what kind of pressure was on the supervisor to ensure that agency policies were followed carefully—after all, she does not appear to have made a big issue of the fact that the nurse knowingly had violated the policy regarding transporting and accompanying the patient to the hospital.

The *agency* had the responsibility to provide health care service; one would wonder how well defined and how limited the service was. Does an agency that forbids its staff members to accompany and/or transport patients to the hospital, even in an emergency situation like this one, really fulfill its ethical and legal responsibilities to provide health care for patients? How does a rule like that one provide an environment within which a nurse can fulfill professional, legal and ethical obligations to patients? It is acknowledged that the assumption of responsibility for the safety of patients who are transported in a staff nurse's car is complex, but where does the agency's responsibility for the meeting of the health needs of patients start and where does it stop?

One could ask what, if anything, the agency had done, beyond what the nurse had done, to pressure community social agencies to take action on the family's social situation. Should a visiting nursing agency take such action? If not, how can its staff members fulfill their ethical obligations as nurses? If an agency takes the position that an action taken by a nurse, which is either contrary to regulations or a bit questionable, is the nurse's responsibility alone, is that agency fulfilling its responsibility for the health care provided? In employing health care professionals, does an agency really employ them to behave as professionals or simply to follow the rules? There are far-reaching ethical implications in this question. If a health care professional agrees simply to follow the rules, even when they are not adequate to a situation and when such following is against the professional's better judgment, is the staff member behaving in an ethical manner? Clearly, the answer is no, if one considers a professional nurse's professional, ethical and, in jurisdictions where standards of practice and ethics are statutory in nature, legal responsibilities to use judgment in accepting and delegating responsibility and to be responsible for his/her own professional behavior. Hence, health care agencies should examine carefully their regulations and their expectations for the behavior of their staff to ensure that these are not in conflict. Results of such an examination should be matched against the objectives of the agency to ensure that, in the light of the policies and practices of the agency, the objectives are achievable. If they are not, either the objectives and/or the policies and practices should be changed in order that the agency can meet its obligations to society.

The *physician* in this situation, as a member of the medical profession, and as either an employee or a "guest practitioner" in the hospital, had an obligation to do what was best for the patient. His examination of the infant appeared to be inadequate and the action that he took was not acceptable. One would wonder why he did not realize that there was more to the situation than was apparent at first glance. A word or two with the mother should have made him question the adequacy of the situation to which he was returning the child. Why did he not see something unusual in the fact that the visiting nurse was with the mother and child? Why did he not realize that the mother was angry and that the nurse was astounded at his decision? If he did realize that, why did he not do more to ensure that his action was appropriate and to support the patient's family and his colleague (the nurse) in health care? One would wonder what kind of pressure was on the physician and what kind of supervision he was receiving. Did he believe that he was fulfilling his responsibility as a health care professional? Did he have any sense of collegiality in his behavior?

The *hospital* had a responsibility to provide health care to patients, in this case the infant, who became a patient as soon as he was admitted to the emergency department. One would wonder whether five minute "once-overs" are typical for that emergency department, particularly in the case of young children who can become very seriously ill in a short time. Does that hospital take any responsibility for providing or making referrals for follow-up care? Where were the hospital nurses in that situation? Who did the teaching of the mother with regard to the care of the sick infant? What kind of admission history was taken?

Society had a responsibility for the well-being of the family involved in this situation. Was there an investigation of the child's death? If there was, was society found guilty? Certainly, the baby did not die because the nurse made a wrong decision. As the nurse noted, he died because of the cold: "the coldness of a social system that forgets that it is social."

This situation is yet another example of the broad mandate and responsibility that nursing has accepted for the well-being of society, at the direct patient care level, the institutional level, the (health care) system level and the broad societal level. Actions were taken by a number of people, but without coordination of them, they were not effective and rights were violated. Neither individuals nor society benefited. Will this happen again? Is it happening right now? What are nurses going to do about it?

NOTES

1. May, William F. "Normative Inquiry and Medical Ethics in Our Colleges and Universities," in David Smith and Linda Bernstein, eds. *No Rush to Judgment* (The Indiana University Foundation, Bloomington, 1978) p. 349.

2. McGarvey, Michael R. "Some Considerations Regarding Ethics and the Right to Health Care," in Elsie Bandman and Bertram Bandman, eds. *Bioethics and Human Rights* (Little, Brown, Boston, 1978) pp. 363–365.

3. Wellman, Carl. *Morals and Ethics* (Scott Foresman and Company, Glenview, Illinois, 1975) p. 20.

4. Fried, Charles. "Equality and Rights in Medical Care," in Joseph Perpich, ed. *Implications of Guaranteeing Medical Care* (National Academy of Sciences, Washington, D.C., 1976) p. 7.

5. Outka, Gene. "Social Justice and Equal Access to Health Care," in Thomas Shannon, ed. *Bioethics* (Paulist Press, New York, New York, 1976) p. 375.

6. *Ibid.*

7. Williams, Bernard. "The Idea of Equality," in Hugo Bedau, ed. *Justice and Equality* (Prentice-Hall, Englewood Cliffs, New Jersey, 1971) pp. 116–137.

8. Nagel, Thomas. "Equal Treatment and Compensatory Discrimination," *Philosophy and Public Affairs,* Vol. 2, No. 4 (Summer 1973) p. 354.

9. Outka, *op. cit.*, p. 380.

10. Ramsey, Paul. *The Patient as Person* (Yale University Press, 1970) p. 248.

11. *Ibid.*, p. 256.

12. Somers, Ann, and Herman Somers. "The Organization and Financing of Health Care: Issues and Directions for the Future," *American Journal of Orthopsychiatry,* Vol. 42, (January 1972) pp. 119–136.

13. Outka, *op. cit.*, p. 385.

14. Outka, *op. cit.*, p. 388.

15. All rights are circumscribed by the rights of others and are subject to the duties of logical and moral correlativity.
16. See Case Study IV, section on Identifying and Clarifying the problem.
17. It would be tedious, if not impossible, to cite the volumes of medical and nursing literature on this subject. However, for those interested, I would refer them to the medical and nursing indexes regarding the nurse–practitioner, the nurse as physician–extender, and so forth.

Case Study II: Extending the Scope of Care

Leah Curtin

INTRODUCTION

In all fairness, it must be recognized that it would be a rare thing indeed for a professional nurse to be faced with only one case situation at a time. As a matter of fact, the nurse in Case Study I had a case load of over fifty families at the time she was caring for Brady and her family. Nurses and other health professionals may envy the luxury of ethicists who can concentrate all of their energies on one case at a time. During part of the time that she was caring for Brady, the nurse also was caring for Mary and her family (Case Study II). Although this case will not be analyzed, a comparison will be made of the decisions faced by the nurse in these two very different situations. Another reason for introducing Case Study II is to point out clearly that ethics are involved in all our interactions with patients—not just those with tragic outcomes!

It was a rainy day in February when the referral slip first came across my - desk. I glanced over the history and physician's orders—a pretty routine case. I don't remember giving the case too much thought as I drove to Mary's house for the first time. Most of my thoughts were directed toward the 16-year-old gravida III who was next on my list for that day. Be that as it may, this was a day to remember—a day when a very pragmatic visiting nurse was to meet a lady with an impossible dream. Dreams are usually ephemeral things and most of us cherish them secretly, never expecting to fulfill them. Mary not only cherished her dream, but fully expected it to become a reality. Further, she expected me to help make it a reality.

"Nurse, I want to walk up the Church stairs on my own two feet and stand there praising God. Will you help me?" This may not seem to be asking much, but the challenges inherent in Mary's dream were appalling. Mary was a 64-year-old diabetic whose right lower limb had been amputated above the knee.

If the referring physician was to be believed, her other leg was soon to go, too. Mary did not follow her diet nor did she properly take her insulin. There seemed to be profound mystery surrounding her urine testing, the only predictable outcome of which was a totally inaccurate test.

This dear, kind lady was overweight and undernourished. Her whole life had been one of working and giving to others. She quite literally had "scrubbed" her ten children through school, making and scraping, laughing and loving, and occasionally nudging them along the ladder of academic success. Consequently, Mary had little time to devote to herself and certainly none to devote to academic pursuits. It was enough for her to know that her children would have a better life. The diabetic charts, exchange patterns, urinanalyses, insulin regulations, and so on may as well have been written in Greek, for she surely did not understand them. But you see, Mary had this dream. . . .

In this particular case, the doctor had referred the patient to our agency and asked us to teach her about her diet, how to run the urine tests, and how to give herself her insulin. I was overworked, harried, harrassed, and pretty realistic, but Mary had her dream and her eyes held mine.

In my professional opinion, Mary's most pressing problem was saving her other leg, a task that the physician had indicated was not likely to meet with success. I had set up bi-weekly visits and bathed her foot, massaged the skin, carefully clipped the toenails, and worked on the cuticles. We exercised every muscle in her leg and foot. The slightest scratch or bruise was treated with the utmost care. If Mary's dream were to come true, we must save this leg!

Of equal importance was the stump of her other leg. We must toughen up the suture line. We must strengthen every muscle. On no account should she permit this stump to become useless. We set up a daily exercise program and Mary learned to lift improvised weights with her stump. Sometimes the pain was excruciating, and it all could have been for nothing, but Mary had her dream and she was willing to work and even to suffer for it.

The second truly major difficulty was the diet. The cooperation of the whole family was necessary here. Even her grandchildren would tattle on her if she ate one forbidden morsel. I would lecture her vehemently for even a minor infraction of her dietary restrictions. With the help of her husband, sons, and daughters, we went over and over the lists. Mary was taught to do her urine tests carefully and to adjust her insulin accordingly. Mary was sure that she could never learn all of these complicated things, but we were equally sure that she could. When she finally did, we were all as proud of her as if she had graduated *summa cum laude*—and she was proud, too.

After six months, even Mary's pessimistic physician admitted that she probably would not lose her other limb and that her diabetes was under control. "But how," said he, "are you going to get her an artificial limb? She doesn't qualify for Welfare and they cost a lot of money. Even if you could raise the money, she can't possibly be taught to use it in the home." It took a lot of persuasion, but we did get him to write the appropriate orders. Nonetheless, Mary came home from the clinic appointment pretty thoroughly dejected. Now we must face practicality: from where was the money to come? What is noteworthy, but somewhat amusing, is that she never doubted for a moment that if she managed to buy the limb, I would be able to teach her to use it in the home.

Clearly, the money was a huge obstacle. It appeared that a family conference was in order. Mary's children, whom she loved so dearly, went to work. We asked local churches and businesses to help. In only two months, we had enough money for Mary's spare part. Mary's husband took her down for the special measurements and we continued the exercise program diligently. Scores of people now shared Mary's dream—it had become almost a community project. Many of the people who helped were poor, even poorer than Mary, and their only reward would be in seeing Mary walk up the stairs of her church to praise God.

Two months later, Mary had her artificial leg. How thrilled she was! The happiness turned to tears when she found that she still could not walk. The limb made her stump sore and it was heavy and awkward. "Thank you, nurse, but this old girl will praise God at home. Pastor said he'd come visit and it won't be so bad." We'd come so far that we had to make it. I was a little harsh with Mary, hoping to make her angry. I told her that I was not about to waste any more of my time on a quitter. If that's the way she wanted it, I'd walk out now and she was on her own.

The next day I was back with one of the finest physical therapists it has ever been my privilege to know— and she just happened to be employed by the Visiting Nurse Association. She had been guiding my steps from the beginning and it was now time for her to appear on the scene. We rolled up carpets, moved furniture, and scavenged lumber. With the help of Mary's husband, we made parallel bars and set to work. In less than three months' time, the impossible dream became a reality. Mary walked up the stairs of Church on her husband's arm and stood there on her own two feet praising God! I didn't get to see Mary climb the steps (I'd been called in that Sunday for a child abuse situation), but I heard that it was quite an occasion. The first hymn the congregation sang that Sunday was "Praise God!" Perhaps impossible dreams aren't too hard to fulfill; it only took a year and a half for this one, but we were lucky.

A COMPARISON OF TWO CASES

The circumstance and the ethical questions presented in Cases I and II are quite similar. The differences between the cases are to be found in the results.

1. The ethos or ethical spirit is the same. That is, the nurse's decision making was based on normative principles in that the dignity, inviolability, and freedom of each human being are regarded as values. Actions are seen as

wrong if they degrade or violate these general principles and right if they enhance the goals extrapolated from the general principles. The nurse acted, whether effectively or ineffectively, on the presupposition that each of the lives involved was of equal value: Brady, her baby, Mary, and so forth. No life was regarded as superior to another: all were regarded as equally valuable.

2. The nurse disagreed with the conclusions reached by the physicians in the respective cases, although she chose different courses of action. In the first case, she objected, but went no farther. In the second case, she persuaded the physician to write the appropriate orders.

3. In both cases, the patients/clients refused further intervention at some point. In the first case, the nurse recognized the factors that might have limited Brady's freedom to choose, but was unsure of the course of action that would not further damage Brady's humanity and still protect the rights of Brady's baby. In the second case, the nurse recognized that the patient was reacting out of pain, discouragement and possibly exhaustion, and took steps to help Mary re-evaluate her decision. Whether her method of dealing with the situation (making the patient angry) was appropriate is problematic, but it appears to have been successful. It should be noted that physical symptoms often are far easier to define and to assess than are psychological ones.

4. The risk of failure was quite high in both cases. The results of failure in Case II, while not as devastating as in Case I, could have profound effect on Mary and her family—one that might be exacerbated by the encouragement given by the nurse in adopting this course of action. It must be noted, however, that the family support system in the second case would both increase the likelihood of success and mitigate the pain of failure. Such a support system was absent in Case I.

5. In both cases, the nurse's responsibilities were not limited solely to the functions designated on the referral slip; rather, her concerns encompassed the total well-being of the patients or clients involved.

Such responsibilities must be viewed in a realistic light. It is not particularly helpful to play Don Quixote de la Mancha and tilt at windmills. It is very helpful to set attainable goals and work toward their fulfillment. In the first case, it is not unrealistic to assume that the nurse eventually might have been able to improve the conditions under which Brady and her family were living, at least to obtain a warmer place for them to live and perhaps a small increase in their welfare allotment. It also is not unrealistic for a nurse to attempt to obtain medical care for a very ill infant. Success in these two areas, in turn, might have increased the potentiality for success in the stabilization of this family.

In the second case, the nurse clearly made a decision to expand her role in serving the patient. However, it was specifically in response to the patient's express wish. The odds against success were very great, but the results of failure were mitigated. It also may be seen that a refusal to respond to Mary's needs would have been a violation of the first principles: to respect the dignity, inviolability, and freedom of each person. If the nurse had refused to respond, Mary would have had little if any chance of attaining her goal.

6. A word must be said also about a nurse's responsibility to society for the expenditure of her time and of public money in both of these cases. It is inappropriate for a nurse to attempt to evaluate the social worth of patients, clients and their families. This statement is predicated on the principles that were articulated at the beginning of this comparison. It cannot be known if Brady would or would not have recovered and become a contributing member of society. It also cannot be known if her baby, had he lived, would have been of value to society. Mary already had worked for many years, but it is unlikely that she would be gainfully employed again in the future. The nurse was concerned with the complex range of human fulfillments that were or could be available to each person. Such actions or measures that are taken must be chosen and undertaken together (patient/client and nurse) as far as is possible. To do otherwise is to violate the humanity of the individuals involved.

COMMENTARY: Case Study II

M. Josephine Flaherty

It is interesting to note that some of the same characters are involved in this situation as played parts in the first case study. Although the probability of success in both situations was not high, the outcomes were quite different.

One of the most important differences was the context in which the action took place. In Mary's case, she started with a positive outlook and did not experience the isolation and negative past experience in terms of social relationships that had been the case with Brady. Mary's periods of discouragement were real but were short-lived, partly because of the "magic" in her view of her "dream" to walk up the stairs of the church. However, a major factor was that although the efforts of the nurse, that in both cases were considerable, were persistent and involved both personal and professional risks for herself as a health professional and as a member of the health care agency, in Mary's case, the combination of Mary's own personal context (the kind of person she obviously was, as indicated by the long years of hard work, both inside and outside her home, that she had devoted to the care of her family) and the social context (her family and the community) in which she lived, provided support that was not available to Brady. The lack of support of society for the money for Mary's prosthesis was similar to society's unwillingness or inability to provide improved economic support for Brady. However, Mary's problems may have appeared more palatable to that society than were Brady's; they formed a picture of a "chronic, disadvantaged multi-problem, unclean (nobody likes cockroaches!), mentally unstable, poor, and altogether unsavory burden on society." Brady's problems would not be solved quickly. Mary's problems were physical and she had a history of being a hard-working, respectable, self-reliant and, to the extent of her means, contributing member of society. Her goal was a challenging one, but a number of people, who put a great deal of effort into the achievement of it, must have believed that it was achievable. One might ask how much effect society's dislike of "poor" and "unstable" individuals who are "burdens" really has on society's ability (or is it willingness?) to take action to change social situations like Brady's.

Mary's family managed to raise the money for the prosthesis. Members of the community helped and derived satisfaction from their part in this "community project." The physician had his doubts, but he did write the orders. The nurse persisted, through all stages of encouragement and discouragement, and took a number of risks. The physiotherapist worked behind the scenes for a long time and made her appearance at the appropriate moment. It is evident that although health care agency rules may not have been broken, they were bent—at least a little.

Perhaps the most important elements in this situation were hope and coordination. There was hope: on the part of (1) the patient who never really gave up, although she was tempted to do so on more than one occasion; (2) the family members who continued to encourage their wife and mother and grandmother, who had been behind all of them for many years; the family found the money for the prosthesis, modified the arrangements in the home to create, in effect, a small physiotherapy department there and monitored the patient's diabetic regime; (3) the physician who wrote the appropriate orders and maintained interest in the patient; (4) the community that pitched in to help; (5) the nurse who really fulfilled the requirements of the nurse–patient interaction that stemmed from her assessment of the patient's needs and resources, the planning and implementation of nursing actions, including cooperation in and coordination of the work of other members of the health care team, and that was directed toward the achievement and maintenance of functional competence by the patient; (6) the physiotherapist who gave ongoing guidance and encouragement to the nurse throughout, and hence indirectly at first and directly later, to the patient and family; and (7) the visiting nursing agency that, implicitly or explicitly, supported these activities by tolerating and not interfering with them.

Cooperation in and coordination of the actions of all players were orchestrated by the nurse, but she could not have achieved these without the other people. The result was a happy one for all concerned, as it was a success story that was worth the agony.

The ethical responsibilities of health care professionals include the requirements for them to supply not only the scientific competence but also the spiritual nourishment that patients need. Cousins has suggested that the most potent medicine available to health professionals is the confidence that patients place in them. The next most potent medicine is the health professionals' ability to harness the natural drive of the human body and mind to overcome its maladies.[1] In Brady's case, there was some of the first but the second was not adequate to the situation. In Mary's case, both types of potent medicine worked in harmony to inspire Mary "to make the special effort necessary to get well."[2] Rights and responsibilities were protected and the objectives of the health care for Mary were realized.

NOTES

1. Cousins, Norman. "Medical Ethics: Is There a Broader View?" *Journal of the American Medical Association*, Vol. 241, No. 25 (June 22, 1979) p. 2712.
2. *Ibid.*

Case Study III: Insubordination—Patient Load

M. Josephine Flaherty

BACKGROUND INFORMATION

About 2230h on February 26, Patient Mason was admitted with irregular breathing and an irregular heart rate to the Emergency Department of a large teaching hospital; various diagnostic tests were done. About 0200h on February 27, Mason went into respiratory arrest and was intubated and ventilated manually. Dr. Brown, physician in charge of the Emergency Department that night, deciding to admit the patient to the Intensive Care Unit, called the I.C.U. to advise the nursing staff of the admission. Nurse Ames, who took the call, said "John, we are very busy. We need more help. Do you want to call Nursing Supervisor Smith or do you want me to call?" Dr. Brown said that he was busy and asked that Nurse Ames call Supervisor Smith and let him know about her response. Dr. Brown called Dr. White, who was in charge of the I.C.U. to apprise him of the patient's condition and the decision to admit him; Dr. White concurred with this action.

Nurse Ames called Supervisor Smith, told her that there was a ventilator patient being admitted to I.C.U. and asked for more nursing staff. Smith said that she could not provide more help, told Ames to "do what you can do" and noted that she would ask the Emergency Department if the patient could be cared for there. She did so and Dr. Brown's response to this request was negative. Smith responded that if this were the case, the physician would have to be responsible for Patient Mason. Dr. Brown replied that he was unhappy with that remark, that he would report Supervisor Smith and that Mason was going to the I.C.U. Supervisor Smith accepted that decision.

Dr. Brown informed Dr. White by telephone that he was having difficulty having Mason admitted to I.C.U. and asked for Dr. White's assistance; White said that he would investigate the matter and call Dr. Brown.

Dr. White called I.C.U., spoke to another nurse, Miss Blank, and reprimanded her for "giving flak" to Dr. Brown. Nurse Blank said that no "flak" had been given and that Dr. Brown had been informed simply that the I.C.U. was at the saturation point in the work load of the nurses. When informed by Dr. White that nurses need only ask for additional help, Nurse Blank noted that Supervisor Smith had been informed and that no help was forthcoming. Neither Dr. White nor Nurse Blank disputed that Patient Mason appeared to need I.C.U. care, but Nurse Blank made it clear that the situation was such that there was no nurse available to care for the new patient. When questioned about this by Dr. White, she said, "No nurse feels capable of accepting the responsibility for another ventilator patient." Dr. White said that he would call Supervisor Smith. He testified later that he had noted to Nurse Blank that he would come in to help with the care of the patient if necessary and that this offer was motivated, not by recognition of the nurses' claim that they could not accept responsibility for more patients, but by recognition that, given the position taken by the nurses, he, as a responsible physician, had no alternative to coming in and providing care. Dr. White called Supervisor Smith and told her that the patient would go to the I.C.U. and that he and Respiratory Technologist Thomas would look after the ventilator so that the nurses could give nursing care. Supervisor Smith telephoned this information to Nurse Clark who replied that the nurses would not care for the patient; Smith told them to try anyway.

At 0520h, Patient Mason arrived in I.C.U. accompanied by Dr. Brown, Dr. Black (an intern), Nurse Evans (Emergency Department Nurse) and Technologist Thomas; they transferred Mason to a bed in an empty I.C.U. room. Nurse Evans attempted to give a report of the patient to Nurse Blank who told Evans that since no I.C.U. nurse would be caring for the patient, she should give the report to the doctors attending to him. Nurse Evans left the I.C.U. At this time, Drs. White and Gold (the intern in I.C.U.) arrived.

The room in which Patient Mason was placed had not been equipped for his care. Those attending him assembled the necessary equipment with the occasional assistance of I.C.U. Nurse Davis (although she was very busy with her own patient who was at least as ill as Patient Mason) and of Nurses Clark and Ames.

Subsequent to these events, Nurses Ames, Blank and Clark were suspended without pay for three days and were warned by the director of nursing that further similar behavior would "jeopardize" their relationships with the hospital as employees. The reason advanced for the suspension was "insubordination," as evidenced by their failure as registered nurses to carry out the following responsibilities:

"—to appoint a team leader or nurse in charge (a policy of the hospital);
—to accept a report and a patient from the Emergency Department nurse;

—to offer to help in the admission of the patient to I.C.U. and in the care given by the medical staff during the remainder of the shift (approximately 3 hours); and

—to report fully the circumstances of the incident to the head nurse at morning report."

Supervisor Smith also was suspended without pay, for five days, because she was "not forceful enough in her supervision of the nurses in question."

What are the ethical problems in this situation?

IDENTIFICATION AND CLARIFICATION OF ETHICAL COMPONENTS

This complex, real-life situation is not illustrative of one discrete ethical issue but involves a complexity of demands, needs, conflicting loyalties, and confusing lines of communication. This incident presents a picture of a health care situation in which the resources in the hospital do not appear to be adequate to the task of the provision of appropriate treatment for a seriously ill patient, a not unusual circumstance in large and small health care agencies today.

There are several types of rights and responsibilities involved:

1. The right of a patient to treatment

2. The rights and responsibilities of nurses as providers of the care

3. The rights and responsibilities of a health care agency to make decisions about who shall admit patients, who shall care for which patients and what the patient–nurse ratios shall be

4. The rights and responsibilities of physicians, as "guest practitioners" in the agency, to admit patients and to make decisions affecting the practice of other health practitioners over whom they have no authority.

Right of a Patient to Treatment. The hospital in question was a public hospital, defined in The Public Hospitals Act of the jurisdiction as "any institution, building or other premises or place established for the treatment of persons afflicted with or suffering from sickness, disease or injury, or for the treatment of convalescent or chronically ill persons that is approved under this Act as a public hospital." Under the same Act, a patient is a "person who is received and lodged in a hospital for the purpose of treatment"; and treatment means "the maintenance, observation, medical care and supervision and skilled nursing care of a patient. . . . " The jurisdiction concerned had a system of universal hospital care insurance by which Patient Mason was covered. Hence, since he was received and lodged in the hospital, Mason became a patient and had the right, by law and by the value system of the society in which he lived, to treatment, including skilled nursing care. A patient who is entitled to skilled nursing care should be able to assume that the nurses will practice competently, will consider the patient's needs paramount, will not harm the patient through acts of commission or omission, and will be faithful to both the patient and to the promises of the profession.

Rights and Responsibilities of Nurses as Providers of Health Care. As registered nurses, the staff members of the I.C.U. had statutory responsibilities to "exercise generally accepted standards of practice for the performance of nursing services." This includes making professional judgments about their ability to accept specific responsibility and the communication of their inability to accept such responsibility to their supervisors. When nurses are expected to practice according to the standards for registered nurses, they have the right to working conditions that make this possible. This includes work loads that are reasonable, including appropriate assistance and supervision. Registered nurses in the jurisdiction concerned are responsible and accountable, by statute, for the "effective supervision of . . . others who contribute to the provision of nursing care," for "the exercise of judgment in delegation of activities, . . . " for collaboration "with other members of the health team in the planning/provision of care," for coordination of "nursing care with other aspects of health care" and for referring and reporting "pertinent information to other members of the health team." The Standards of Nursing Practice also include responsibilities for collaboration with other nurses and for seeking help and guidance when nurses are unable to perform competently. All of the nurses in this situation shared these responsibilities. One might ask how effectively they collaborated and communicated. Was the action of the supervisor appropriate? Should other nurses have been sent to the I.C.U.? Should the Emergency Department nurse have behaved differently? Do nurses have the right to "civil disobedience" in health care?

The Rights and Responsibilities of a Health Care Agency to Make Decisions About Who Shall Admit Patients and Who and How Many Persons Shall Provide Care. By admitting physicians to practice privileges in a hospital, either as full staff physicians or as resident or junior interns, does a hospital delegate *carte blanche* responsibility to these physicians to admit patients and to decide the wards or departments to which patients will be sent, in the absence of consideration of the occupancy and staff situations in the hospital? Does the hospital have the obligation to admit all patients needing care to its own wards or could Patient Mason have been sent to another public general hospital? In the city core area involved, there are several hospitals with a combined total of well over 3,000 beds, within a two-mile radius of the hospital to which Mason was admitted. Does a hospital have a right to permit extremely heavy patient loads in patient care areas?

The Rights and Responsibilities of Physicians as "Guest Practitioners." Do physicians have the right to make decisions that affect directly the practice of members of another health discipline over which they have neither statutory nor organizational line authority in the work situation? Are physicians obliged to collaborate with institution managers and with other health professionals? Do physicians have the right and the qualifications to assess nursing care needs of patients as opposed to medical care needs?

ANALYSIS OF THE SPECIFIC SITUATION

Background Information

1. Mason was in need of intensive care including a ventilator. The ward of choice was the I.C.U.

2. The I.C.U. was staffed inadequately for its patient load. There were six nurses on duty, two of whom were relief nurses without experience in the I.C.U. and whose special care unit competence was limited. There were eight patients, five of whom were on ventilators or respirators and all of whom had monitoring equipment and/or indwelling tubes, drains, and so forth. One patient was on isolation technique for infection.

3. The nurses were on a twelve-hour shift that was supposed to include time for meals and coffee breaks. None of the nurses had a meal break; some had a cup of coffee in the Unit.

4. The nursing supervisor had a nondirective style of supervision and rarely gave direct orders.

5. No team leader had been appointed although the appointment of one was required by hospital policy. Since the supervisor had received reports from each of the nurses on the unit, she was aware of this breach of policy. The supervisor made no attempt to redistribute patient assignments.

6. The Emergency Department nurse who accompanied the patient to the I.C.U. returned to the Emergency Department without giving a report on her patient to the I.C.U. nurses.

7. The I.C.U. nurses requested additional help; they were refused help and were told to "do the best you can."

8. Hospital policy states that ventilated patients cannot be left unobserved or unattended.

9. No direct order or directive was given to all or any of the six nurses in the I.C.U. to care for Patient Mason.

10. Although the director of nursing had authority to hire more nurses, she noted during an arbitration hearing related to this incident that she had not done so because she had a budget to follow.

INDIVIDUALS INVOLVED IN DECISION MAKING

1. Physicians

A physician in the Emergency Department decided to admit the patient. The physician in charge of the Intensive Care Unit concurred. The Emergency

Department physician notified the I.C.U. that the patient was coming and was informed that the nurses could not handle another patient. He asked an I.C.U. nurse to telephone the nursing supervisor about this. He informed the I.C.U. physician that he anticipated difficulties with the admission of his patient.

Although the Emergency Department physician had admitting authority, he also had responsibility to ensure that the area to which his patient would be admitted was appropriate. One would question how appropriate the I.C.U. was on this occasion when it was clear that there was a shortage of nurses. The I.C.U. physician telephoned the I.C.U. nurses and reprimanded them for "giving flak" to the Emergency Department physician. He said that he would talk with the nursing supervisor but the outcome of that conversation, if it did take place, is not known. He did volunteer to come in to look after the patient if necessary but noted that this decision was motivated only by his responsibility as a physician and not by his recognition that the nurses needed help.

That four physicians and one respiratory technologist attended the patient in the Intensive Care Unit is indicative that they were aware of the complexity of the care demanded and of the fact that the nurses were unable to deal with this situation. In view of the fact that five persons were caring for one patient, one wonders why the physicians felt qualified to assert that the I.C.U. nurses should have been willing and able to care for this patient in addition to the other patients in the Unit. Since the two senior physicians involved were cognizant of the number and nature of patients in the Unit and the extent of the nursing staff on duty, one would question why they did not take action to ensure that additional nursing help was made available. Dr. White had noted that nurses who needed extra help need only ask for this. He was aware that such a request had been refused and yet he insisted that the patient be admitted to the I.C.U. and he believed that the nurses had been incorrect in their refusal to assume responsibility for this additional patient.

Why did physicians in this situation have the power to affect so directly the conditions of work for nurses—members of another health discipline over which they had neither statutory nor organizational responsibility? What was the quality of the communication between the physicians and the nurses in this agency, where a nursing supervisor was told that she would be reported for telling the physician that if he admitted the patient to the I.C.U. he would have to assume responsibility for the patient and where the same physician reprimanded a nurse in the I.C.U. for what he alleged was "flak" given to another physician by another nurse?

As health professionals, did the physicians have the responsibility to reassess the admission of the particular patient to their hospital in view of staffing problems that were apparent? Were the physicians exercising their responsibility to provide treatment, which by definition includes skilled nursing care, when they knew that this was not possible in that Unit?

2. The Nursing Supervisor

The nursing supervisor knew the conditions in the Intensive Care Unit on that shift as she had received reports on all patients at approximately 2200h in the evening. She was aware that no team leader had been chosen and she made no attempt to deal with this obvious breach of hospital policy. Although she had visited the Unit at 2200h, apparently she made no attempt to return to the Unit later to give nursing assistance to the staff and to see the new patient who had been admitted. In a conversation with the I.C.U. physician, she had told him that if he admitted the patient to the Unit, he would have to be responsible for the patient. When she was told that he would admit the patient anyway and report her for her comment, she accepted that decision.

When she was asked for nursing assistance by the I.C.U. nurses, she instructed them simply to "cope" and "do the best you can." At no time did she give a direct order to all or any of the nurses to care for the new patient. She noted later that her style of supervision recognized the fact that registered nurses are professional people with the responsibility to make professional judgments. However, there is no clear indication that she supported nurses in their resolution to refuse to accept responsibility for the new patient. There is no indication of the extent to which the supervisor communicated with the Emergency Department nurse. The fact that subsequent to these events, the nursing supervisor was suspended by the hospital for five days indicates that the hospital believed that the supervisor did not fulfill the responsibilities of her job on that occasion. It should be noted that the supervisor must also have been aware of the fact that although it was hospital policy that no ventilated patient be left unobserved or unattended, there were more ventilator patients in the Unit than there were nurses qualified to care for them. One would wonder also why the supervisor did not spend more time in the Unit that night when she was aware of the fact that carrying heavy patient loads were two relief nurses, neither of whom was an experienced or qualified I.C.U. nurse.

3. Nurses in the I.C.U.

There is no evidence to indicate that the nurses had asked for additional nursing help before the question of the admission of a new patient arose, even though they were understaffed for the patient population in the Unit. The nurses did explain to the physician who notified them about the new patient that no nurse was capable of assuming responsibility for the new patient. The nurses did contact the supervisor and ask for help. When the new patient was brought to the I.C.U., the nurses made clear that they would not accept the new patient and assume responsibility for him. Their reasons were related to the patient load they already were carrying. Although they claimed later that they were concerned about their responsibility for the provision of safe care for patients already under their care, apparently they did not make an issue of the safety factor on the evening concerned. While they might be faulted by some observers for this, it would seem reasonable to assume that they were extremely busy trying to do what needed to be done without becoming philosophical and providing detailed rationales for the stand they were taking.

The nurses were faulted by the hospital for failing to appoint a team leader according to the policy of the hospital. However, it was noted later (and this was not challenged) that the practice of failing to appoint a team leader had been going on for some time. The supervisor was aware of this and apparently did nothing to correct the situation.

The nurses acknowledged later that they gave limited help to the physicians involved in the care of Patient Mason. A physician noted that the nurses had "taken time to have a cup of coffee and yet they did not have time to care for the new patient." The nurses noted that one or two of them had drunk a cup of coffee at the nursing station while they were charting or speaking on the telephone. The nurses were faulted for not reporting details of the incident in the morning report when they went off duty. Their response was that they believed the situation had been handled and that their supervisor was aware of it and hence that a further report was not necessary. One would question their judgment on this issue in view of their professional responsibility to communicate appropriately with other members of the team.

It seems obvious that these nurses were aware of their professional responsibility to make judgments, to take action, and to be accountable for that action. Apparently they believed they were acting appropriately. It should be noted that they did not make a point of their legal responsibilities related to the abandoning of patients during the night in question. However, it cannot be assumed that this matter was not in their minds.

4. Emergency Room Nurse

In accordance with hospital policy, emergency room Nurse Evans accompanied Patient Mason to the Intensive Care Unit and attempted to give a report on him to one of the nurses present. When that nurse refused to take the report, because she was refusing to assume responsibility for the patient, apparently Nurse Evans left the Unit without giving a report. One would question why this nurse did not fulfill this responsibility and/or notify the supervisor that a report had not been given. It is not known how many other nurses were in the Emergency Department that night or how many other patients were there. However, there is little evidence that the Emergency Department nurse did anything in the Intensive Care Unit except assist the four doctors and one respiratory technologist to transfer the patient to an I.C.U. bed. Apparently she did not assemble equipment for the I.C.U. patient room. It may be that she was pressed to return to the Emergency Department immediately or that she was not aware of where some equipment was kept. One would wonder how much attempt she made to assist with the settling of the patient in the I.C.U. One cannot assume that she did not make attempts to do this. In view of the fact that the Emergency Department nurse failed to carry out her reporting responsibility and apparently failed to discuss this with her supervisor, one would wonder why the hospital did not discipline her for failure to carry out her responsibilities.

5. Hospital Authorities

This large general hospital was experiencing, no doubt, the same fiscal restraints that confront all health care institutions in these times. During a later arbitration hearing, the director of nursing acknowledged that she had been aware of the state of staffing in the hospital and in the Unit in question. One would wonder why she had permitted the Intensive Care Unit to be staffed as this one was. In view of hospital policy in relation to responsibilities of nurses in special care units, why were two of the six nurses totally inexperienced in intensive care unit work? By that policy, they were limited in their practice in that situation, because relief nurses who are not certified for specific procedures may not administer intravenous drugs and perform certain other activities related to hemodynamic monitoring. Why was a supervisor not available to monitor the work of these inexperienced nurses?

Although the director of nursing admitted later that she did have authority to hire additional nurses, she said she did not do so because she had a budget to follow. One would question the professional responsibility of a nurse manager who knowingly allows conditions to exist that threaten or make impossible the provision of skilled nursing care and the fulfillment of the standards of nursing practice in the agency. It is acknowledged that emergency situations in staffing can arise and this may well have been one. However, it must have been known for a great many hours before the new patient was admitted that there were too few nurses who were qualified to care for ventilator patients in that Unit. One would wonder why additional nurses could not have been found between the hours of roughly 1930h when the shift began and 0520h the next morning when the new patient was admitted to the I.C.U. One would question whether this situation had occurred before, whether it was one of long standing and whether it would continue. It is known that shortly after the occurrence of the incidents described in this situation, additional nurses were hired for the hospital and for the I.C.U. This and the disciplining of the nursing supervisor suggest strongly that the hospital was aware of its inadequacy. One would wonder, then, why the hospital felt justified in the disciplining of the I.C.U. nurses who took action that they believed was appropriate for professional nurses.

6. The Collective Bargaining Agreement

In this hospital, the nurses were covered by a collective bargaining agreement that was developed under the labor relations laws of the jurisdiction.

It is recognized that the management level of an organization, including a hospital, has the right to decide what shall be done by whom in that organization and to regulate the distribution of resources, physical and human, within the institution. Hence, management has the right to assign responsibilities to members of the staff and this can lead to problems. For example, when members of the staff, such as nurses, are professionals who are accountable to the statutory body for the quality and scope of their practice, to the employer for carrying out the responsibilities of the job, to the patients who receive care, and to themselves for the character of their practice, which is carried out according to standards of nursing practice, statutory regulations, and the code of ethics of the profession, there may be conflicts between the nurses' loyalty to the employer and their loyalty to the profession and to the recipients of care.

It has been said for some time in the nursing profession that it is nurses who should make judgments regarding nursing practice and the nursing needs of patients. In this situation, it appears that physicians assumed the responsibility for making such judgments and this is not unusual in health care today. Nurses of the eighties believe they are qualified to make decisions about the nature and extent of nursing responsibilities that they can assume and, indeed, in the jurisdiction in which the situation under question occurred, the taking of responsibility for professional actions by nurses and their being accountable for their actions both are required by statute. One would wonder whether nurses have a right to "civil disobedience" in health care. Labor relations laws, largely in the industrial setting, allow for an *obey and grieve rule,* the rationale behind which is to give disaffected employees an opportunity to challenge a particular management decision in a way that recognizes both the interests of the employer in having work assignments carried out and the interests of the employee in obtaining a just disposition of his or her complaint. To allow employees to practice insubordination in light of their disagreement with a work directive could threaten the right of an employer to manage the organization. In the collective agreement at the hospital in question, there is a section that defines very clearly that the management of the hospital and the direction of working forces are fixed exclusively in the hospital and shall remain solely with the hospital, except as specifically limited by particular provisions of the agreement. The assignment of responsibilities to employees such as nurses rests with the hospital. Disaffected employees are expected to *obey* at the time and *grieve* later.

However, under the labor relations laws of the jurisdiction involved, there are several exceptions to the *obey and grieve* rule. These include the right of employees to disobey if they are asked to carry out a task that is unsafe or reasonably believed to be unsafe or if they are asked to do something illegal. It is noteworthy that under that law, although an employer cannot expect workers to do something that is unsafe for them, there is no provision for employees to refuse to do something that is unsafe for the recipient of their care. Hence, because of the failure of the law to deal specifically with the third set of interests, those of the patient, in a health care situation in the jurisdiction involved, it seems that the threat to safety of a patient is not sufficient to allow health care employees to disobey. It is partly for this weakness in the law that the charge of insubordination of these nurses was upheld by an arbitration board and later by judicial inquiry.

If the nurses in this situation consciously had believed and had stated that by obeying the apparent directive to care for Patient Mason, they could be found guilty of abandoning other patients and hence of professional misconduct, or that they could be found to be incompetent because they had displayed in their professional care of patients a lack of judgment or a disregard for the welfare of patients, they would have pointed to their explicit responsibilities as professional nurses under the statutes that govern registered nurses in their region of the country. In this situation, they could have claimed that assuming responsibility for the new patient would have constituted an illegal act for them and their insubordination could have been upheld under the *obey and grieve* rule. It should be noted, however, that not all nursing statutes are as strong and as explicit as the ones in the jurisdiction in which these incidents took place.

It is important to distinguish between two dimensions of nurses' behavior: their professional responsibility and their obligation to their employer. Since nurses' main obligation to the employer is to behave as competent professional nurses if that employer has hired them to work as professional nurses, it is difficult to separate the two dimensions because nurses' obligation to the employer and their professional responsibility are one and the same. It could be suggested, then, that in refusing to take on the additional patient and thus acting as responsible professionals, these nurses in fact were fulfilling their responsibility or obligation to their employer to behave as competent professionals.

ETHICAL IMPLICATIONS

It appears that in this situation, there were several options or possible courses of action that might have been chosen by the persons who played parts in the decision making. Apparently, each of these decision makers acted the way he or she believed was right. One could wonder, however, if those people really did believe that their actions were right or whether some, pragmatically, were "going by the book" or were evading honest confrontation with reality. Although the actions taken may appear to be simply decisions based on facts, clearly they involve an ethical problem because the solution does not rest solely within science, it is perplexing to some or all of the people involved, and it has implications that touch many areas of human concern. That there are several types of rights and responsibilities involved has been acknowledged. It is questionable whether each of the actors in the situation projected fully the consequences of each possible course of action and identified fully the good and/or harm that could result.

It seems obvious that none of the possible options—refusal to admit Patient Mason and referral of him to another hospital, retention of him in the Emergency Department for care, the transfer of him from there to a unit other than the I.C.U., the assignment of nurses from another unit to either the Emergency Department or the I.C.U. to care for him, the co-opting of the nursing supervisor to care for him, the "calling in" of additional nurses to the hospital, *et al.*—was acceptable to all of the decision makers involved. However, there is little evidence that genuine attempts were made by any or all of them to explore the possible options in cooperation with the others. All persons and groups involved seemed to be determined to follow their own decisions for action, even though the issue had been reported to both a senior physician and a senior nurse. Some decisions (those of the physicians) seemed to be based on recognition of Patient Mason's human need for care without full enough consideration of the needs of other patients in the I.C.U. Other decisions (the nurses') did not deny Patient Mason's need for care, but appeared to be based on their recognition of other patient's needs, of their duties and obligations to provide care for them, and of their inability to fulfill those duties in addition to the new ones that would be imposed by the extra patient. Other decisions (the nursing supervisor's) appeared to be derived from the recognition that since she had spoken with the admitting physician and received no satisfaction, she should instruct the I.C.U. nurses simply to do their best, on their own, without her formal assistance. Her lack of action, and the hospital administration's, in the face of their knowledge about the level of staffing in the I.C.U. on the night in question, that clearly was in contravention of hospital policy with regard to number and qualifications of nurses assigned to the I.C.U., and their awareness of the failure of the nurses (on more than this one occasion) to appoint a team leader suggests evasion of honest confrontation with reality.

This particular situation required shared decision-making activity. There seems to be little evidence of sharing of deliberations and discussion of options. There is no clear evidence of recognition, by all persons involved, of the locus of authority for the decision making. The result was a series of incompatible decisions, with little indication that there was understanding of why dissenters were not in agreement with the decisions of other people. In this situation, there was confusion within and among the social expectations, held by some members of the hospital, for nurses to obey and conform, for physicians to make decisions that affect other disciplines over which they do not have line authority and responsibility and for the nursing supervisor to manage. There was confusion also in relation to the legal or statutory responsibilities of physicians as professionals and "guest practitioners" in the hospital, of nurses as professionals and employees, of the nursing supervisor as a professional nurse and an administrator, and of the hospital as a provider of treatment that included skilled nursing care.

The situation was a puzzling one but not a rare one. Each decision that was made had an element of right action that was perceived by the decision maker, and an element of wrong action that was demonstrated in the consequences. The situation provides an example of failure on the part of a number of health care professionals, all of whom perceived themselves to be competent and ethical, to behave in a collegial manner in the effort to find a solution for a practical and ethical problem. Mutual respect and cooperation and responsible leadership by both of the professions involved would have led to a more satisfactory solution. Nurses and physicians would do well to reflect on how they would or could have responded in this or a similar circumstance, on whether situations like this one will be repeated, and on what can be done to prevent them.

COMMENTARY: CASE STUDY III

Leah Curtin

The most important point Flaherty makes in her analysis of this case study is " . . . nurses' main obligation to the employer is to behave as competent professional nurses . . . [thus] nurses' obligations to the [hospital] and their professional responsibility are one. . . . " This simple and powerful statement provides a sound framework for nurse–employer relationships. The hospital has the authority to hire and to fire nurses, but it does not have the authority to coerce nurses to act contrary to their professional judgments. To attempt to do so is not a legitimate use of institutional power and is an unjustifiable interference with professional practice. The hospital has the authority and responsibility to articulate administrative policies and to insist on the maintenance by nurses of approved standards of practice and of professional behavior. Hence, it cannot reprimand or discipline nurses whose conduct in fact is in keeping with institutional policies and established standards of practice. That is, an institution cannot give lip service to its own policies and standards while insisting that its employees act contrary to these policies and standards. In this situation, the hospital disciplined the nurses for behavior that was in keeping with standards of practice and statutory obligations in the jurisdiction.

In addition, the hospital, as an employer of professionals, has an obligation to permit and to facilitate professional practice. Among other things, this obligation includes the provision of space for the making of discretionary professional judgments. As Flaherty points out, administrative authorities were aware of the short staffing in the Intensive Care Unit. Six nurses were on duty, two of whom were relief nurses who had no previous I.C.U. experience, and there were eight patients, five of whom were on respirators or ventilators and all of whom had monitoring equipment and/or indwelling tubes, drains and so forth. One of the patients required isolation technique for infection. In the nurses' professional judgment, they were not sure that they could care adequately for the patients already in the I.C.U. and they certainly could not care adequately for another seriously ill patient.

Although the nurses clearly communicated this judgment to their supervisor and to the physicians involved in the case, they apparently were not as clear about the rationale for their decision. Communication probably would have been enhanced considerably if they had followed hospital administrative policies and designated one nurse to act as team leader or charge nurse. That they did not do so, as Flaherty notes, weakened their position in this conflict.

The physician did communicate clearly both his decision to admit Patient Mason to the Intensive Care Unit and his rationale for the decision (the patient was critically ill). However, he failed to take into account the nurses' assertion that the care the patient needed could not be provided in the I.C.U. at this time. Apparently, the physician thought that he was competent to make decisions about the nursing care needs of patients and the amount of time a nurse would have to devote to this patient to care for him adequately—an interesting but invalid assumption.

Evidence is presented in the case study that it took four physicians and one respiratory therapist to care for Patient Mason; therefore, it reasonably could be assumed that one nurse who already was caring for other seriously ill patients could not safely assume the responsibility of caring for this incoming patient. Of course, one can question the competence of the physicians to practice nursing. Physicians are not prepared educationally or experientially to practice nursing and this could account for the extraordinary number of physicians required to deliver nursing care to this one patient.

Apparently the physicians learned nothing from this experience. They did not demonstrate an appreciation for the complexity and demands of nursing care because they maintained in a subsequent investigation that the nurses could and should have accepted the patient in the I.C.U.

In summary, the I.C.U. nurses made a professional judgment and there is evidence to support the validity of that judgment. The hospital and nursing administration, by allowing an Intensive Care Unit to be staffed in that fashion, exhibit a lamentable disregard for institutional policies and standards of nursing practice. What is astounding is that the arbitration board upheld the hospital's decision to discipline the nurses for acting in a manner that, in their judgment, was consistent with their obligation to protect their patients.

Case Study IV: Consent, Conflict, and "Euthanasia"

Leah Curtin

A seventeen-year-old boy was riding in the back of a pickup truck when it went off the road and turned over in an embankment. He was thrown from the truck into a wooded area and a small branch was forced through his skull. He was rushed to a local hospital emergency room, comatose and near death. His parents and a well-known neurosurgeon were called: I don't know in which order.

A tracheotomy was performed in the emergency room and the patient was placed on a respirator. Subsequently, he underwent emergency surgery. To maintain his nutrition, hyperalimentation was started post-surgically in the Intensive Care Unit. Surprisingly, except for contusions and abrasions, there was no damage other than that caused by the head wound. Although an EEG revealed some brain activity, all vital signs were absent. His pupils were dilated and unresponsive to light, he had no deep reflexes, and he did not respond to stimuli of any kind. The heat-control mechanism in his brain was affected and his temperature varied widely from severe hypothermia to severe hyperthermia.

Three weeks after surgery, the boy still was in a deep coma and still was in the Intensive Care Unit. The parents maintained a constant vigil and were consulted about all major decisions, including procedures that required written consent and those that did not. Decisions about continuing the respirator, continuing hyperalimentation, and about whether or not to resuscitate the boy if he experienced cardiac arrest were among these decisions.

The parents experienced increasing anxiety and depression during this period. The mother suffered from recurrent nightmares and the father was in a car accident that destroyed the family's only auto. They had four other younger children who also had problems and needs. To make matters worse (if possible), a major storm hit the area and a large tree in their front yard fell, crushing their garage and damaging the roof of their house; fortunately, no one was hurt. However, their child's apparent suffering and the seeming

219

hopelessness of his case increased their suffering, and the hospital staff felt a conflict over their duty to the boy as a patient and to the parents as patients. It sometimes seemed that the boy's continued existence was harmful to the parents' and siblings' well-being, and the parents began requesting that all the machines be disconnected in the hope that the boy would die.

The nursing and medical staff members were divided over the resolution of this situation. A significant number believed that all treatment should be stopped and that the boy should be allowed to die. On the other hand, a large number thought that the boy still had a chance to live and that to deny the boy this chance would be unjust—it would be an act of euthanasia.

IDENTIFICATION AND CLARIFICATION OF THE PROBLEM

Many relevant ethical problems are raised in this situation, the first of which is, "What is euthanasia?" Another common and recurring problem is, "Under what circumstances, if any, can one person make a decision for death for another?"

Certainly, few would question the parents' right to make decisions for their incompetent, minor child, but what are the health professionals' roles if those decisions seem to be in the best interests of the parents rather than in the best interests of the child? Before this analysis can proceed, the two major ethical issues presented by this situation must be explored and clarified.

EUTHANASIA: A CLARIFICATION

The issue of euthanasia is a matter of public concern today. Health professionals inevitably are drawn into this controversy by virtue of their role and function in society and by virtue of the fact that various pieces of legislation introduced in numerous states specifically name the physician and the registered nurse as the "implementors" of euthanasia. While the debate rages between opponents and proponents, it becomes increasingly clear that there is mounting confusion with regard to what this term means and its potential implications for individuals, health professionals, and society at large.

The function of language is to facilitate communication, that is, to clarify, to convey meaning and thought accurately. "To understand a word is to grasp how it is used in the language game."[1] The meaning of a word "does not consist in the objects it names, but rather in the way it is used in a language."[2] What is the meaning of the word euthanasia and how is it used in the English language?

Certain expressions do occur for which better substitutes could be found[3] and, in this case, ought to be found. The word euthanasia is unfamiliar to many persons, equivocal and ambiguous in meaning, ill-chosen as being general where it should be specific, often allusive where the allusion is not known or obvious, and often a malapropism or a misnomer. Those who defend the use of the word euthanasia may respond with claims that this is a perfectly good word that conveys the concept of a happy or painless death (Gr. *eu*-well, and *thanatos*-death). This claim is justified only if one assumes that the meaning of a word is derived strictly from its etymological origins rather than from its use in the language. The use of the word euthanasia does not, in fact, always reflect accurately its etymological origins.

A happy or good death has been defined by Daniel Callahan of the Institute of Society, Ethics and the Life Sciences as one in which an individual has 1) lived out his normal life span; 2) fulfilled those goals in life that he set for himself; 3) fulfilled all of his obligations and responsibilities; 4) not suffered excessive or prolonged pain; and 5) experienced death that was brought about by natural rather than artificially induced means (*e.g.,* the individual was not shot or run over by a truck).[4] The dictionary definition of euthanasia, that is, "the painless inducement of death for merciful reasons,"[5] does not meet these criteria. To induce death implies that some artificial means are taken; otherwise, death would occur naturally and there would be no need to induce it. Therefore, when death is induced there is no reason to suppose that the individual has lived out his normal life span. Whether the individual has fulfilled his obligations and responsibilities or goals in life is a moot point that certainly is not addressed in the dictionary definition. The definition implies that the intention must be merciful, but it does not specify for whom the decision is merciful, that is, for an individual suffering pain, for the family or friends of that individual who cannot bear to see his pain, or for society that often must bear the painful burden of the expense of his care. The word euthanasia certainly is ambiguous in its meaning. This ambiguity may have been tolerable if further muddying of the semantic waters had not occurred.

Today the word euthanasia is used to signify a number of practices that vary widely in their significance and impact, although all have one thing in common: the death of an individual human being. A brief analysis of those practices, all bearing the somewhat ambiguous title of euthanasia, will now be attempted.

1. The word euthanasia may be used to refer to voluntary mercy killing. This practice most closely conforms to the dictionary definition of euthanasia and refers to the direct killing of a person, on that person's request. One might think that the term "assisted suicide" would be more appropriate; however, there is a subtle shade of difference. The phrase "voluntary mercy killing" implies that some physical disorder, which results in the imminence of death and which probably is associated with increasing deterioration of the person and/or pain of a greater or lesser amount, is the motivation for the request to be put to death.[6] The phrase "assisted suicide" carries with it no such implication, but merely signifies that an individual, for any of a variety of reasons (dishonor, disgrace, despair, *etc.*), may request assistance in the act of suicide.

An example of voluntary mercy killing is the case of George Zygmanik. Mr. Zygmanik was a patient in the intensive care unit of Jersey Shore Medical Center in Neptune, New Jersey. He had been paralyzed from the neck down in a motorcycle accident and he begged his brother, Lester, to kill him. Lester smuggled a sawed off shotgun into the intensive care unit and fatally wounded George.[7]

2. The word euthanasia may be used to refer to the practice of directly inducing death with the prior authorization of the individual, that is, prior to the onset of the disease or disability, and provided that the person no longer is capable of expressing his/her wishes, the person executes a document authorizing someone to put him to death.[8] It seems that the phrase "mercy killing with prior authorization" is a more accurate description of this practice than is the word euthanasia.

An example of legislation permitting such a practice was introduced in the Idaho State Legislature (H.B.143) in 1969.[9]

3. The word euthanasia may refer to the practice of directly inducing death in an individual without the person's consent, but with the permission of those empowered to act in his/her behalf. Such a practice is referred to as noninvoluntary euthanasia.[10] The word "noninvoluntary" needs some clarification. The word voluntary means "brought about by one's own free choice."[11] The word involuntary means "not by choice, not consciously controlled."[12] The prefix non means "not . . . and is used to give a negative force, especially to nouns, adjectives, and adverbs; non- is less emphatic than in- and un- which often give a word the opposite meaning."[13] The word noninvoluntary, although not found in any dictionary of the English language, has been manufactured to describe those situations in which a proxy authorization is obtained for mercy killing. The word proxy means "the agency or function of a deputy; the authority to act for another"[14] and seems to be a most appropriate descriptive word for this practice. The phrase "mercy killing with proxy authorization" is a more accurate description of this practice than are euthanasia and noninvoluntary euthanasia.

An example of "mercy killing with proxy authorization" is the administration of an overdose to a child in the final stages of Tay Sachs Disease on the authorization of the child's parents.[15]

4. The word euthanasia may refer to the practice of directly inducing death for merciful reasons without the consent of the individual or anyone empowered to act in his/her behalf.[16] Some may feel that the practice could be described more accurately by the word "murder," but there are significant differences. The word "murder" means "the unlawful and malicious or premeditated killing of one human being by another."[17] The definition of mercy when used in this context appears to conform to the fourth definition of mercy that is presented in *Webster's New World Dictionary:* "kind or compassionate treatment; relief of suffering."[18] The qualifying adjective "mercy" precludes the use of the word "murder" to describe this practice, as the inclusion of the one (mercy) precludes the other (malice). Perhaps a more accurate description of this practice would be involuntary mercy killing.

An example of involuntary mercy killing was described as follows:

> ... "a mass of broken cranial and cerebral tissue emerged, the head was born to everyone's horror and the emaciated fetus began to cry—everyone was equally horrified. The mother would soon come out of the anesthetic and demand to see the baby. I undertook to bathe the baby myself ... I ... immersed the baby head first ..."—Lord Segal of England, describing how he drowned a newborn baby who had been mutilated at birth.[19]

5. The word euthanasia also is used in the contemporary English language to refer to the voluntary withholding of artificial life support mechanisms or treatments when such mechanisms or treatments offer little if any hope of benefit to the individual.[20] This practice involves consideration of the benefits (or lack of them) of treatment for a given patient. Once in possession of the known facts regarding his/her physical condition, the patient freely opts for no treatment. Such a practice more accurately could be described as a patient's right to refuse treatment, even though such refusal may result in death or the hastening of the moment of death.

One example of this practice could be the person with kidney failure who refuses to undergo dialysis or the individual with oat-cell carcinoma of the lung who refuses chemotherapy.

6. The word euthanasia often is used to refer to the withholding of artificial life support mechanisms and treatments with the prior voluntary authorization of the individual. That is, prior to the onset of the disease or disability and provided that the individual no longer is capable of expressing his/her wishes, the person executes a document authorizing the withholding of artificial life supports and treatments under certain conditions. Generally, this is the practice referred to in the Living Will.[21]

7. The word euthanasia may refer to a "noninvoluntary" withholding of artificial life support mechanisms or treatments when such mechanisms or treatments offer little if any hope of recovery.[22] Such a practice might be referred to accurately as proxy authorization to withhold treatment.

An example of proxy authorization to withhold treatment is a decision not to treat a newborn with significant defects on the authorization of the parents. One such example was described as follows:

> The hospital gave the baby no treatment other than pain killers—no antibiotics to fight infection and no oxygen therapy to aid his breathing. Just good nursing care and a diet of milk. As the baby lost strength, the nursing staff became so upset the hospital speeded up the hours of rotation. Peter couldn't hold down his food, so at his death, dehydration was severe. Meningitis had reoccurred .... Severe retardation, a mindless existence, would have been certain.[23]

8. The word euthanasia may refer to the involuntary withholding of artificial life support mechanisms or treatments when such mechanisms or treat-

ments offer little if any hope of recovery or when such treatments might prove to be excessively inconvenient to the family.24 Such a practice infers that there was no consent from the individual even though he or she was capable of giving consent. Such a practice should be referred to as the involuntary withholding of treatment.

An example of the involuntary withholding of treatment is as follows:

> The night before surgery, the woman's son-in-law called, reminded the doctor that he had performed approximately the same surgery on the woman several years earlier and asked him to cancel the surgery. If the physician operated the next day, the family savings would be wiped out and they would have to go without a color television, a second car and a larger home. He (the physician) explained that the few extra years she would gain from this operation would hardly justify the privation to which this young family would be subjected.25

9. The word euthanasia may be used to refer to the practice of the voluntary withdrawal of treatment or artificial life support mechanisms when such mechanisms or treatments a) have not significantly benefited the individual, b) no longer are effective in the treatment of the individual, c) prove to be excessively painful to the individual, or d) offer little if any hope of recovery to the individual. Such a practice should be referred to as the patient's right to withdraw from treatment.26

An example of the patient's right to withdraw from treatment is illustrated by a kidney dialysis patient who refuses to undergo further dialysis or who refuses to follow the diet regimen.

10. The word euthanasia may refer to prior authorization to withdraw treatment or artificial life support mechanisms under the same conditions listed above and provided that the individual is unable to communicate his/her wishes. Certainly the phrase "prior authorization to withdraw treatment" is more accurate and more specific than is the general term euthanasia.

An example of prior authorization to withdraw treatment is the removal of a respirator from an individual who has executed a Living Will and who is now comatose.

11. The word euthanasia commonly is used to refer to the practice of "non-involuntary" withdrawal of artificial life support mechanisms when such mechanisms have not significantly benefited the individual, no longer are effective in the treatment of the individual, prove excessively painful or offer little if any hope for recovery. Such a practice, however, could be described more accurately as proxy authorization to withdraw treatment than as euthanasia.

An example of proxy authorization to withdraw treatment is the celebrated Karen Ann Quinlan situation, in which the parents authorized the removal of a respirator from their apparently irreversibly comatose daughter in the full expectation that it would hasten the moment of her death.

12. The word euthanasia may be used to refer to the involuntary withdrawal of treatment or artificial life support mechanisms[27] under the same conditions listed in Number 11. Such a practice more accurately could be described as "involuntary withdrawal of treatment."

One example of involuntary withdrawal of treatment is the following:

> About four times in the past year, doctors at the Maryland Institute for Emergency Medicine turned off the respirator that was maintaining the life of a quadriplegic patient whose body was completely and irrevocably paralyzed—but whose brain was functioning. . . . The quadriplegics are never told their respirators are going to be turned off, and their families are told only obliquely, according to Dr. William Gill, clinical director of the Institute. . . . Their spinal cords have been severed at the base of the skull, usually in an accident, and they cannot live without mechanical aides. . . . They can think, see and hear. . . ."[28]

13. The word euthanasia may come closest to conforming to its etymological origins when it is used to refer to the care and treatment of dying patients as epitomized by St. Christopher's Hospice in Sydenham, England.[29] Such a practice, for clarity's sake, should be referred to as humane and reasonable care for the dying patient.

14. The word euthanasia may be used to describe a practice in which those who "would be certain to suffer any social handicap—for example, any physical or mental defect that would prevent marriage or would make others tolerate his company only from a sense of mercy."[30] are put directly and painlessly to death. The principal concern in this practice is not the individual; rather it is the aesthetic sensitivities of other persons in society. An aesthete may be defined as "a person highly sensitive to art and beauty; a person who exaggerates the value of artistic sensitivity or makes a cult of art or beauty."[31] The "goodness" of this death or the "mercy" exercised is for the aesthetic values of society, a society that places the highest value on youth and beauty. Therefore, it would seem more appropriate to refer to this practice as aesthetic killing. Some may think that murder would be a more accurate term, but there is a subtle difference. By definition, murder implies a malicious intent. The intent here is not strictly malicious; rather, it is characterized by a sincere desire to spare society the "pain" of viewing or supporting "those whom some persons would have difficulty in recognizing as human."[32]

A second motive for aesthetic killing may be to promote the improvement of the race,[33] in which case "eugenic killing" is a more accurate term than is euthanasia.

15. The word euthanasia may be used to describe a practice in which those who have little or no hope of recovery and who appear to be of little or no benefit to society are refused treatment.[34] The individual's potential and probable contribution to society is stressed; his/her wishes or potential for human fulfillment are not really factors in the decision making.[35] In such a

practice, the concern is clearly for the welfare of society as a whole rather than for the individual or for the individual's family. Such a practice, that is, "the selective utilization of medical resources [that are] inadequate to care for all those in need,"[36] more accurately could be described as deliberate medical triage than as euthanasia.

An example of deliberate medical triage well might be Dr. Walter Sackett's 1974 proposal in Florida for Death With Dignity.

> Sackett wants to include retarded citizens, especially profoundly retarded ones (he calls them grotesques), in the category of "terminally ill" people. He thinks the second and especially the third provisions of his bill would permit Florida to extinguish the lives of 90 percent of the 1,500 most retarded people in state hospitals. This, he says, would save billions of dollars that could be used for "good social purposes."[37]

16. The word euthanasia has been defined recently as "institution of therapy that it is hoped would hasten death."[38] The word therapy is a derivation of the word therapeutic, which is defined as "serving to cure or heal; curative; concerned in discovering and applying remedies for diseases."[39] The word death is defined as "the act or fact of dying; permanent cessation of life."[40] It is contradictory to use the word "therapy" in conjunction with the hastening of death unless there is redefinition either of death (as a cure for disease) or of therapy (as serving to kill, killing; concerned with hastening death), or possibly of both. For this reason, this contemporary definition is rejected as paradoxical and nonsensical.

In summary, then, the word euthanasia, as used in the contemporary English language, may refer to any one or all of the following: voluntary mercy killing, mercy killing by prior voluntary authorization, mercy killing with proxy authorization, involuntary mercy killing, the patient's right to refuse treatment, prior authorization to withhold treatment, proxy authorization to withhold treatment, involuntary withholding of treatment, the patient's right to withdraw from treatment, prior authorization to withdraw from treatment, proxy authorization to withdraw treatment, involuntary withdrawal of treatment, reasonable and humane care for the dying, aesthetic killing, eugenic killing, and/or deliberate medical triage.

The word euthanasia asserts diverse and widely divergent propositions related only because they all imply the death of an individual human being. The method or means (if any) used to induce death, the reasons for the inducement of death and the ramifications of the acceptance of these various practices are so dissimilar that the continued use of one term (euthanasia) to apply to all of these promulgates confusion rather than clarity. Therefore, the word euthanasia should be eliminated and replaced with the appropriate descriptive terminology. Such a course of action would allow for a more cogent exploration of the various ethical, legal, social, and medical factors inherent in the various practices and would promote rational discussion among those who are most seriously concerned about or most directly involved in such practices.

In the particular situation in question, that of the young man with the head injury, the practice involved can be described most accurately as "proxy authorization to withdraw treatment" and not as "euthanasia" by any other definition. This clarification now allows us to consider the second major ethical question raised by this case study, that is, "Under what circumstances may one person make a decision for another?"

THE SCOPE AND LIMITS OF PROXY CONSENT

To approach adequately the question of proxy consent, one first must examine four aspects of consent in general. First, consent is something that is peculiar to each person. It cannot be transferred. It applies to all human interactions, as is exemplified by the ancient law of battery that allows no unconsented touchings.[41] However, it also is true that once a patient is admitted to the hospital, health professionals cannot avoid touching the patient.[42] That is, physicians and nurses are not legally or morally free to do whatever they want once they have assumed the care of a patient: they must act and their actions necessarily include touching the patient—sometimes very invasive or intrusive touching. This is not to say that such touching is illegal or even wrong; it is to point out that the touching, although it may be authorized, is unconsented. Hence, in the situation under consideration, the parents may authorize action, but they really cannot consent for their son.

The particular mix of these factors and the relative importance attached to each can become quite complex; not infrequently, judicial clarification is sought. It is important to note that in cases of proxy consent, the courts most often put emphasis on health professionals' obligations to act in the best interests of patients or clients. In cases regarding the consent of competent adults, the courts usually favor the patients' decisions *even if they are not in their own best interests.*

Second, for consent to be valid, it must be both uncoerced and informed.[43] If operations or procedures are offered without discussion of their relative risks and benefits, consent is meaningless.[44] The problems of informing patients and their families are relatively insignificant when they are considered next to the proviso that consent (or authorization) be uncoerced, because few things are as coercive as the threat of suffering and death, or conversely, the threat of continued life in a state of profound disability.

Third, consent frequently is uninformed even when health professionals conscientiously try to share relevant information.[45] If the problems were due solely to power lust on the part of health professionals or even to poor communication with patients and their families, definitive steps could be taken to correct the deficiencies. Unfortunately, the problems involved in the adequate informing of patients are far more complex: they include a mix of fear, pain (physical and psychological), trauma, dependence, social and institutional pressures, guilt, anxiety and, occasionally, the desire to escape.

Fourth, "Consent may be a necessary but not sufficient condition for doing something to someone, particularly when death is involved."[46] For example, free and informed consent does not justify homicide.[47] If consent is not sufficient to justify homicide, is parental (or spousal, *etc.*) authorization sufficient to justify causing death indirectly through the withdrawal of artificial means of sustaining life?

With this brief discussion of some of the problems of consent as a background, one can approach a discussion of the conditions necessary for voluntary consent to the withdrawal of treatment when death is the expected outcome. If it is not morally permissible for a rational adult to consent to the withdrawal of treatment under such circumstances, it would be difficult, if not impossible, to defend a decision to withdraw the treatment that is necessary to sustain someone else's life.[48]

For voluntary withdrawal from treatment under these circumstances (*i.e.,* life and death circumstances), to be justified, three conditions would have to be met. First, a conscious decision to participate in one's own premature death would have to be justifiable. It should be noted that the death would not be premature if no interventions were undertaken. There are significant differences between suicide and not doing everything possible to prolong one's life. In the latter case, the person is not refusing to save his life—he is refusing to prolong the process of his dying. What is at stake, then, is not a "right to die" but rather the rights to bodily integrity and self-determination, both derivatives of the right to life. Such a decision involves an acceptance (or rejection) of the conditions imposed on human life and a conscious decision to participate in or control a most significant event in one's life—its end. In view of imminent and inevitable death, and given a respect for the rights to bodily integrity and self-determination, a conscious patient not only has a right to make decisions, but he also may have a duty to make his own decision.[49] That is, it is justifiable for a patient to make a conscious decision to withdraw from treatment, even if it results in his premature death.

Second, if it is justifiable for a rational, adult patient to refuse treatment under these circumstances, it also would have to be justifiable for nurses and physicians to cooperate with or to participate in such a decision.[50] But, is it ever justifiable for health professionals to cooperate with a person's decision to end his life prematurely by refusing treatment? In other words, may health professionals help people to participate in or control the conditions surrounding their dying?

Although one thrust of the health care endeavor is to resist death, another is to relieve suffering. In the exercise of either of these activities, health professionals are obliged to respect the human rights of patients. Moreover, in the face of a patient's near and inevitable death, health professionals are not required by law or by ethical concern to intervene in a natural process—

particularly when such intervention is unwanted, inappropriate and, ultimately, ineffective. Hence, it is justifiable for health professionals to cooperate with a patient's decision to refuse treatment under these circumstances.

Third, it would have to be demonstrated that the criteria for informed consent could be met when a person is dying. If patients often are uninformed under less trying circumstances, is it likely that truly informed consent for death could be demonstrated? Certainly, conscious patients and their families almost universally understand the meaning of the word death. If health professionals tell them that death will come sooner if some medication is omitted or some treatment is withdrawn, they generally understand what is said. Such explanations surely are not as complex as discussions of what is involved in a coronary by-pass or abdominal–perineal resection. Moreover, even though the condition of being near death often is associated with an inability to make rational judgments, this is not always the case. However, the problem of coercion is omnipresent. To be offered the choice, "Do you want to die or do you want to suffer and then die?" certainly does not present agreeable alternatives. Unfortunately, such options may be the case for the patient. Although health professionals cannot eliminate pain, suffering or death, they should make it clear (no matter which choice a patient makes) that suffering can be mitigated and that death can be delayed but not prevented. Reality, presented as gently as possible, can be understood. Perhaps the coercion is still there, but it is nature's coercion, not ours.

If one can accept the premise that a person justifiably can participate consciously in his own premature death under certain circumstances, with the cooperation of health professionals, one now can approach the question, "Under what circumstances may one person decide to withdraw life-sustaining treatment for someone else?"

One way to approach this problem is to use what is called the principle of substituted judgment. That is, an ideal observer[51] must ask what this person might want under these circumstances if he were competent to decide for himself. Even if one assumed that all people have a natural desire to live, nearly everyone would agree that there are some circumstances that would make continued existence intolerable. Moreover, if one were offered a long life in a deep coma (given that the diagnosis was sound and the prognosis was clear), it is difficult to understand why anyone would want to be so maintained.[52] The more deeply comatose a person, the less likely it is that he could "want" anything in the sense of being able to formulate a wish to die—or even to live. However, if a person were to substitute his judgment for someone else's,[53] he might superimpose an alien value structure on that person or family. This factor is particularly significant when disability or death is the projected outcome of a decision. There also is an added risk that one might confuse his own suffering or the suffering of others with the patient's suffering.[54]

If an individual is not suffering, there seems to be no persuasive argument that, in a moment of lucidity, he certainly will wish to die. In short, it cannot be concluded definitively that, unless the comatose state is irreversible, one confidently can allow an individual to die using the notion of substituted judgment.

The justifications put forth for allowing incompetent patients to die can be divided roughly into three arguments, each seeking to maximize the interests of a different group: society, the family or the patient.

The societal arguments usually emphasize the cost of care for such a person. Also, a concern is expressed for social justice in the distribution of health resources. Aside from the implication in this argument that an individual's life should be subject to the economic considerations of the community, there are other objections to it. First, society is inconsistent in its application of cost–benefit analyses. Irreversibly retarded, irreversibly mentally ill, irreversibly aged and irreversibly and completely handicapped people are maintained by society. Why should any particular type or group of persons be excluded? Certainly, some people call for the elimination of all unproductive persons, but is this an acceptable alternative? Moreover, society preserves and maintains the lives of criminals who have deliberately damaged others because many thoughtful persons disagree about the legitimacy of the death penalty for even the most heinous of crimes. How, then, can one justify the denial of life to someone who has done no wrong and whose only "crime" is a debilitated body or mind?

Although it is both necessary and proper for a social body, such as a legislature, to establish guidelines for the distribution of health resources, is it proper for individual health providers to make clinical decisions about individual patients *vis à vis* whether a person will be of benefit to society? Are doctors and nurses competent to make such decisions? By what criteria? According to whose values? The notion that health professionals should withdraw or withhold their services according to a personal assessment of the social utility of patients or clients is rejected categorically.

A second justification that is put forth for allowing an incompetent person to die is that it best serves the interests of his family.[55] In short, health professionals should allow incompetent patients to die so that their families will not be burdened. Several considerations are involved in this premise. If one holds the position that this course of action can be taken only if the family agrees to or demands it, then one must presume that professionals are not moral agents, that is, that they bear no responsibility for their actions, and they are merely the instruments of the decisions of others. Such a position also infers that parents or other family members "own" the patient and may dispose of this person as they see fit. The third is that the family members' (parents', *etc.*) interests always should take precedence over the best interests of the patient. There is no clear reason why this must be so, other than perhaps a utilitarian calculus that infers many other premises in addition to this one.

On the other hand, if one holds the notion that health professionals alone should determine what action is in the patient's best interests, one not only risks the imposition of an alien value structure on patient and family, but also denies the legitimate authority and concern of the patient's family. Such a posture is both presumptuous and arrogant.

While the court decision regarding Karen Ann Quinlan appears to give support to the notion that parents have absolute control over the destiny of their minor or incompetent children,[56] there are many court decisions that indicate otherwise. The New Jersey Supreme Court gave custody to Karen Ann's parents only on the presumption that withdrawal of treatment was in *her* best interests.[57] In addition, the Court made it clear that this decision could be made only if a hospital committee composed of numerous persons from various disciplines agreed with it.[58] *The court did not say that the decision to discontinue care was justified on the grounds that it served her parents' interests.* Finally, the central ethical commitment of health professionals is primarily to patients or clients and only secondarily to families. These priorities ought not to be confused.

A third justification for allowing someone to die is based on the presumption that it is in the person's best interests. Such a presumption naturally leads one to inquire how the best interests of an incompetent patient should be defined. Four guidelines could be used:

1. Any such decision should be based on as much information as possible.

2. The rights and duties of all persons involved in the decision making should be weighed and balanced carefully. This must include consideration of the patient's values (if known), the family's wishes, the laws of the state or province and the professional, ethical, and legal obligations of health care providers (personal and institutional).

3. The socially cherished obligations to preserve life and to relieve suffering cannot be discounted. The consequences of alternative courses of action must be projected and weighed carefully. The health professionals must keep in mind at all times that they are substituting their judgments for that of the patient in very critical decisions.

4. Given the fact that many people are involved in such decisions in the modern hospital and that each of these people must bear moral and legal responsibility for his/her actions, it is not permissible for one person to make a unilateral decision for the death of another person. This position was given recognition and support by the New Jersey Supreme Court's decision regarding Karen Ann Quinlan. The court rejected the notion that such decisions were solely a medical prerogative and recognized and protected her parents' right to participate in decisions regarding her medical care. However, the court stated that the decision to withdraw treatment would be valid only if it were approved by a hospital committee,[59] that is, that such a decision would not be a prerogative solely of a physician and family. Another acknowledgement of the shared nature of such decisions can be found both in the *Report of the Critical Care Committee of the Massachusetts General Hospital*[60] and in the Beth Israel Hospital of Boston's document, *Orders Not to Resuscitate*.[61]

In summary, proxy decisions regarding the withdrawal of care are limited by several circumstances: (1) The decision must be informed. (2) The decision must be demonstrated to be in the best interests of the patient. (3) The decision must not be unilateral, that is, it must be a shared decision.

ANALYSIS

Complex problems do not lend themselves to simplistic solutions. The introduction of serious ethical problems increases stress at a time when parents, nurses and physicians are under great tension. At times, it may seem that professional therapeutic duty to the family can be fulfilled only at the expense of the patient—or conversely, that therapeutic duty to the patient can be fulfilled only at the cost of the family's suffering. Although it is very difficult to engage in serious ethical reflection at such times, often it can offer alternatives.

Neither an absolute policy that requires maximal treatment for all incompetents nor a totally permissive policy that allows family members alone to decide can be defended. The former leads to the ridiculous and inhumane practice of trying to keep everyone alive forever. The latter implies that a family's authority over its members is absolute—and includes the right to engineer the death of an ill member if his or her existence threatens the happiness of other members of the family. An ethically defensible resolution to the apparent dilemma presented in this case must be found in the difficult ground between these extremes.

Families may misunderstand relevant data. Their decisions may be affected by feelings of guilt or fear. Moreover, families as well as health professionals may reach decisions that are based on ill-begotten notions of compassion and, indeed, may confuse both issues and priorities. Although attempts to find an ethically defensible solution can increase tension for all people involved, the consequences of the ignoring or the obscuring of the ethical issues may be irreversible and the harm done may be incalculable.

A careful reading of this case study highlights three major points: (1) the boy's condition was critical but not yet hopeless; (2) the parents seemed to confuse decisions regarding custody with decisions regarding care; and (3) the medical and nursing personnel experienced a conflict between their compassion for the parents' problems and their obligations to the young patient. For the sake of clarity, each point will be addressed separately.

1. What is *known* about this seventeen-year-old accident victim is as follows: (a) He is in good health apart from the injuries that resulted from his accident. (b) Despite the fact that all other vital signs are negative, an electroencephalogram indicates that there still is brain activity. It also should be noted that, given the severity of the trauma, it is not unusual (though certainly not desirable) for the patient still to be in a deep coma. (c) The extent of damage to the patient's brain cannot be assessed accurately until the swelling subsides— provided that he survives that long. The health professionals at least ought to know that all the data are not in yet—and they should so inform the parents.

To act rashly, precipitously, and irreversibly on a scanty data base is neither professionally nor ethically defensible—however much one might sympathize with the parents' burdens.

2. Families can and do have a right to participate in decisions regarding the care and treatment of their members. However, their moral and legal authority is not absolute. Moreover, the unconscious motivations that may enter into the act of relieving oneself of what may appear to be a lifelong burden to care for a totally dependent person cannot be discounted. Such a prospect could overwhelm almost anyone.

Therefore, decisions about care and custody can and must be separated.[62] Decisions about care often are urgent and irrevocable. Decisions about custody (if it should become an issue) not only are not urgent, but are reversible. Not only will the separation of these two issues allow families to distinguish urgent decisions from less immediate concerns, but it also will provide more time for data collection. Thus, future decisions can be grounded more firmly and based on sound information.

The separation of decisions about care and decisions about custody may reduce the conflict of interests between the family and a (possibly permanently) disabled patient. It acknowledges the fact that the continued existence of the patient may threaten the emotional, social and financial well-being of the family and it helps to reduce tensions: families no longer have to choose between authorizing death or committing themselves to life-long care.

3. Finally, the effect of the emotional and professional conflicts that nurses and physicians experience cannot be underestimated. Health professionals are human beings, too, and the emotional drain of experiencing human tragedy on an almost daily basis can be devastating. Nurses and physicians who experience the pressure of knowing that their efforts on the patient's behalf are increasing the suffering of a family may lose perspective and judgment. Whether the family's request is implicit or explicit (as in this case), health professionals must be astute enough to recognize the quandary. If the tension is acute, health care professionals should withdraw from the treatment of one or the other. This does not mean that either (or both) the patient or family is to be abandoned, but merely that steps must be taken to reduce the conflict.

This can be accomplished in a number of ways, one of which is to request a psychiatric clinical nurse specialist, family therapist, or social worker to intervene. Such an alternative requires institutional support and interdisciplinary cooperation. Both nurses and physicians must learn to recognize the limits of their psychological strength. Indeed, it may not be possible for one person or even one group of professionals to care for the whole family.[63] When this is the case, all may be better served by recognizing the problems and taking steps to see that the needs of individuals are met (as far as possible) by those who are most capable of meeting them. That is, individual professionals must learn to use effectively the resources that are available to them. This proposal may seem radical (how dare one suggest that nurses or doctors *cannot* do everything!), but it offers a realistic method of approach to tension-filled, conflict-laden, emotionally draining situations.

Certainly, there are situations in which it is fully appropriate to withdraw care, but decisions to do so should be reached carefully in the light of as much information as possible. Moreover, clinical decisions should be based on what is in the patient's best interests, whether or not the decisions are in accord with the best interests of the family. In this particular situation a number of actions should be taken:

1. A case conference should be held to share information and to discuss the ethical problems raised in this situation.

2. Care and custody decisions should be separated for the parents, and other realistic options should be presented.

3. The health professionals already caring for the patient should request intervention from others who can concentrate their energies on caring for the family.

4. The time that is gained by these actions should be used to collect more information.

OUTCOME

The final events in this case are dramatic and instructive. The swelling of the brain decreased and the boy returned to consciousness. The use of the respirator no longer was required and, in due course, hyperalimentation was discontinued. Brain damage appeared to be minimal, although the boy seemed to have "lost" all his education, (*e.g.,* he was unable to read, to count, to write or to spell). The parents' increasing anxiety throughout these necessarily prolonged events was alleviated by the intervention of a psychiatric nursing clinical specialist. In her discussions with the family, the possibility of relinquishing custody on either a permanent or temporary basis was raised. Although the parents did not choose this option, the knowledge that it was available served to alleviate some of the pressures on them. The stress on the medical and nursing staff was decreased as the parents no longer requested that their son be allowed to die. The boy's positive response to the treatment and his return to consciousness encouraged all people who were involved. Hence, when he developed a brain abscess and died following emergency surgery, everyone was shocked and upset.

The essentially tragic nature of this situation was alleviated for the staff members by the development of a spirit of mutual comfort and support and, perhaps, by the development of an understanding of their own limits and needs for assistance. They acquired some new resources to help them survive the pathos of their professions. The parents who lived through this tragedy have returned to a more normal life. They remember the courage and the suffering of their son more than the trials and hardships that caused their own suffering. Moreover, all persons involved know that they did the best they could in the face of uncertainty and finitude.

COMMENTARY: CONSENT, CONFLICT, AND "EUTHANASIA"

M. Josephine Flaherty

The ethical implications of euthanasia are addressed in considerable detail in Curtin's discussion of this situation, and many aspects of the question are explained and illustrated. The pressures on different people involved are highlighted and clarified. In many respects, in spite of the young man's dramatic death, the outcome is not an unhappy one.

One aspect of the situation that is particularly significant is the recognition by the participants of both their responsibilities for and limitations in the caring dimension of their roles in the planning and implementation of the patient's therapeutic regime. The separation of the custody and care dimensions was of great value, not only to the family but also to the members of the health care team. As was mentioned, the daily contact with devastating medical conditions, which is experienced by health care professionals in special care units, and the far-reaching emotional and social effects of these situations on the families, on the health care institutions and their staff members, and on society can (and do) drain the strength of even the strongest human beings. That the health professionals and the family members recognized this, sought and accepted the specialized skills and care of another health care professional, the psychiatric clinical specialist nurse, was a commendable example of the true "caring quality" and teamwork of medical and nursing practice behavior. It had happy consequences for those concerned, all of whom were strengthened by it and were thus more capable of dealing with the situation.

This case study is not only illustrative of the complexity of the question of euthanasia, but is illustrative of the necessity for genuine teamwork and for thoughtful and informed reflection by the group of people—health care professionals and lay persons alike—who are involved in the critical care of patients. It is an example of one of the realities of health care of the eighties—that although incredible scientific and technical advances have been made in medicine and in health care, no amount of technology will ever be a "substitute for sobriety, common sense and discernment in the search for the patient's (and the family's) good."[64]

NOTES

1. Passmore, John. *A Hundred Years of Philosophy* (Penguin Books, New York, 1968) p. 427.
2. *Ibid.,* p. 428.

3. Ryle, Gilbert. "Systematically Misleading Expressions," in Morris Weitz, ed. *Twentieth Century Philosophy: The Analytic Tradition* (The Free Press, New York, 1966) p. 183.

4. Callahan, Daniel. In a lecture presented at the International Institute of Health Care, Ethics and Human Values held at Mt. St. Joseph College, Mt. St. Joseph, Ohio, July 1976.

5. *Webster's New World Dictionary.* Unabridged, Second Edition (World Publishing, New York, 1966).

6. Anonymous. *A Plan for Voluntary Euthanasia,* Second Revised Edition (Euthanasia Society of England, 1962).

7. Mitchell, P. *Act of Love: The Killing of George Zygmanik* (Alfred A. Knopf, New York, 1976).

8. Mannes, Marva. *Last Rights: A Case for the Good Death* (William Morrow and Company, New York, 1974).

9. In this act, euthanasia is defined as the painless inducement of death. Introduced in the Idaho State Legislature in 1969, this bill did not pass. However, the summary of the bill read "An act declaring the administration of euthanasia lawful, subject to the provisions of this act; defining terms; providing for the signing of a declaration in the presence of two witnesses and for the administration of euthanasia in accordance with the terms of the declaration; providing the time when a declaration becomes effective and for the holding of the declaration; providing for the revocation of a declaration; providing the form for a declaration; providing for reports on the condition of hospital patients who have made declarations and providing that physicians or nurses shall not be required to assist in the administration of euthanasia; providing for the administration of drugs; providing that physicians who administer euthanasia are not guilty of any offense; providing for the notification of the county coroner; providing that physicians and nurses who take part in the administration of euthanasia shall not be deemed to have breached any professional oath or affirmation; providing penalties; providing for regulations by the State Board of Health; providing severability, and providing a short title." Entitled the "Voluntary Euthanasia Act of 1969."

10. Kole, Marvin, ed. *Beneficent Euthanasia* (Prometheus Books, New York, 1975) p. 143.

11. *Webster's, op. cit.*

12. *Ibid.*

13. *Ibid.*

14. *Ibid.*

15. Fletcher, Joseph. "Ethics and Euthanasia," *American Journal of Nursing,* Vol. 73 (April 1973) pp. 670–675.

16. *Ibid.*

17. *Webster's, op. cit.*

18. *Ibid.*

19. "Mercy Killing: When Doctors Play God," *The News,* Zalienpole, Pa. November 3, 1973.

20. *Interim Hearing on the Rights of the Terminally Ill,* California State Assembly, San Francisco, California, October 8, 1974, p. 8.

21. Both "Living Will" and "The Christian Affirmation of Life" state sets of beliefs and delineate circumstances under which individuals do not want their dying prolonged by the use of artificial means of sustaining life. A copy of "Living Will" can be

obtained from the Society for a Good Death, 250 West 57th Street, New York, New York 10019. Copies of "The Christian Affirmation of Life" are available from the Publication Department of the Catholic Health Association, 1438 South Grand Boulevard, St. Louis, Missouri 63104.

22. Duff, R. and A. G. M. Campbell. "Moral and Ethical Dilemmas in the Special Care Nursery," *New England Journal of Medicine,* 289, (October 25, 1973) p. 894.

23. Pell, Roger. "The Agonizing Decision of Joanne and Roger Pell," *Good Housekeeping* (January 1972) p. 35.

24. Hall, Elizabeth and Paul Cameron. "Our Failing Reverence for Life," *Psychology Today* (April 1976) p. 106.

25. *Ibid.*

26. Fletcher, *op. cit.*

27. Colen, B. D. "Doctors Decide Life Support End," *Washington Post,* March 10, 1974.

28. *Ibid.*

29. Morrison, Robert S. "Dying," *Scientific American* (September 1973) pp. 55–61.

30. Will, George F. "Death With Dignity?" *Cincinnati Post,* May 20, 1974.

31. *Webster's, op. cit.*

32. Will, *op. cit.*

33. Alexander, Leo. "Medical Science Under Dictatorship," *Child and Family,* Vol. 10, No. 1 (1971) p. 40.

34. Wertz, Richard, ed. *Readings on Ethical and Social Issues in Biomedicine* (Prentice-Hall, New York, 1973) p. 146.

35. *Ibid.*

36. *Ibid.,* p. 154.

37. Will, *op. cit.*

38. Williams, Robert H. "The End of Life in the Elderly," *Postgraduate Medicine,* Vol. 54 (December 1973) p. 58.

39. *Webster's, op. cit.*

40. *Ibid.*

41. Prosser, W. L. *Law of Torts* (West Publishing Company, Minneapolis, Minnesota, 1972).

42. Robertson, J. A. "Involuntary Euthanasia of Defective Newborns," *Stanford Law Review,* Vol. 27 (1975) pp. 213–269.

43. Beecher, Henry K. *Research and the Individual* (Little, Brown, Boston, 1970) pp. 30–31.

44. *Canterbury v. Spence* 464 F2D 772 (1972).

45. *Cf.* Fletcher, John. "Realities of Patient Consent to Medical Research," *Hastings Center Report,* Vol. 1 (1973) pp. 39–49.

    Gray, H. B. *Human Subjects in Medical Experimentations* (Wiley Interscience, New York, 1975).

    Ingelfinger, Franz J. "Informed But Uneducated Consent," *New England Journal of Medicine* Vol. 287 (1972) pp. 465–466.

46. Frost, Norman. "Proxy Consent for Seriously Ill Newborns," in David Smith and Linda Bernstein, eds. *No Rush to Judgment* (Indiana University Foundation, Bloomington, 1978) p. 4.

47. LaFave, W. and A. Scott. *Handbook of Criminal Law* (West Publishing Company, St. Paul, Minnesota, 1972).

48. Frost, *op. cit.,* p. 5.

49. All rights carry with them corollary duties. If a person has a right to determine his own future and to determine what will happen to his body, the person also has the corollary moral duty to make such decisions. Conversely, others have a duty to respect this person's decisions and, at the very least, not to interfere with this person in the exercise of his right or duty. To the degree that a person is incapable of fulfilling the duties of moral correlativity, others assume this duty for him.

50. Frost, *op. cit.,* p. 5.

51. For a thorough discussion of this matter see: Firth R. "Ethical Absolutism and the Ideal Observer," *Philosophy and Phenomenological Research* Vol. 12 (1952) pp. 317–345. Firth suggests that an ideal judge should have the following qualities: (1) omniscience, (2) omnipercipience, (3) disinterest, (4) dispassionateness, and (5) consistency.

52. Frost, *op. cit.,* p. 7.

53. Robertson, *op. cit.,* p. 48.

54. Cooke, Robert E. "Whose Suffering?" *Journal of Pediatrics,* Vol. 80 (1972) p. 906.

55. *Cf.* Duff, R. S. and A. G. M. Campbell. *op. cit.,* pp. 890–894.

   Gustafson, J. "Mongolism, Parental Desires, and the Right to Life," *Perspectives in Biological Medicine,* Vol. 16 (1973) pp. 529–557.

56. *In the matter of Karen Ann Quinlan, An Alleged Incompetent.* Supreme Court of New Jersey, A-116, March 31, 1976.

57. *Ibid.*

58. *Ibid.*

59. *Ibid.*

60. "Optimum Care for Hopelessly Ill Patients: A Report of the Critical Care Committee of the Massachusetts General Hospital," *The New England Journal of Medicine,* Vol. 295, No. 7 (August 12, 1976) pp. 362–364.

61. Rabkin, Mitchell, George Gillerman and Nancy Rice. "Orders Not to Resuscitate," *The New England Journal of Medicine,* Vol. 295, No. 7 (August 12, 1976) pp. 364–366.

62. Frost, *op. cit.,* p. 15.

63. *Ibid.,* p. 16.

64. Kass, Leon R. "Ethical Dilemmas in the Care of the Ill," *Journal of the American Medical Association,* Vol. 244, No. 17 (October 24/31, 1980) p. 1946.

Case Study V: Abortion, Privacy, and Conscience

Leah Curtin

In 1974 Mary Jane S. was the head nurse on a gynecology ward in a large metropolitan hospital. Following the 1973 U.S. Supreme Court decision on abortion, many saline abortions were performed in the hospital. Although the saline was injected in the operating room, the patients were transferred to the gynecology floor where the nurses usually delivered the dead fetuses in the patients' rooms. The entire nursing staff of the gynecology ward was upset about this situation.

Moreover, the nurses questioned the validity of the patients' consent to this procedure for two reasons: (1) many patients thought the procedure would be completed when the saline was injected—they did not know that they would have to go through labor and delivery; and (2) if the patients happened to see a fetus (and many of them did, despite the precautions taken by the nursing staff), they expressed shock at the size and form of the fetus.

To exacerbate matters further, the hospital administration determined that, to relieve the heavy schedule of the operating room, the saline injection was to be performed in the treatment room on the gynecology ward. The head nurse and staff nurses objected on two grounds: (1) the treatment room was not equipped with oxygen or other emergency equipment to cope with complications that might arise; and (2) although they had cared for patients after injection of saline, they refused, on grounds of conscience, to participate directly in the destruction of the fetus. The head nurse sent a written statement to the nursing office, signed by each staff nurse and by her, that stated that they would not comply with this directive, listed their reasons and expressed the nurses' concerns about the lack of informed consent for this procedure. In response, the director of nursing informed them in writing that they must comply or lose their jobs.

239

At the root of this situation is the issue of abortion and the complex moral questions that it raises for society, for women who seek abortions and for those who perform or assist in the performance of abortions. In addition, this case study raises questions about relationships among professional nurses' personal values, their professional ethics, their obligations to the institutions that employ them, and their statutory rights and obligations. The questions raised by the issue of abortion are: (1) "What actually occurs in an abortion and why would anyone object to participating in an abortion procedure?" (2) "Is there a legal right to abortion and, if so, do health personnel have a legal obligation to provide abortions?" Other questions raised in this case study can be phrased as follows: (1) "What are the legal and moral rights of abortion patients to nursing care?" (2) "What is the role of the nurse, if any, in obtaining informed consent for abortion procedures?" (3) "What are the legal and moral rights and obligations of the staff nurses in this situation?" (4) "What are the legal and moral rights and obligations of the administrative nurses?" and (5) "What are the legal and moral obligations of the hospital?"

ABORTION AS AN ISSUE

Moral philosophers are in considerable disagreement (as are nurses) about what actually occurs in abortions and, particularly, in late abortions.[1] Nearly every serious moral commentator, "whether pro-abortion or anti-abortion, recognizes that fetal life is (1) life, (2) a necessary precursor to what everyone agrees is a morally relevant state of being, and (3) once ended, some possible person will not exist. Put in another way, nearly everyone recognizes that killing a fetus at any stage [of development] is killing, ending or preventing someone just like us from being, and that only a moral idiot would suppose that the fetus is better off for not having been born."[2]

Most thoughtful commentators also recognize that pregnancy and child-rearing can involve serious hardships for women and families. "Specific and direct harm, medically diagnosable even in early pregnancy, may be involved. Maternity, or additional offspring, may force upon the woman a distressful life and future. Psychological harm may be imminent. Mental and physical health may be taxed by child care. There also is the distress . . . associated with an unwanted child, and there is the problem of bringing a child into a family already unable . . . to care for it. In other cases . . . the additional difficulties and continuing stigma of unwed motherhood may be involved."[3]

What is at issue in the abortion debate is the status of the fetus as a member of the human species when the existence of the fetus poses a threat to the physical, psychological or social well-being of a pregnant woman and/or other family members. At the crux of the anti-abortion argument is the humanity of the fetus and the danger to all persons that is posed by a public policy that permits or promotes the destruction of any human being according to age or stage of development. At the crux of the pro-abortion argument is the pregnant woman's right to self-determination and the sociopolitical problems posed by unwanted parenthood.

In essence, the abortion debate involves questions of value rather than questions of fact. Serious advocates of abortion do not deny either the existence of the fetus (by claiming that it is only a potential, not an actual being) or the fact that a human fetus is a member of the species *homo sapiens*.[4] What they do claim is that even though the fetus is a human being in the earliest stages of development, it is not yet a person in terms of the characteristics that usually are ascribed to personhood (*e.g.,* awareness of existence, cognition, emotion, etc.).[5]

Pro-abortion commentators argue that their position allows for recognition of the evolving, changing, maturing aspects of human life and does not deny the reality of the present. That is, they acknowledge the fact that the fetus is a member of the human species but they claim that the fetus does not have human rights because it is not fully a person and only human persons possess human rights. Therefore, if there is any conflict between the well-being of the fetus (human being) and the well-being of the woman (human being *and* person) who carries that fetus, the woman's interests always should prevail.

In answer to such claims, anti-abortion commentators point out that such a position is based on opinion and not on fact. The biological facts indicate that the fetus is a member of the human species; they claim that one human being should not be destroyed merely because a second human being may suffer social, emotional, or even physical harm because of the first human being's existence. Moreover, an anti-abortion commentator will claim that many human beings (*e.g.,* infants, the mentally retarded, the comatose, the mentally ill, the senile, and so forth) do not demonstrate all of the characteristics usually ascribed to personhood. The pro-abortionists' argument separates humanhood from personhood by ascribing human rights only to persons and by denying them to some members of the human species. The anti-abortionists claim that this is both arbitrary and dangerous because it places all human beings who do not meet certain standards of excellence at risk of death if their existence threatens the well-being of the elite who do meet such standards.

Although many anti-abortion commentators would allow destruction of a fetus as part of a procedure intended to save the life of a pregnant woman, they would not permit abortions in situations in which pregnancy results from incest or rape. Although many pro-abortion commentators would limit abortions to the first trimester of pregnancy, many others hold the position that abortion is acceptable at any time throughout the pregnancy. Some people hold the position that abortions are morally acceptable only if they are undertaken for such serious reasons as rape, incest, or deformity of the child; others hold that abortions done for personal or psychological reasons are morally acceptable because the fetus is not a person and therefore its status is determined solely by the value the mother chooses to place on it.

MORALITY AND LEGALITY

Arguments, debates, discussions, and articles about abortion frequently confuse two separate and distinct issues—to wit, the morality of abortion and the legality of it. Both opponents and proponents of abortion obscure these issues with emotional rhetoric, appeals to compassion, and contradictory claims. However, they seem to hold at least one point of view in common— that whether abortion should be legal or illegal hinges on its morality. They assume that what is moral must be legal and, conversely, that what is immoral must be illegal. This equation of legality and morality may lead to a dangerous form of legal positivism that grants absolute moral authority together with legal authority to the state, usually through the court system. The position taken is that rights are what the courts say they are: there are no rights except those enforced by law. Thus, prior to court decisions, no rights exist; there are only claims and counterclaims. Therefore, legal positivists claim that "there are no 'rights' in the abortion issue at all until the conflicting claims of fetal life and maternal privacy have been resolved by the courts, and then there shall be only those rights the courts assign."[6]

Although rarely addressed or even recognized in abortion debates, this assumption constitutes a serious threat to both parties, in that it denies that either the woman or the fetus has inherent rights. It extends the power of the state to such an extent that no one has a right to life, a right to self-determination, a right to privacy, or any other right unless the state chooses to grant such rights. According to this view, no human being has a just claim against the state unless the state chooses to recognize that claim. Therefore, not only are the actions of any state legal, but they also are right, good, and proper because the state has been invested with all moral as well as legal authority. Individuals, when faced with the power of the state, are stripped of human rights and "legitimately" may be used to advance the interests, concerns, or goals (temporary or permanent) of the state. Thus, for example, in the area of abortion, women could be forced by the state to have abortions when the state judges it to be in its best interests or, conversely, they could be ordered by the state to carry pregnancies to term when it is in the state's interests.

The blind assumption that what is legal must be moral is one of the most significant issues in the abortion debate because it strips all human beings of human rights. With this in mind, one can analyze the legal status of abortion and its ramifications for health professionals.

ABORTION AND LEGAL RIGHTS

The courts traditionally and legitimately have served both as protectors of rights and as arbiters in conflicts of rights situations. Although contemporary court decisions have tended to recognize fetal rights in some circumstances,[7] they also always have made distinctions about what legal rights pertain to individuals according to age, marital status, mental competence, and so forth.

In recent years, the courts and, in particular, the U.S. Supreme Court, have recognized and slowly developed protections for certain zones of privacy— whether or not the actions occurring in those zones be commendable or reprehensible.[8] In fact, the U.S. Supreme Court's decision on abortion rested heavily on the articulation of a Constitutional right to privacy. The majority opinion read:

> The Constitution does not explicitly mention any right of privacy. In a line of decisions, however, going back perhaps as far as *Union Pacific v. Botsford,* 141 U.S. 250, 251 (1891), the Court has recognized that a right of personal privacy, or a guarantee of certain areas or zones of privacy, does exist under the Constitution. In varying contexts the Court or individual justices have indeed found at least the roots of that right in the First Amendment . . .[9] in the Fourth and Fifth Amendments . . .[10] in the penumbras of the Bill of Rights . . .[11] in the Ninth Amendment . . .[12] or in the concept of liberty guaranteed by the first section of the Fourteenth Amendment. . . .[13] These decisions make it clear that only personal rights that can be deemed 'fundamental' or 'implicit' in the concept of ordered liberty . . .[14] are included in this guarantee of personal privacy. They also make it clear that the right has some extension to activities relating to marriage . . .[15] procreation . . .[16] contraception . . .[17] family relationships . . .[18] and child rearing and education . . .[19]

In reaching its decision about abortion, the U.S. Supreme Court found that the Constitution does not define "person" clearly and, that as most court decisions applied the term "person" to the fetus only postnatally, the fetus is not protected by the Fourteenth Amendment. Therefore, in weighing the conflicting claims of the protagonists the Court determined that "the right of privacy, however based, is broad enough to cover the abortion decision; that the right, nonetheless, is not absolute and is subject to some limitations; and that at some point the state interests as to protection of health, medical standards, and prenatal life, become dominant."[20]

In addition, the Court recognized the place of conscience and explicitly protected freedom of conscience among health professionals.[21] In summary, the U.S. Supreme Court did not proclaim a right to abortion; rather it placed such a decision under the protection of a qualified right to privacy.

ABORTIONS AND THE LEGAL DUTIES OF HEALTH PROFESSIONALS

Do health professionals have a legal duty to provide abortions for women who seek them? To answer this question, one must look to the nature of the court decisions regarding abortion as well as to the collective decision of society in this regard, for it is on these bases that society's expectations of health professionals are predicated. These legal and social expectations form a framework on which the social duties and responsibilities of health professionals are built and indicate the legal bounds within which decisions must be made.

Some proponents view abortion as a positive benefit right, that is, something that society must provide; thus, they claim that health professionals have a duty to perform abortions. Other proponents claim that abortion is a negative freedom right, that is, a right to do or not to do something (in this case bear children) with no substantive duty for society or health professionals to provide for or to perform abortions. Essentially, the U.S. Supreme Court has held that the decision to abort falls under the protection of the right to privacy, that is, it did not create a legal right to abortion. In subsequent decisions it has held: (1) that no one may interfere with a woman's decision—not even her husband (if the woman is married) or her parents (if the woman is a minor); and (2) that neither a state nor the federal government has an obligation to fund abortion.[22] As a result, a woman is legally free to seek an abortion from those who are willing and able to fulfill her wish; health professionals are legally free to assist with or to perform abortions (depending on their own view of this procedure); and society may or may not provide abortions through funding according to the collective decision of its citizens. If the U.S. Supreme Court had created a right to abortion, a woman would be free to seek an abortion, society would be obliged to provide abortions (through appropriate funding) and health professionals could be required to assist with or to perform abortions if they wished to remain in their respective positions in society.

It should be noted that, at the present time, health professionals have no legal obligation to assist with or to perform abortions. In fact, provincial, state, and federal statutes provide legal protection for those who, on the grounds of conscience, will not assist with or perform abortions. That is, individual health professionals do not have a legal duty to provide abortions for women who seek them. However, health professionals who work in facilities that provide abortions have certain obligations to their employers and to the women who come to these facilities to have abortions.

LEGAL AND MORAL RIGHTS AND OBLIGATIONS OF NURSES

Abortion is a serious ethical issue about which responsible persons of undoubted scholarship and integrity disagree profoundly. As human beings and as professionals, nurses are obliged to act in accord with their sincere convictions. Health professionals cannot be considered to be merely means to attain the ends of others. Moreover, they are not simply observers, but are active participants in abortion procedures. For them, abortion is as much a moral decision as it is for the pregnant woman. If an individual professional (physician or nurse) sees the abortion procedure as the taking of innocent human life, it is unlikely that he or she would (or should) participate in this operation. The professional must not sacrifice personal integrity and certainly must never be required by policies, laws, or social expectations to do so.[23]

It should be remembered also that since health professionals are not under the same kinds of pressures as are women who are seeking abortions, they may regard the procedure differently. Even if one does not believe that the abortion procedure involves the destruction of a human person, repeated exposure to abortion procedures (particularly those in the second and third trimester) can have a very negative effect on the health professionals involved.[24] Further, the nurse, who must spend more time with the patient than do other health workers, literally lives through each procedure with her. Although it is true that the nurse does not experience abortion in the same way as the woman who undergoes the procedure, he/she is exposed repeatedly to the taking of life (whatever the status or value of that life may be).

Nurses who work with abortion patients by choice or by chance must judge carefully their personal views of the abortion procedure, the rights and needs of abortion patients, the demands of their professional codes, and their obligations to the institutions that employ them. Indeed, nurses and other health care workers have a legal right to refuse to participate in abortion procedures,[25] but this right is not absolute. It is limited by their legal and moral obligations to patients and their professional and ethical obligations to employers.

No institution, agency, or person may attempt to force a nurse to participate in an abortion procedure.[26] Moreover, institutions or people in authority may not discriminate in any way against any person who performs, or who refuses to perform or assist in the performance of, an abortion. However, nurses who have conscientious objections to participation in abortion procedures have legal and moral obligations (1) to avoid working in areas or facilities where large numbers of abortions are performed routinely;[27] (2) to make these objections known to the director of nursing services in writing;[28] and (3) to care competently and humanely for any abortion patient with whom they do have contact.[29] Moreover, a nurse may not abandon abortion patients in mid-treatment or mid-shift, but must see to it that the health and safety needs of these patients are met.[30]

Although no particular nurse has an overriding legal or moral duty to choose to take care of abortion patients, all nurses have a duty to treat any patient with dignity, respect and understanding. At the core of this argument is the distinction between one's duties and obligations to others and to oneself and attempts to assess the moral character or worth of individual persons. Assessments of moral character or worth rest on philosophical notions of human nature and its excellence.

In contrast, determinations of one's duties and obligations to others are based on commitments made and roles assumed. The obligations of one person relate directly to the rights of another. As human beings, nurses have an obligation to respect the humanity of all persons. As citizens, nurses have an obligation to respect the legal rights of other citizens, including the abortion patient's legal right to privacy in making and carrying out her decision to abort. As professionals, nurses have an obligation to provide competent nursing care to all who receive their services.

On occasion, nurses who have moral objections to abortion inadvertently may become involved in the performance of abortions—preoperatively, operatively, or postoperatively. If this occurs, the nurses must care for the patients safely and humanely (if there is no one to take their place) and, later, lodge objections with the nursing and hospital administration. Nurses may not endanger the patient's physical or emotional safety.

LEGAL RIGHTS AND OBLIGATIONS OF HOSPITALS

In *Roe v. Wade* and *Doe v. Bolton,* the U.S. Supreme Court recognized the existence of "institutional conscience." That is, the Court provided that hospitals owned and operated by religious groups that have conscientious objections to abortion *do not* have an obligation to provide for the performance of abortions in their facilities.[31] However, public hospitals may have a legal obligation to provide abortion services to the communities that they serve.[32] Although public hospitals may have an obligation to provide abortion services, they are prohibited by statute from using any form of coercion or discrimination against anyone in their employ who participates or who refuses to participate in abortion procedures.[33] Thus, hospitals that provide abortion services are obliged to seek out health professionals and others who are able and willing to perform or assist in the performance of abortions.

Implementation of conscience clause legislation can pose some difficult administrative problems. "Still, moral persons need social space. Otherwise, outward behavior and job descriptions will drive professional, moral and religious ideals or beliefs into irrelevant inwardness, and personal integrity will be destroyed."[34] Preservation of the moral integrity of health professionals benefits society and health care institutions as well as individuals. However, hospitals have the right to expect that health professionals who knowingly accept employment in positions and areas in which abortions are done will, in fact, fulfill their contractual obligations. Moreover, hospitals have a right to expect that health care workers who seek to be employed by them or who are employed by them will notify administration in writing if they have objections to participation in abortion procedures. A New Jersey court decision affirmed a hospital's authority to transfer health care workers who have objections to abortion to areas of the hospital in which they will not, or are unlikely, to come into contact with abortion patients.[35]

RIGHTS OF ABORTION PATIENTS

Women who seek abortions do not have a legal right to abortion; rather, they have a limited legal right to privacy that, in most instances, encompasses the decision to abort. They also have a right to information about the nature, complications, possible benefits, and alternatives of abortion. The same criteria for informed consent apply to abortion as to other surgical procedures. The physician who performs the procedure has the nontransferable legal obligation to obtain informed consent. If, prior to surgery, nurses suspect that the patient does not understand the procedure, they have a moral and legal obligation to inform the physician and to refuse to sign or witness consent forms. If, after the procedure has been performed, patients ask questions that indicate that they did not understand what was involved in their abortion procedures, nurses also should inform the physician.

Although patients have a moral and legal right to information, the legal position of nurses in the provision of such information is ambiguous. The law does not prohibit nurses from giving information to patients, but it also does not explicitly permit it. Even though the American Nurses' Association's Division of Maternal–Child Health's *Statement on Abortion* holds that "The nurse has a responsibility to give the patient objective information . . . before, during and after a voluntary interruption of pregnancy."[36] Nurses may have difficulty in fulfilling this obligation if physicians object or if it is contrary to institutional policies. This does not relieve nurses of their responsibilities to provide information to abortion patients, but it does point out the difficult positions in which nurses may find themselves (see Case Study X).

All patients have a right to expect competent and courteous care from all nurses. They have a right to be respected as persons and they have a right to expect all health care personnel with whom they may come in contact to respect the privacy of their decisions.

Nurses may or may not approve of abortions or they may or may not agree with a patient's reasons for choosing an abortion (if she divulges them—and she often does). However, the provision of competent, compassionate, and understanding nursing care, while it does not require agreement with the patient's decisions about care, does require sensitivity to the physical and emotional needs of others. Being nonjudgmental does not require that nurses make no judgments; rather, it implies an acceptance of human beings as they are and not as others may think they ought to be.

If nurses are not sensitive to the physical and psychological needs of abortion patients, they will be unable to respond to their needs.[37] Nurses who hold the position that abortion is wrong owe it to themselves to act responsibly to protect their integrity. Generally, it is in the best interests of both abortion patients and nurses for nurses who oppose abortion to refrain from all involvement with abortion patients. However, if such nurses do come in contact with abortion patients, the patients have a right to expect nurses to protect them from physical and emotional harm and to withdraw their nursing services only if other qualified professionals are available to care for them.

CASE ANALYSIS

Mary Jane S. and the staff nurses were within their legal, moral, and professional rights to refuse to participate directly in the saline abortion procedures. Neither the hospital nor the director of nursing service was justified in attempts to force the nurses to act contrary to their consciences. Moreover, the attempt to coerce the nurses, by the threat to fire them, was both illegal and unethical; even government does not have authority to violate the conscience of an individual citizen. The nurses did not refuse to care for the abortion patients and they did not abandon them. Indeed, their objections were based, in part, on consideration of the health and safety of the patients and of the rights of patients to informed consent.

DENOUEMENT

The nurses involved sought legal counsel and, on the advice of counsel, they presented copies of the State and Federal Conscience Clauses to members of the administrative staff of the hospital. As a result, the hospital reversed its decision to perform abortions on the gynecology ward; the saline continued to be injected in the operating room. The problems regarding consent were not resolved.

COMMENTARY: CASE STUDY V

M. Josephine Flaherty

This situation, as Curtin has pointed out, involves a number of issues and concerns. The whole question of abortion—if, when, where, and by whom it can or should be performed—has been discussed a great deal in Canada and in the United States and different policies and practices now exist in various jurisdictions. It is clear that most health professionals have given at least some thought to the question and many have made decisions about whether or not they will participate in all or any procedures that relate to abortions. Changes in practices in some agencies have put strain on some of these professionals such as the nurses described in this case study, who were faced with new policies that affected their day to day practice.

These nurses were aware that abortions were being done in the hospital and they were caring for post-abortion patients. Many of them were upset by the fact that they were caring also for patients, following saline injections in the operating room, who were in the process of aborting in their rooms on the wards. Hence, it was obvious that the nurses were not comfortable with their participation in this much of the abortion procedure. There is no evidence, however, that the nurses made formal complaints to nursing administration authorities about this. Can it be concluded that they had decided to go along with the practice even though it was distasteful to them?

Curtin has noted that they also were concerned about the validity of the patients' consents to the saline procedure because the nurses believed that the patients really did not understand the nature of the procedure and the fact that they would experience labor and delivery of the fetus. The case study indicates that the nurses "questioned" the validity of the consent but it does not specify how this questioning was done and whether or not it was put in writing.

The hospital's decision to do the saline injections on the ward precipitated the submission of a formal, written complaint to the nursing office that included a refusal by the nurses to participate in the saline injections in the treatment room for reasons related to the adequacy of the equipment for emergency situations and to the conscientious objections of the nurses to "direct" participation in the abortion procedure.

Some observers would wonder why the nurses were prepared to care for post-saline injection patients and indeed to assist with the delivery of the fetus, when they were not willing to act in a way that they saw as meaning to "participate directly in the destruction of the fetus." One could understand the puzzlement of a director of nursing who might not be able to understand why one of these types of activities by nurses was less "direct" than the other in terms of the destruction of the fetus, because, presumably, a physician or other person would be injecting the saline in both the operating room and the treatment room. The nurses' rationale for the invoking of a conscience clause type of objection for one of these situations and not the other is not clear.

It may be that the nurses were just as unhappy about caring for the post-saline injection patients from the operating room as they were for the patients who were to be injected on the floor but that they did not have sufficient strength or support to object formally until the procedure was to be brought to the gynecology ward. Had the nurses been more consistent, their position would have been strengthened and might have been more clear to the nursing administrator.

Curtin has noted that the nurses were within their legal, moral, and professional rights to refuse to participate directly in the saline abortion procedures. This argument could be challenged, however, because the nurses did not make clear what they meant by "direct" participation in the procedure. It could be suggested that the continuing care of a patient during a hospital induced abortion-related labor and the delivery of the fetus is as direct a type of participation as is assistance to another health care professional in the injection of saline in an operating room or a treatment room. The nurses failed to identify where their conscience began and ended. If the nurses were upset about their care activities for post-saline injection patients, why did they not refuse to care for them?

The second basis for the nurses' opposition to the treatment room procedure related to the lack of appropriate equipment for emergency situations, and this provided a strong argument that seemed to be relatively free of personal bias or opinion. It is surprising that the director of nursing and other administrative personnel were not persuaded by this argument in light of their personal, professional and institutional responsibilities for the provision of adequate and safe care for patients. It is equally surprising that physicians were prepared to carry out the procedure in a less than adequately equipped room. The heavy operating room schedule did not relieve either hospital administrators or physicians of their responsibilities to ensure that practice and care were safe; hence, neither group should have agreed to use of the treatment rooms, if indeed they were not equipped adequately.

The case study description does not indicate that anyone challenged the nurses' assertions about the adequacy of the treatment room equipment. Hence, it is astounding that the nursing director would instruct the nurses to work in what could be unsafe circumstances and thus act in contravention of professional standards of nursing practice, codes of nursing ethics and presumably, hospital policies.

The director's behavior appeared to be unreasonable and irresponsible from the point of view of her professional, ethical, and institutional responsibilities. She was hardly a worthy role model as a professional nurse and an administrator. Further, as Curtin pointed out, the attempt to coerce the nurses to comply by threats of dismissal was unacceptable behavior for the director and the hospital, and the nurses' action in response to this was justified.

Another of the nurses' objections related to the validity of the patients' consents to the procedures. The nurses did take action in the expression of their concerns—apparently both verbally and in writing. Curtin noted that this problem was not resolved. It should be emphasized that while physicians in some jurisdictions may have explicit responsibilities for informing patients about the nature of treatment and the implications of consent, both hospitals and nurses—individually and in groups and positions in the decision making and administrative hierarchy—share the responsibility for ensuring that patients understand what is happening to them. Apparently, the problem of abortion patients' understanding of the saline procedure was well-known in the hospital. Since it was not resolved, all parties involved—hospital authorities, physicians, and nurses—were guilty of failure to fulfill their responsibilities as practicing professionals and as persons who were committed to carry out hospital policies regarding informed consent. All three groups should take immediate action to solve this problem if the hospital and its care-givers are to live up to their contracts with society and their legal responsibilities for informed consent.

Perhaps what is most disturbing about this case study is that the behavior of professional health care workers and hence the service delivered by a health care agency resulted (and apparently continues to do so) in an inadequate level of quality in the health care provided. Each group of professionals involved demonstrated some irresponsible behavior.

Physicians were not thorough in their informed consent for patients practices. The hospital made new rules apparently without appropriate investigation and consultation. The nursing director demonstrated unsound and unprofessional management procedures. The nurses were concerned about their patients and their practice and took some appropriate action; however, they were not consistent in their own positions on the issues.

Any hospital that does procedures that are as controversial as are abortions should recognize the problems that may occur and take action to deal with them. In this situation, the policies and procedures should be examined and evaluated for their appropriateness and clarity and modified or reinforced as necessary. Nurses and hospital administrative authorities should review the nature of their contracts with each other, clarify their respective responsibilities and obligations, discuss openly the variety of aspects and points of view of the abortion question that are found in the situation and agree on how the various groups will behave in relation to them, in order to achieve the goal of quality of patient care.

The administrative group—nursing and other—should review its methods and styles of communication, as should the nursing staff, with a view to adopting more effective mechanisms for exchange of information and discussion of issues. Considerable effort should be put into the improvement of the affective climate of the institution and the relationships between management and staff.

NOTES

1. Many articles and books could be cited here, for example: Perkins, Robert, ed., *Abortion: Pro and Con* (Schenkman Publishing, Cambridge, Massachusetts, 1974).
2. Baumrin, Bernard. "Toward Unraveling the Abortion Problem" in Elsie and Bertram Bandman, eds. *Bioethics and Human Rights* (Little, Brown, Boston, 1978) p. 110.
3. *Roe v. Wade* 314 F. Supp. 1217 Supreme Court No. 70-18.
4. For further information on the physiological beginnings of human life, please see: Quimby, I. N. "Introduction to Medical Jurisprudence: An address delivered by the Chairman of the Section on Medical Jurisprudence at the 38th Annual meeting of the A.M.A., June 10, 1887," *J.A.M.A.* Vol. 9 (August 6, 1887) pp. 161–66. "In physiology a cell or cellule constitutes the origin or commencement of every plant and animal and the elementary form of every tissue, in fact the entire organized human body may be considered to be made up of a congeries of cells, each set having its own life and appropriate functions. From these cells the embryo and foetus is developed. This is a truth so well settled that no well informed physician would care to deny it. Should we not then assert most positively that the life of the foetus commences at the moment conception takes place, and therefore the destruction of the foetus, at any period of gestation, should constitute murder?"

Patten, B. M. *Human Embryology,* 2nd Edition (The Blakiston Company, Inc., Toronto and New York, 1953) p. 52. "There is perhaps no phenomenon in the field of biology that touches so many fundamental questions as the union of the germ cells in the act of fertilization; in this supreme event all the strands of the webs of two lives are gathered in one knot, from which they diverge again and are rewoven in a new individual life-history . . . The elements that unite are single cells, each on the point of death; but by their union a rejuvenated individual is formed, which constitutes a link in the eternal procession of LIFE."

Arey, C. B. *Developmental Anatomy: A Textbook and Laboratory Manual of Embryology* (W. B. Saunders, Philadelphia and London, 1965) p. 55. "The union of the male and female sex cell 'definitely marks the beginning of a new individual'."

Shettles, C. B. *Journal American Medical Association,* Vol. 214 (December 7, 1970) p. 1895. "By . . . definition a new composite individual is started at the moment of fertilization. However, to survive, this individual needs a very specialized environment for nine months . . . From the union of the germ cells, there is under normal development a living, definite going concern. To interrupt a pregnancy at any stage is like cutting the link of a chain; the chain is broken no matter where the link is cut."

Gordon, Hymie. "Genetical, Social and Medical Aspects of Abortion," *South African Medical Journal* (July 20, 1968) pp. 721–30. ". . . from the moment of fertilization, when the deoxyribose nucleic acids from the spermatozoon and the ovum come together to form the zygote, the pattern of the individual's constitutional development is irrevocably determined; his future health, his future intellectual potential, even his future criminal proclivities are all dependent on the sequence of the purine and pyrimidine bases in the original set of DNA molecules of the unicellular individual. True, environmental influences both during the intrauterine period and after birth modify the individual's constitution and continue to do so right until his death, but it is at the moment of conception that the individual's capacity to respond to these exogenous influences is established. Even at the early stage, the complexity of the living cell is so great that it is beyond our comprehension. It is a privilege to be allowed to protect and nurture it."

Guttmacher, A. F., *et al. Planning Your Family* (Macmillan Company, New York and London, 1964) p. 36. "After explaining the process of fertilization, he stated: 'Fertilization, then, has taken place; a baby has been conceived. After conception occurs, the egg attaches itself to the wall of the womb where it grows nine months until the baby is ready to be born'."

Heisler, J. C. *A Textbook of Embryology for Students of Medicine,* 2nd edition (W. B. Saunders, Philadelphia and London, 1901) p. 38. "Fertilization is that peculiar union of spermatozoon and egg-cell which initiates the phenomena resulting in the formation of a new individual."

McMurrich, J. M. *The Development of the Human Body: A Manual of Human Embryology,* 7th Edition (P. Blakiston's Sons, Philadelphia, 1929) p. 31. "It is perfectly clear that the reduction of the chromosomes in the germ cells cannot very long be repeated in successive generations unless a restoration of the original takes place occasionally, and as a matter of fact, such a restoration occurs at the very beginning of the development of each individual, being brought about by the union of a spermatozoon with an ovum."

Gilbert, M. A. *Biography of the Unborn* (Williams and Wilkins, Baltimore, 1938) pp. 2–5. "Not until the 19th century did men finally realize that the union of the sperm with the egg creates a new human being. Life begins for each of us at an unfelt, unknown, and unhonored instant when a minute, wriggling sperm plunges headlong into a mature ovum or egg . . . It is at this moment of fusion of the ovum and the sperm (a process called fertilization) that a new human being is created."

Hamilton, W. J., *et al. Human Embryology Prenatal Development of Form and Function* (Williams and Wilkins, Baltimore, 1945) p. 1. "There are no essential differences between prenatal and postnatal development; the former is more rapid and results in more striking changes in shape and proportions but in both the basic mechanisms are very similar if not identical."

Dodds, G. D. *The Essentials of Human Embryology,* 3rd edition (J. Wiley and Sons, New York, 1946) p. 2. "This fertilized egg is the beginning of a new individual."

Davies, J. *Human Developmental Anatomy* (Ronald Press, New York, 1963) p. 3. "Human development may be said to begin with the union of the male and female germ cells in the art of fertilization."

Langman, J. *Medical Embryology,* 2nd edition (Williams and Wilkins, Baltimore, 1969) p. 3. "The development of a human being begins with fertilization. . . ."

Gesell, A. *The Embryology of Behavior* (Harper Brothers, New York, 1945) p. 172. "Our own repeated observation of fetal infants (an individual born and living at any time prior to 40 weeks gestation) left us with no doubt that psychologically they were individuals. Just as no two looked alike, so no two behaved alike. One was passive, when another was alert. Even among the youngest, there were discernable differences in vividness, reactivity and responsiveness. These were genuinely individual differences, already prophetic of the diversity which distinguishes the human family."

5. Abstracted from Joseph Fletcher. "Indicators of Humanhood: A Tentative Profile of Man," *Hastings Center Report,* Vol. 2, No. 5 (November, 1972). According to Joseph Fletcher, the fifteen positive human criteria are: 1) Minimal intelligence; 2) self-awareness; 3) self-control; 4) a sense of time; 5) a sense of futurity; 6) a sense of the past; 7) the capability to relate to others; 8) concern for others; 9) communication; 10) control of existence; 11) curiosity; 12) change and changeability; 13) balance of rationality and feeling; 14) idiosyncrasy; 15) neo-cortical function. The five negative human criteria are: 1) man is not non- or anti-artificial; 2) man is not essentially parental; 3) man is not essentially sexual; 4) man is not a bundle of rights; 5) man is not a worshiper.

6. Newton, Lisa. "No Right at All: An Interpretation of the Abortion Issue," in Elsie and Bertram Bandman, eds. *Bioethics and Human Rights* (Little, Brown, Boston, 1978) p. 115.

7. *Scott v. McPheeters,* 33 Cal. App. 2d. 629, 92P. 2d 678 (1939), petition for rehearing denied, 93P. 2d 562 (1939); *Bombrest v. Katz,* 65 F. Supp. 138 (D.D.C. 1946); *Amann v. Faidy,* 415 Ill. 422 (1953); *Daley v. Meier,* 33 Ill. App. 2d 218 (1961); *Sinkler v. Kneale,* 401 Penn. 276, 164 A. 2d. 93.

8. *Roe v. Wade,* 314 F. Supp. 1217 Supreme Court No. 70-18.

9. *Stanley v. Georgia* 394 U.S. 557, 564 (1969).

10. *Terry v. Ohio* 392 U.S. 1, 8–9 (1968); *Katz v. United States,* 389 U.S. 347, 350 (1967); *Boyd v. United States,* 116 U.S. 616 (1886), see *Olmstead v. United States,* 277 U.S. 438, 478 (1928). (Brandeis, J. dissenting)

11. *Griswald v. Connecticut,* 381 U.S. 479, 484–485 (1965).

12. *Ibid.,* at 486 (Goldberg, J. concurring).

13. *Meyer v. Nebraska,* 262 U.S. 390, 399 (1923).

14. *Palko v. Connecticut,* 302 U.S. 319, 325 (1937).

15. *Loving v. Virginia,* 388 U.S. 1, 12 (1967).

16. *Skinner v. Oklahoma,* 316 U.S. 535, 541–542 (1942).

17. *Eisenstadt v. Baird,* 405 U.S. 438, 453 (1972), id., at 460, 463–465 (White, J. concurring).

18. *Prince v. Massachusetts,* 321 U.S. 158, 166 (1944).

19. *Pierce v. Society of Sisters,* 268 U.S. 510, 535 (1925) and *Meyer v. Nebraska, supra.*

20. *Roe v. Wade,* 314 F. Supp. 1217 Supreme Court No. 70-18.

21. *Ibid.*

22. The recent (June 1977) Supreme Court decision regarding abortion funding illustrates this point of view.

23. *United States v. Seeger,* 380 U.S. 163, 170 (1965).

24. This problem has been referred to in a number of articles, among which are:

   Connor, E. J. "Therapeutic Abortions," *Audio Digest Ob. Gyn.,* Vol. 17, No. 16 (August 18, 1970).

   Peters, D. R. "N. Y. Nurses Quit Over Abortions," *National Catholic Reporter* (November 6, 1970).

   LeRoux, R. (Moderator). "Abortion," *American Journal of Nursing,* Vol. 70 (1970) pp. 1919–1925.

   Marder, L. "Liberal Therapeutic Abortion: Cure or Cause of Mental Illness," *Audio Digest Ob. Gyn.,* Vol. 16, No. 17 (September 2, 1969).

Kibel, H. D. "Staff Reactions to Abortion, A Psychiatrist's View," *Obstetrics and Gynecology,* Vol. 39 (January 1972) pp. 128–133.

McDermott, J. F., and W. F. Char. "Abortion Repeal in Hawaii: An Unexpected Crisis in Patient Care," *American Journal of Orthopsychiatry,* Vol. 41 (July 1971) pp. 620–26.

Snider, A. J. "Helping Do Abortions Puts Strain on Nurses," *Chicago Daily News Service* (May 16, 1972).

Denes, Magda. "Performing Abortions," *Commentary* (Published by the American Jewish Committee, New York, October 1976) pp. 33–37.

Kessler, Kenneth, and Theodore Weiss, "Ward Staff Problems with Abortions," *International Journal of Psychiatry in Medicine,* Vol. 5, No. 2 (1974) pp. 96–103.

25. *Cf.,* Mich. Comp. Laws sec. 331.552, §2; Ky. Rev. Stat. sec. 311.800 §11; Cal. Health and Safety Code sec. 25955(a); Fla. Stat. sec. 458.22(5); Mass. Gen. Laws Chap. 122, sec. 121; N.Y. Civ. Rights Law (Consol.) sec. 79-i (I).

26. *Cf.,* American Nurses' Association's Division of Maternal and Child Health Nursing Practice's *Statement on Abortion,* adopted by the Maternal–Child Health Division Executive Committee, June 12, 1978.

27. *Ibid.*

28. *Cf.,* footnote 25.

29. *Cf.,* footnotes 26 and 27.

30. American Nurses' Association's Division of Maternal and Child Health Nursing Practice's *Statement on Abortion, op. cit.*

31. *Roe v. Wade,* 314 F. Supp. 1217 Supreme Court No. 70-18. and *Doe v. Bolton* 319 F. Supp. 1048 Supreme Court No. 70-40.

32. *Poelker v. Doe,* No. 75-442 45 LW (June 21, 1977) pp. 4794–97. In this decision, the Court determined that (contrary to the Schoening case) all public hospitals do not have to provide abortion services.

33. The federal Conscience Clause Act, 42 U.S.C. 300 a-7. Mich. Comp. Laws sec. 331, 552, §2; Ky. Rev. Stat. sec. 311.800, §11; Cal. Health and Safety Code sec. 25955 (a) and (b); Fla. Stat. sec. 458.22(5); Mass. Gen. Laws Chap. 122, sec. 121; R.I. Laws sec. 23-16-10.1; N.Y. Civ. Rights Law (consol.) sec. 79-i (I), and so forth.

34. Ramsey, Paul. *Ethics at the Edges of Life* (Yale University Press, New Haven, 1978) p. 69.

35. Beverly Jazelik, a nurse in New Jersey, objected to participation in abortion procedures. Subsequently, the hospital transferred her to another area of the hospital. Ms. Jazelik objected and sued the hospital. The Court decided in favor of the hospital's right to transfer the nurse to another area.

36. American Nurses' Association's Division of Maternal and Child Health Nursing Practice, *op. cit.*

37. For a discussion of one method developed to assist abortion patients, please see the questionnaire on pp. 92–93 of Anderson, Claudia, Barbara Clancy, and Ruth Hassanein, "Psychoprophylaxis in Midtrimester Abortions," *J.O.G.N. Nursing* (November-December 1976) pp. 29–93.

Case Study VI: Nurse–Physician Conflict—Telephone Orders

M. Josephine Flaherty

Ann Marie C, a newly graduated baccalaureate nurse, received the notification that she had passed her state board examination on the same day she was scheduled to be in charge of the evening shift for the first time. When she arrived on the unit, she jubilantly shared her good news with the other staff members before she started to work. Later that evening (2135h), she entered Mr. B's room to check his vital signs (blood pressure, temperature, pulse, and respirations). She noted that his blood pressure had fallen from 160/100 to 110/40. She also noted that his respirations were shallow, rapid, and labored. He was pale and perspiring profusely. His temperature was 98.6° F.

Ann Marie C returned to the nurses' station and called Mr. B's physician. She reported these observations to the physician and asked him to come in to see the patient. She was uncomfortable because Mr. B's vital signs had changed dramatically and she thought he might be going into shock. The physician told her to monitor the patient closely (vital signs q 15 min.) and to call him again in an hour. Ann Marie duly noted this conversation on the patient's chart in the nurses' notes. At 2230h, she again called the physician and reported that the patient's blood pressure had fallen slightly to 105/40 and that his respirations were 15—shallow and labored. He still was pale and perspiring. The physician again told her to observe the patient closely and to call him again if there were any significant changes in the patient's condition. Again, the nurse noted the interchange on the patient's chart in the nurses' notes. At 2305h, the patient experienced a cardiac arrest and a code was called. Mr. B responded to cardiopulmonary resuscitation and was transferred to the Intensive Care Unit. His physician was notified by telephone. The night supervisor called Mr. B's family and they rushed to the hospital. When the family arrived, Mr. B's physician was there. Among other things, the physician told them, "If only the nurse had called me sooner, all this could have been avoided."

The family members were quite upset. Mr. B's daughter (who was a registered nurse) thought that Ann Marie C had been derelict in her duties. Subsequently, the family lodged a complaint against Ann Marie C with the hospital's administration. Ann Marie was called to the nursing office and asked if she had observed any symptoms or signs indicative of impending cardiac arrest and if so, why she had not notified the attending physician. Ann Marie said that she had noted the changes in the patient's vital signs; she asserted that she had called the physician—not once but twice. Morever, she said that she had recorded in the nurses' notes the times of the calls, the content of the calls, and the physician's response. The director of nursing checked Ann Marie's story and found that the patient's chart provided written evidence to support her claims. However, the family members were not satisfied; they demanded a full investigation.

During the course of the investigation, the physician asserted again that Ann Marie C had not called him. Moreover, he suggested that she had falsified the nursing notes because she was afraid of what would happen. There was enough time between the time Mr. B experienced his cardiac arrest and the time he was transferred to intensive care for her to do this. Since it was a possibility, the director of nursing felt obliged to determine whether this was what actually had happened. Ann Marie categorically denied the physician's allegation; it was Ann Marie's word against the physician's word.

OUTCOME

The outcome of this situation is not known to the authors.

IDENTIFICATION AND CLARIFICATION OF ETHICAL COMPONENTS

This case study raises interesting problems. For example, what is the position of the nurse who takes "orders" over the telephone? What happens to interprofessional cooperation when members of either discipline are dishonest? Would Ann Marie be justified in defending herself to the patient's family? What responsibility do nurses in administrative positions have to protect staff nurses who take telephone "orders" from physicians?

This situation, which is not unusual in health care today, involves not one, but several ethical issues that arise from a series of conflicting demands, needs, loyalties, lines of communication, and perceptions of the above series of events. It presents a picture of a hospital that should have been able to respond appropriately to an incident involving a patient but in which at least one, and perhaps more than one, of the health care professionals involved apparently failed to fulfill the responsibilities for which they were accountable.

A number of rights and responsibilities are involved; they include:

1. The right of a patient to appropriate nursing and medical care

2. The right of a family to be able to expect that their relative will receive expert care and that they will be notified appropriately of his progress or lack of it

3. The rights and responsibilities of a nurse as a provider of health care

4. The responsibilities of a health care agency to ensure that patients receive adequate and appropriate care and that staff members and physician "guest practitioners" demonstrate generally approved standards of performance

5. The right of the agency to expect that licensed and/or registered health professionals will practice accordingly

6. The rights of nurses and physicians to make decisions regarding patient care

7. The rights of a family to complain about the nature of the health care given

8. The responsibility of a health care agency to respond to concerns and complaints of patients, and/or families, by investigating the complaints and by taking appropriate action.

Each of these points is addressed in the following paragraphs.

The right of the patient to appropriate care. That the patient had been admitted to the hospital is evidence of the hospital's commitment to provide adequate and appropriate treatment. Society recognizes the hospital's commitment and the patient's right to treatment, by law and by the value system of the society. The patient also has the right to skilled nursing and medical care and the right to assume that the health care professionals will practice competently, will consider the patient's needs to be paramount, will not harm the patient through acts of commission or omission and will be faithful to the patient, to the promises of their professions and to the policies of the hospital.

The rights of the family to expect expert care for their relative and to be notified appropriately of his progress. The family was familiar with the patient's physician and had a right to expect that he would provide sound medical care and that the hospital would provide sound nursing and other health care, would coordinate all care that the patient received and would keep the family appropriately informed.

The rights and responsibilities of the nurse as a health care provider. The nurse, as a registered nurse, had the responsibility to exercise the standards of nursing practice for which her registration made her accountable. This involves application of the nursing process that includes assessment of patients' health needs, planning and implementation of nursing care, collaboration with other members of the health care team, adherence to the policies and practices of the employing agency, communication with appropriate other persons through verbal and written means and the exercise of judgment in the acceptance and delegation of responsibility. At the same time, the nurse has a right to working conditions that make possible the implementation of the standards of nursing practice; such conditions include reasonable work loads, appropriate assistance and supervision, open and effective lines of communication with other workers, and the right to be respected for professional skills and abilities.

The responsibility of a health care agency to ensure that adequate care is provided for patients by competent professionals and the right to expect adequate standards of practice from health care workers. Since the administration of a health care agency is responsible for everything that happens in the agency, the administration is obliged to ensure that adequate and safe care is provided for patients. This responsibility is implemented through screening, selection, and supervision of health care workers and monitoring of the effects of hospital care. The agency should have a system through which significant changes in patients' conditions will be reported to a responsible agent in a senior or supervisory position. The agency should be able to be confident that the health care professionals involved will provide a high quality of service and will act within statutory and institutional regulations. The agency also should have the right to expect integrity from the health professionals who practice there; this involves truth-telling, documentation of and accountability for their behavior, and the subjection of it to the scrutiny of peers.

The rights of nurses and physicians to make decisions about the care of patients. As professionals, physicians and nurses have rights to make medical and nursing decisions, respectively. It is assumed, however, that such decisions are based on appropriate data about which the health professionals feel confident. Should physicians make medical decisions without seeing patients, particularly if the communicator (here, the nurse) of information has concern about the patient involved? If medical decisions are made under such conditions, does a nurse have the right and/or responsibility to seek another opinion? If the nurse does have such a right, to what other authority can and should an appeal be made?

The responsibility of a health care agency to take action on concerns or complaints of patients or families. The agency, with its commitment to provide health care service, is required to investigate, immediately and fully, complaints of patients and/or families and to take appropriate action. This includes verification of data, including testimony of the persons involved about the situations, clarification and modification as appropriate of policies and practices, confrontation if necessary of health care professionals whose information is conflicting and/or whose behavior appears to be questionable, and the taking of disciplinary action that is indicated.

ANALYSIS OF THE SPECIFIC SITUATION

Background Information

1. Ann Marie C was notified about her success in the state board examinations and shared the good news with colleagues as she was beginning her first experience in charge of the unit on the evening shift.

2. At 2135h, she discovered that Mr. B's blood pressure had fallen from 160/100 to 110/40, that his respirations were shallow, rapid, and labored, that he was pale and perspiring, and that his temperature was 98.6°F.

3. She called Mr. B's physician to report her findings and asked him to come to see the patient. The physician told her to watch the patient (to check vital signs *q 15 min.*) and to call him in an hour. She noted the conversation on the chart.

4. At 2230h, she called the physician, telling him that the patient's blood pressure had fallen to 105/40, that his respirations were 15 and shallow and labored and that he was pale and perspiring. The physician told her to observe the patient and to notify him again if there was a significant change. She noted the conversation on the chart.

5. At 2305h, the patient had a cardiac arrest and, after cardiopulmonary resuscitation, was taken to the intensive care unit.

6. The physician was notified by telephone. The night supervisor informed the family who came to the hospital.

7. The family members were upset and their conversation with the physician resulted in their belief that the nurse had not notified the physician soon enough for him to intervene.

8. The family filed a complaint against the nurse. The hospital investigated it.

9. During the investigation, it was noted that the chart corroborated the nurse's story. However, the physician suggested that she had had enough time to falsify the chart and that she might have done so because of her fear of what might happen as a result of the incident.

THE INDIVIDUALS INVOLVED IN THE SITUATION

1. The Nurse

Although Ann Marie was a new graduate, she had been successful in the state board examinations and hence was recognized by the statutory body as competent to be registered to practice nursing. The hospital had enough confidence in her to place her "in charge" on the evening shift. As soon as she noticed a change in the patient's condition, she decided that it was serious enough to warrant a visit by the physician; she notified him accordingly and noted this on the patient's chart. She also noted the telephone orders that were given to her and she followed these orders. When she called the physician the second time and was told to notify him again if there were " any significant change in the patient's condition," she was confronted with the making of a decision about what was a "significant change." It is not known whether and if so, to what extent, she asked the physician for clarification of this. She had thought that the original drop in blood pressure was significant enough to warrant a visit from the physician; however, he did not agree and told her to watch the patient and to call him in an hour. Although there was some change during that period, the physician did not believe that it was serious enough to warrant his coming to the hospital. It is probable that even though the patient's blood pressure had not dropped a great deal during the hour, the fact that the patient was not much, if any, better was alarming to the nurse. It is not known whether Ann Marie called the evening nursing supervisor at this point, but it would have been wise for her to do so, particularly because she was worried that the patient was not improving and because she was not a very experienced nurse. She also might have sought assistance with clarification of the meaning of "significant change." It is assumed that there were no other physicians available in the hospital (such as residents or interns) who might have been consulted by the nurse.

Apparently, when the cardiac arrest occurred, appropriate and successful action was taken and appropriate recording was done by the nurse. The night supervisor became involved. It is assumed that she was satisfied with Ann Marie's behavior, as there is no evidence that the latter was censured by her superiors, or even questioned at length, until the family filed the complaint.

There is no evidence to suggest that Ann Marie falsified the nursing records. Her notification of the evening supervisor about her concern for the patient would have strengthened her position in the face of the physician's conflicting version of what happened. It is unfortunate that the evening supervisor did not check with Ann Marie earlier to verify that all was well on her first evening in charge. One could ask whether this relatively inexperienced nurse should have had more supervision in this situation.

Ann Marie was correct in maintaining the position that she had taken appropriate communication action—in her calls to the physician and in her charting—but she should be counseled to notify a nursing supervisor in situations like this one. Her handling of the verbal telephone orders seemed to be appropriate but one would wonder what was the nature of the hospital's policy about such orders. Ann Marie would be justified in defending herself to the patient's family if there were a face-to-face meeting with the family. However, her accountability for her behavior was first to the patient, through her care and her records and reporting, and then to the nursing department; her behavior in these accountabilities was appropriate. In the face of a difference of opinion and/or lack of honesty by another health professional, a nurse has the responsibility to subject her behavior to the scrutiny of her peers and Ann Marie did this. A nurse has the right to be supported by her nursing peers and superiors for her correct behavior in the face of accusations by another professional.

2. Nursing Administrative Staff Members

The nursing administrative staff members are responsible for ensuring that adequate nursing care is given. Hence, a nursing supervisor should monitor the various situations during each shift and should be particularly conscious of the amount of experience and skill that is possessed by the nurses. One would wonder whether, and how many times, the supervisor had visited and/or communicated with Ann Marie's unit during the shift and how well informed the supervisor was about all patients' conditions. It is assumed that the supervisor was not concerned about Ann Marie's behavior, because she did not initiate disciplinary action against her. The supervisor was accountable for the events of the evening and should have been involved, in defense of her staff member's actions, in the investigation being conducted by the director of nursing.

3. Director of Nursing

The director of nursing responded appropriately to the complaint of the family; it is assumed that data were gathered from appropriate sources. It is assumed (although this is not clear in the case study description) that the director believed that Ann Marie's charts reflected accurately her behavior. In the light of the physician's conflicting testimony, one would hope that the nursing director would have asked for consultation with senior medical staff about the physician's position on the issue. It would be interesting to know whether the particular physician was in the habit of coming to the hospital as soon as he was called, whether he was likely to behave as he did on this occasion, and whether there had been other incidents in which his testimony was in variance with that of the nurses. It is unfortunate that he said things to the family that apparently he had not said to Ann Marie; or, did he confront the nurse himself about her behavior? If he had been concerned and had believed that she did not call him twice during the evening, why did he not discuss this with the director of nursing and/or the night supervisor? Why did he feel the need to blame the nurse entirely for the situation? Did he have no feeling of collegial responsibility for the care of his patient? It appears that the physician was not telling the truth in the situation. It is unfortunate that he found it necessary and appropriate to suggest to the director of nursing that Ann Marie's records were not honest and even to suggest reasons why she might have falsified them.

4. The Family

The family was justified in its approach to the director of nursing, particularly when its early investigation suggested that there was a failure by the nurse to provide adequate care. In the face of conflicting testimony, the family would be hard pressed to know whose word could be trusted. However, because of past knowledge of the physician, if his behavior had appeared satisfactory, the family might be inclined to trust his word, because he is much more experienced than is a newly graduated nurse.

5. *The Hospital*

The hospital is responsible for the verification of the competence, through evaluation of their behavior, of the persons who practice there. One would hope that this agency had a review and auditing system that was being implemented. The policy of the hospital about telephone orders should be examined, evaluated and modified if necessary, for the protection of the patients, the staff and the agency. Nurses in administrative positions should be prepared to ensure that such policies are relevant and practicable and that they are followed by all persons concerned. Since nurses are responsible to the nursing department, the latter should be prepared to defend staff nurses against attacks by other professionals, if the nurses have followed agency policy and/or behaved in accord with the policies and practices of the profession. If there are doubts about whether physicians will use complete candor in their telephone ordering behavior, the orders can be recorded on tape and kept for reference, at least until the telephone orders are signed by the physicians issuing them. There is precedent in Canada for use of tape recorders for telephone orders; in that country, for example, at least one court decision was made in favor of a nurse in the light of tape recordings of the telephone orders. At all times, physician's telephone orders should be written and identified as to time, date, physician giving the order, and nurse receiving it.

CONCLUSION

Interprofessional cooperation and collaboration can be destroyed in the absence of respect, consideration, and honesty on the part of all concerned. If these conditions do not exist, nurses should refuse, with justification, to receive and to take action on telephone orders. Working under conditions in which it is not possible to practice according to the standards of nursing practice for which they are accountable constitutes a breach of ethics for nurses. Hence, administrative personnel in hospitals and other health agencies must ensure that the conditions under which cooperative and collaborative care can take place do exist in the agency. Otherwise, the quality of patient care will be threatened as it was in this situation, and the health care agency will not be able to fulfill its responsibilities to patients.

COMMENTARY: CASE STUDY VI

Leah Curtin

A situation such as the one described in this case study threatens the credibility of health care institutions and health care professionals. The patient, Mr. B, if he was conscious, may have feared death or a damaged life. His family shared these fears and bore the added burden of anxiety imposed by the physician's communication which inferred that Mr. B did not receive good nursing care. Considering that Mr. B was placed in the intensive care unit of the same hospital and needed considerable nursing care, the family well may have feared that the nurses caring for him there also were incompetent. The professionals involved (nurse, physician, supervisory nurse, administrative personnel) may have feared legal liability, loss of income, and loss of prestige.

One of the problems presented in a situation like this one is that people will react to their fears rather than react or act to meet the needs of the patient, his family, and the personnel involved. A responsible institution will move to reduce fear and moderate the stresses imposed on family and health personnel by the situation and by the physician's and nurse's conflicting claims. The hospital can realize these goals through its policies and practices and through the behavior of its leaders. To promote excellence in both medical and nursing practices, institutions must provide a continuous flow of education, support, and correction. Clearly, questions of policy and practice were involved in this situation and its appropriate resolution should have included elements of education, support, and correction.

Flaherty rightly points out that the hospital was obliged to ensure that patients received adequate and safe care and was responsible for the care given (or not given) to patients. To meet this obligation, institutions not only must articulate and implement policies and select only qualified people for employment, but they also must provide adequate staffing, support, and supervision where necessary. Ann Marie was a newly graduated nurse and yet she was placed in charge of a floor. Moreover, there was no evidence presented that other professional nurses were working on the floor during that shift. In addition, even though the supervisory nurse(s) must have know that Ann Marie C never had been a charge nurse before, there was no evidence to indicate that the supervisor visited that floor to offer the support and guidance that is the primary function of the position. Although it could be argued quite rightly that Ann Marie C should have called the supervisor, it could have been that Ann Marie trusted the physician's medical judgment about the care of his patient—if one assumes that, indeed, she did call him as she claimed and did document that she had done so. There certainly was no evidence that Ann Marie C disagreed with the physician; rather she followed his telephone instructions to observe the patient closely and she reported back to the physician within a reasonable amount of time. Appropriate questions to be raised are whether Ann Marie C should have agreed with the physician, or, whether she had enough self-confidence and experience to disagree with him. The former question raises the issue of nurses' competence to question physicians' medical judgments when physicians are not present to observe the patients involved. The latter question raises a problem frequently addressed in the nursing literature, that is, the adequacy of the socialization process to which women in general and nurses in particular are subjected.

At any rate, Ann Marie C was placed in a position of considerable responsibility by the hospital and she obviously accepted the responsibility when she agreed to be the charge nurse. If Ann Marie throught she was not equal to the task, she had a responsibility to so inform the nursing supervisors. However, supervisory personnel also have a responsibility to assure that those whom they place in responsible positions are capable of fulfilling the responsibilities. In addition, supervisory personnel are obliged to provide the resources that are necessary for the fulfillment of those responsibilities—personnel, administrative support, and materials. There is some evidence to indicate that some of these resources were not provided.

The physician's conduct in this case is highly questionable. As Flaherty notes, there is considerable evidence that the nurse did inform him of the patient's condition and no evidence (other than the physician's word) that she did not notify him. Moreover, his remark to the family about the nurse's conduct was ill-timed and ill-judged. It appears to have been an attempt to exculpate himself by attempting to place blame on another professional. Family members, awakened unexpectedly in the middle of the night and apprised of the critical condition of their relative, do not need to hear that their loved one's condition was a result of poor care. Indeed, if Ann Marie C had not reported the patient's condition to the physician, he would have been justified in taking action by informing her superiors of the situation. However, the physician did not do so; rather, the family brought the complaint to the attention of hospital authorities. If the physician had known that Ann Marie C had failed to notify him and, in addition, had falsified the nursing notes, why did he not report the situation? Was he so concerned about Ann Marie C that he was willing to protect her at the expense of accurate and honest records, safe care, and his own professional reputation? If this had been the case, the physician's conduct was irresponsible. If this was not the case (as Flaherty notes) it appears that the physician's conduct was dishonest.

Dishonest conduct among health professionals results in distrust and fear. It undermines the basis of patient–professional relationships, damages the credibility of health care institutions and destroys interprofessional relationships. Consequently, the hospital, through such bodies as the medical executive committee and the nursing council, should have taken immediate steps to uncover the truth and, subsequently, initiated appropriate action that may include censure of the conduct of a professional. In addition, it is hoped that the hospital kept Mr. B's family fully informed about the progress and findings of the investigation and of any corrective actions that were taken. The tendency in such situations often is to gloss over or cover up the facts in the belief that this may prevent the family from initiating legal action. Indeed, if appropriate support and guidance were lacking and if staffing were inadequate, and if Ann Marie were not qualified to be in charge, the hospital's position would be tenuous at best. However, this family and this patient already have been subjected to dishonesty (on someone's part). Family members clearly were upset and further attempts to conceal information or to distort the truth could have led to more fear and justifiable anger. To earn and to maintain the trust of individuals and of the community, a hospital must convey a sense of reliability and honesty. This incident threatened the trust relationship between this hospital and the people it serves. Although the authors do not know the outcome of this situation, they hope that appropriate action was taken to preserve the community's trust in the hospital.

Case Study VII: Refusal of Treatment for Minors

Leah Curtin

The scene is a local community hospital. The patient is a twelve-year-old girl suffering from serious injuries caused by a traffic accident. Her hemoglobin has fallen to four and she is in need of blood transfusions before surgery can be done. The child's parents refuse to permit a blood transfusion because their religious convictions forbid it.[1] The child's physician is well known in the area for his willingness to practice medicine in accord with the religious beliefs of this particular group and his practice consists largely of many members of this religion who drive up to a hundred miles to see him. The physician postponed the surgery and decided to try conservative therapy in the hope that the child would survive without surgery until she was able to replenish her own blood supply.

The members of the nursing staff caring for the girl were concerned. The child was in shock and near death. There was every indication that she was bleeding internally and no indication that the hemorrhage had stopped. They respected and admired the physician and they understood the sincerity of the parents' religious beliefs. Some of the nurses thought that they should act to protect the patient by notifying the hospital administration of this situation. Other members of the nursing staff thought that nurses should not interfere— that the physician should determine the course of medical treatment and should assume the responsibility of notifying the hospital administration of any unusual steps he chose to take. The head nurse called the physician's office to notify him of the child's deteriorating condition, but he did not choose to alter his course of action. It was clear that the physician chose not to notify administration and that the girl's condition was deteriorating rapidly; therefore, the head nurse decided to act: she notified the supervisor who apprised the nursing administrator of the situation.

The nursing administrator notified the hospital administrator who immediately contacted the physician. The physician refused to change the course of

265

treatment by ordering blood transfusions. The hospital administrator then contacted the chief of staff who examined the patient and determined that the child's only chance of survival was surgery and that blood transfusions would be necessary if surgery was to be performed. The child's primary physician was contacted again both by the chief of staff and the hospital administrator.

The primary physician had recontacted the parents to apprise them of their daughter's condition and the parents remained adamant: their daughter was not to receive a blood transfusion. Therefore, when the chief of staff and the hospital administrator called him, he again refused to order blood transfusions and to undertake surgery. The hospital administrator, on the advice of the hospital's lawyer (advice based on the chief of staff's appraisal of the child's condition), sought legal intervention. A judge appointed the administrator the child's temporary guardian; the administrator immediately authorized physicians to undertake whatever steps that were necessary (including blood transfusions) to save the child's life. However, the child died before there was time either to give the transfusions or to perform surgery. It must be noted that all of these events took place within an eight hour period.

As a consequence of this case, the hospital threatened to revoke the physician's privileges unless he promised in writing to authorize blood transfusions under similar circumstances in the future. In response, the physician has taken the hospital to court alleging that its action constitutes an unwarranted intrusion on his practice of medicine and deprives him of his livelihood.

There are many factors in this situation that bear examination. Were the parents acting appropriately by, in a sense, imposing their religious beliefs on their minor child under these circumstances (*i.e.*, life and death circumstances)? Was the physician acting responsibly in respecting the parent's wishes? Did the nurses interfere inappropriately in the physician–family relationship by notifying the hospital administration of this situation? Did the hospital administrator and the chief of staff act appropriately? On what basis did the judge intervene in the private decision making of the physician and family? Did the hospital act appropriately in demanding that this physician promise in writing to authorize blood transfusions in similar circumstances in the future?

THE PARENTS' POSITION

The parents' position is complex. Parents have a duty to protect and nurture their children and to promote their children's well-being in all ways that are open to them. Their religious belief is that blood transfusions violate God's law and that transgressors will be punished eternally. From their perspective, it is far better for their daughter to lose her temporal life than to spend her eternal life in hell. Therefore, the parents think that acting in the best interests of their child consists of refusing transfusions even though their daughter may die as a result. Although others may consider their decision unwise or even foolish, there is no reason to accuse the parents of malicious intent or of neglect. Their beliefs should be respected, certainly, as they apply to themselves; their actions should not be maligned as they are acting, according to their own lights, in the best interests of their child.

On the other hand, even if one accepts the beliefs as true, how could this child or any other child be held responsible by a just God for actions that are performed on her without her knowledge or consent? Could the parents be more concerned about saving their souls than their daughter's soul? If so, it still is a legitimate concern; but can it be exercised at the price of their daughter's life? Would the assumption by someone other than the parents, of authorization of the blood transfusions, offer a viable alternative to parents who are caught in such a bind? The parents probably would not be held responsible by God or by the community of believers for actions that are taken without their consent and that are against their expressed wishes. The question is: can or should parents be permitted to apply their religious beliefs to a minor child whose life hangs in the balance? Are there limits to parental rights?

The right of parents to direct the future of their children is cherished by society but it is not absolute, that is, parental rights do not include a right to abandon or to endanger their children or to let their children die when readily attainable assistance is available.[2] Parental control over children has been absolute in the past, but it has been diminished considerably in modern times. For example, today parents must provide an education for their children and they may not sell them into slavery or put them to work in factories or in fields at a tender age. Although parents may administer an estate for a child, they may not assume ownership of the child's property. Moreover, children's rights to protection from physical, sexual, and emotional abuse as well as from neglect that is motivated by nonreligious reasons have been recognized and protected by law. If someone claimed a religious reason for abusing children in any of these areas, would this abuse suddenly become acceptable as an act of religious freedom? Would or should the law then protect such actions? Although one may choose to die for his religious convictions, may he choose death for another person for these same convictions if the person is not a child? Does the fact of being a child change this situation? Today, people would balk at the idea of the human sacrifice of a child to a deity; is not the situation described in this case study somewhat analogous to such a sacrifice?

On the other hand, one is drawn to the notion of respect for the sincerely held religious convictions of other people. It is unjust to malign people because their religion forbids them to accept one type of medical care. In most circumstances it also would be unjust to oppose or to obstruct the efforts of a physician who is doing his best to respect his patients' religion despite the risks. Generally, it is inappropriate to take steps to remove a child from parents' custody when they sincerely believe they are acting in the child's best interests.

In the case of a consenting adult, the rights to self-determination, integrity, inviolability of the person, and to religious freedom all militate for noninterference[3] However, parents' right to refuse, on religious grounds, life-saving treatment for their children is challenged. The right to be and to remain alive is the most fundamental right of any person, a precondition for the existence and exercise of all other rights, including the right to exercise one's religion. Although the courts generally have recognized that individuals may choose to sacrifice their own right to life for something they value more highly (*e.g.*, religion), courts almost uniformly have prohibited parents from exercising their rights to religious freedom if it endangers the lives of their children. Therefore, although responsible persons may disagree about the moral right of parents to infringe on their children's right to life for any reason (including religious reasons), their legal rights are far less ambiguous. Generally speaking, parents may not refuse life-saving treatment for their children even if such treatment violates their religious beliefs.

THE PHYSICIAN'S QUANDARY

The physician in this case has a large practice consisting principally of members of this religious group. Therefore, it is necessary for him to take certain risks, or at least a greater degree of risk than he would encounter ordinarily in the practice of medicine. He was attempting by all means short of blood transfusions to preserve this child's life. He apprised the parents of their daughter's critical condition and of her need for blood. Some members of this religious group would rather die than receive a blood transfusion; others are not as scrupulous. Apparently, the parents were not of a liberal persuasion and they refused permission for the blood transfusions. The child was in a critical condition and might not have survived even if she had been given blood transfusions. The physician knew that if he acted in accord with the parent's wishes, the child would be at an even greater risk of death. However, if he acted at variance with their wishes, he would be: (1) condemning their daughter to hell according to the parents' beliefs; (2) breaking faith with the parents who came to him because he was known to respect their religious scruples; and (3) breaking faith with the entire community of believers who had come to rely on him for their medical care. He could not risk surgery without the forbidden transfusions and so he postponed surgery and attempted to use conservative therapy only. Does the increased risk to the child justify violation of the trust of the parents and the community of believers? Apparently, the physician either reached the conclusion that it did not—or he might not have believed that blood transfusions would alter significantly the course of events. That is, perhaps he believed that the child's injuries were so extensive that both blood transfusion and surgery would not save her life and, therefore, that it would serve no purpose to upset the parents further.

The physician perceived that his duty was to respect the parents' beliefs and to keep faith with the community of believers. Although he was aware of the fact that such a course of action would reduce the child's chances of survival, he also might have thought that the child would not survive even if blood transfusions were given and surgery were undertaken. He did not abandon the girl; instead, he proposed to try to save her life with less than optimal tools. There is no doubt that at least one physician, the chief of staff, disagreed with him and was convinced that in critical situations, the best tools available should be used to give the patient the best possible chance to survive.

THE NURSES' POSITION

Nurses, both as professionals and as hospital employees, have specific obligations to protect patients from harm[4] and to report unusual incidents or behavior to appropriate authorities. They have the duties of loyalty to the patient and of contractual obligations to the hospital. They have no obligations to the physician other than those imposed by a collegial relationship. Although nurses frequently carry out the physician's medical regimen, a physician does not have line authority over hospital nurses. Therefore, he does not have the authority to tell them *not* to report an incident or to act contrary to hospital policy or patient well-being.

Although sensitive to the sincerity of the parents' religious convictions, the nurses were aware of the direct threat that these convictions posed to the girl's life. While the nurses recognized that people have a right to free exercise of religion, they questioned whether this right should be exercised to the detriment of another person. Moreover, nurses' ethical obligations focus on the welfare of those who are entrusted to their care. This child was entrusted to their care; her parents were not. In addition, the patient, both by virtue of age and the damage she had sustained, was far more vulnerable to abuse than were her parents. As patient advocates, the nurses were obliged to consider her rights first.

The nurses, as colleagues of the physician, had an obligation to collaborate with him in the care of patients. They also had an obligation to share their concerns with him and to apprise him of any course of action that they might take that would affect his medical regimen. From the case study presented, it is not clear whether the nurses told the physician that they felt obliged to report this situation to administrative authorities. If they did not, they should have done so. However, it is clear that they did apprise the physician of the girl's deteriorating physical condition. If the physician truly believed that the child could not benefit from blood transfusions and surgery, he should have informed the nurses of this. Given the gravity of the child's condition and the significance of the right involved (the right to life), the physician's assertion that the wishes of the parents must be followed was not sufficient justification for a choice to use less than optimal tools in the attempt to save her life.

Although physicians assume the primary legal and moral duty to prescribe a medical regimen, nurses also have legal and moral duties with regard to the medical as well as the nursing regimen. They have both a moral and legal duty to question the medical regimen if they have reason to believe that it is not in the patient's best interests or that it may harm the patient. Even though nurses may not prescribe a medical regimen, they can appeal a medical decision through appropriate channels. Such a course of action need not be disrespectful or officious. It is possible to respect others (physician and parents) and, at the same time, to disagree with their proposed course of action.

In summary, the nurses chose a responsible course of action under the circumstances. Their professional duties to the patient and their contractual obligations to the hospital were fulfilled.

THE POSITION OF ADMINISTRATION

Once notified of this situation, members of the administrative team took immediate action. The first action was to verify the facts of the situation and the hospital administrator with the assistance of the chief of staff, did so. Given that the child's condition was critical, the administrator and chief of staff contacted the primary physician to elicit his cooperation. When this was not forthcoming, they consulted the hospital's legal counsel who advised them to seek court intervention as quickly as possible. The rationale for the lawyer's decision probably was twofold: (1) there is legal precedent for this action, that is, the courts usually intervene in cases where minors are deprived of life-saving medical treatment[5] and (2) the hospital could be accused of criminal negligence if it failed to take what a court or a jury determined to be reasonable steps to save a patient's life. Blood transfusions usually are considered reasonable (*i.e.*, not heroic) medical measures that should be used when necessary to save life.[6] In summary, the initial actions taken by the hospital administrator were reasonable and responsible in view of the legal and moral obligations of hospitals to patients.

The course of action chosen by administrative authorities following the death of the child, however, are problematic. In this particular case, the child died before any direct physical intervention was possible and the hospital understandably would prefer to avoid other such cases in the future. A hospital has an obligation to provide at least reasonable care for patients and to maintain at least the minimal standards that are expected by the community. To be sure, a hospital must require that the physicians to whom it grants privileges practice medicine at an acceptable level and it should not grant privileges to those who practice substandard medicine. However, is not this situation a special case? Even though all medical signs indicated that the child should have received the transfusions, was the physician acting contrary to the minimal standards criterion in this particular set of circumstances? It could be argued that these peculiar circumstances would exempt this particular case from the minimal standards criterion.

There is no reason to believe that the physician would not order transfusions for those patients who had no religious prohibitions in this regard. Moreover, the right of competent adult patients to refuse medical intervention (totally or in part) has been upheld by the courts. Adult members of this religious group cannot be presumed to be incompetent merely because of the religious convictions they hold. If a court upholds the hospital's right to withdraw privileges from this physician *in toto,* it is quite likely that other hospitals also will withhold privileges because of their understandable desire to avoid being placed in such a situation themselves. Such an action could be tantamount to (1) denying the physician the right to practice medicine and thereby removing from him his ability to earn his living, and (2) denying medical care to a not insignificant portion of the population merely because their religion forbids one aspect of care. The latter action seems to be an unjust interference with religious freedom.

The hospital's stipulation that the physician promise in writing to order blood transfusions in similar cases in the future may seem to be reasonable. Yet such a requirement would obligate the physician to break faith with this community of believers at least with regard to the treatment of its children. Moreover, no other physicians are required to sign such a document even though they also might have minor patients who are members of this religious group. It is discriminatory to require this physician to sign a pledge merely because he is known to respect the religious beliefs of patients when others are not required to sign such a pledge.

THE COURT

Judicial intervention to secure life-saving medical treatment in cases involving minors whose parents voice religious objection to blood tranfusions or operations is common. In these situations in the United States, the courts uniformly have upheld state interference with parents' control in order to safeguard children.[7] The courts justified this interference by invoking the *parens patrie* doctrine, that is, the state's legitimate interest in the welfare of children and its right and duty to protect those who are unable to care for themselves. The *parens patrie* doctrine usually is embodied in child neglect statutes and authorizes the state to intervene when parents fail to provide necessary medical care.[8] Even without specific legislation, there have been indications that such interference would be forthcoming.[9] Given the long history of judicial intervention, the court would appoint a temporary guardian for the purposes of medical decision making who would have the authority to authorize blood transfusions.

Docs such state interference impose undue hardship on parents or interfere with their constitutional rights to privacy? If the state removed itself completely from the area of family decision making, the consequences could be far-reaching. For example, if parents sincerely believe that their child would be better off dead than continuing to live in a damaged condition, should this belief be respected? If so, how damaged should a child be for the wishes of the parents to be respected? If parents sincerely believe that the continued life of a child will infringe unjustly on their financial and emotional resources or cause hardship for other siblings,[10] should their decision to withhold treatment from their child be respected? At least one California court decision seems to support this position.[11]

Few would agree that parents should have absolute authority over their children. The notion that parents own their children and may do with them as they please is not acceptable in modern times,[12] but the right and duty of parents to act in the best interests of their child has been recognized, respected and fostered.[13]

In summary, it can be concluded that the state has a legitimate interest in the welfare of children and certainly has both the authority and the duty to protect children when necessary.[14] In cases that involve medical treatment, the state's authority usually is exercised by the courts and most court decisions favor the provision of life-saving medical treatments even when such treatments are contrary to the religious beliefs of the parents.

CONCLUSION

All health professionals have a duty to respect the clearly expressed wishes of competent patients with regard to their care. However, the obligations of health care professionals to families of patients is secondary to their obligations to the welfare of the patients. Health professionals should not confuse a family's value system with a patient's value system. In cases of conflict, therefore, the needs of an incompetent patient usually must take precedence over the wishes of the family. Whenever possible, of course, these interests should be balanced.

In the case study situation, there seems to be no other decision that the parents could have reached, given the sincerity of their religious convictions. The course of action chosen by the physician is problematic, but he was faced with a serious problem that he handled in good faith. The nurses were justified in their intervention as were the hospital and the courts. However, the actions taken by the hospital subsequent to the child's death seem to be discriminatory and the physician is justified in his attempts to prevent the hospital from withdrawing his privileges unless he signs a written statement to the effect that he will order blood transfusions in similar cases in the future.

OUTCOME

At the present time, this case is still in litigation.

COMMENTARY: CASE STUDY VII

M. Josephine Flaherty

As has been noted, this situation has interesting and far-reaching implications. A number of observations can be made about the actions that were taken.

The case study indicates that the physician decided to postpone surgery, but it does not note whether he consulted colleagues about his decision to use conservative treatment for the present time. There is no indication of how the physician had behaved in similar situations in the past or even if he had faced similar situations. There is some evidence to indicate that the parents had been approached about the possibility of blood transfusions and that they had refused because they "were not of a liberal persuasion." It is not known whether, if at all, concern about his relationships with the other members of the patient's religious persuasion affected the physician's decision to withhold the transfusions. This may not have been a major factor; his decision may have been predicated solely on his respect for the patient and her family and on his belief that conservative therapy might be successful. It is unlikely that the physician would have acted in this way, on his own, without consultation with colleagues, if he had not had some belief in the possibility of success with the conservative treatment. Hence, he cannot be accused, without further evidence, of practicing poor medicine or of performing illegal or unethical acts from which his patient should be protected. There is no doubt that the physician was taking risks; however, it must be assumed that his professional judgment was involved in his decision to take the risks. Even though one might not agree with that decision, a licensed professional has the right to be respected for his professional judgment.

If the physician agreed to the transfusions only because a higher authority decreed that they be given, he still would be confronted with a decision to continue to be the physician in charge of the patient, to work with the parents and to carry out a plan of care that was contrary to or at least different from his plan. He might be prepared to do this but it cannot be said definitively that in doing this, he would not be breaking faith with the family and with the rest of the religious group. In the final analysis, the physician is responsible and accountable for his decision.

The position of the nurses was understandable; they were responsible for the nursing care of their patient and that care included patient advocacy. However, it is not clear whether they had discussed their concerns with the physician, whom they respected, and/or with the family. As members of the health care team, nurses are required to communicate appropriately with significant others, including fellow professionals—both physicians and nurses—and the patient's family. One would wonder whether there had been a patient care conference of any kind before the director of nursing and administrative personnel were notified and whether a chaplain or counsellor had been consulted.

In reporting the situation to administrators, did the nurses talk with their head nurse or supervisor? Were they motivated by the positive welfare of the patient, the *summum bonum,* or by protection of her from harm, the *summum malum,* thinking of child abuse or neglect on the part of the parents, in their action of reporting to superiors?

There is no clear evidence that failure to report the incident would have constituted unethical conduct by the nurses unless they believed that such failure was in direct contravention of their patient advocacy role. The major aspect of their responsibility was the nursing care of their patient; they could give physical, social, spiritual, and emotional care without blood transfusions. However, their ethical and advocacy responsibilities did require them to communicate their concerns. What is not clear is whether they communicated with all of the relevant people and what was the nature of the nurses' disagreement about whether administrative personnel should be notified. Certainly, the nurses' decision to report their concerns to a higher authority, an action that resulted in that authority taking action that interfered with the physician's proposed plan of care, cannot be thought to constitute interference by the nurses in the physician–family relationship. If anyone interfered with that relationship, it was the courts and the hospital administration, but it is doubtful that either of these could be accused of interfering with the relationship.

The questions related to the nurses' (and other workers') respect for the religious beliefs of patients and families are complex. Nurses and other health professionals are becoming increasingly conscious of the significance that religious, cultural, and personal differences among patients have in the resolution of ethical and professional patient care problems. Although health care is thought to be a service oriented activity, nurses and other health care professionals are expected to exercise judgment in their service and care. If they sacrificed this judgment completely to the wishes of their patients, they could move from serving patients to being slaves of patients and thus they would be failing to exercise part of their professional role. On the other hand, if health care professionals imposed their will or ideas completely on patients, they would be making decisions for patients rather than with them and hence, could be accused of denying patients their autonomy. As has been suggested, there is need for a delicate balancing of points of view. This is accomplished usually through collegial decision making. In this case situation, it is not clear how much, if any, consultation there was between the physician and the administrative personnel before the matter was taken to judicial authorities. It is hoped that this action was accompanied by appropriate discussion and shared decision making by all people involved.

It is not clear whether the administrative decision was made by one or by several people and whether it was the result of discussion with a group of responsible persons. The speed with which the matter was referred to the judiciary for a court order suggests that the administrators' decision might have been made rather quickly and with relatively little consultation. One would wonder why the administrative personnel had not been aware of the situation earlier.

Certainly the hospital's action should not have been motivated only by the thought of the sparing of the staff from stress and turmoil, although these factors would contribute to the nature and extent of the staff's motivation to take extraordinary action—if notification of senior personnel about concerns can be thought to be extraordinary.

Curtin's conclusion that the various people's and groups' decisions were justified is reasonable. What is astounding, however, is that the hospital attempted to coerce the physician to sign an agreement about how he would handle specific situations in the future and that this action by the hospital was accompanied by the threat to revoke his privileges if he did not comply. Hence, one can understand why the physician is going to court over the matter.

It is reasonable to assume that the hospital is required to provide the minimal level of care that is expected by the community. However, a significant part of the community involved in this situation believed that the physician was acting according to appropriate standards of practice. By refusing to provide care to patients that would permit patients to refuse blood transfusions, the hospital would be infringing on the rights of the members of the particular religious group concerned and thus it would not be responding to their needs. By requiring a physician to sacrifice his professional judgment to a hospital general rule, the agency would be denying him the right to practice according to his beliefs and according to his professional qualifications. His behavior cannot be labelled as "substandard medicine" unless his statutory (licensing) body decides, on behalf of the medical profession, that he was not demonstrating generally accepted standards of practice. Hence, the hospital's proposal that the physician signify in writing that he will behave according to a hospital dictum, that may or may not have been developed by medical colleagues, is not reasonable. It could open the door to other kinds of conditions and methods of practice being required of physicians and other health professionals and invalidate the strength of professional autonomy—at personal, professional and statutory levels. This could destroy the concept of professional medical and health care practice.

NOTES

1. While not objecting to medical treatment in general, Jehovah's Witnesses believe that blood transfusions violate Biblical injunctions against eating blood (Acts 15:28–29; Deuteronomy 12:32; Genesis 9:3–4; Leviticus 17:10–14).

2. Larsen, G. "Child Neglect in the Exercise of Religious Freedom," *Kent Law Review,* Vol. 32 (1954) p. 283.

3. Cantor, Norman L. "A Patient's Decision to Decline Life Saving Medical Treatment: Bodily Integrity Versus the Preservation of Life," *Rutger's Law Review,* Vol. 26, No. 2 (winter 1973) pp. 231–234.

4. *The Code for Nurses With Interpretive Statements.* American Nurses' Association (Kansas City, Missouri, 1976).

5. Larsen, *op. cit.*

6. *Ibid.*

7. See People *ex rel. Wallace v. Labrenz,* 441 Ill. 618, 104 N.E. 2d 769, *cert. denied,* 344 U.S. 824 (1952); *State v. Perricone,* 37 N.J. 463, 181 A. 2d *cert. denied,* 371 U.S. 890 (1962); *Morrison v. State,* 252 S.W. 2d 97 (K.C. Ct. App. 1952); *People v. Pierson,* 1976 N.Y. 201, 68 N.E. 243 (1903).

8. Larsen, *op. cit.*

9. *State v. Perricone,* 37 N.J. 463, 475, 181 A. 2d 751, 759 (1962); *In re Clark,* 21 Ohio App. 2d 86, 87, 185 N.E. 2d 128, 129 (Ohio Common Pleas 1962).

10. Annas, George J. "The Limits of Parental Authority," *The Hastings Center Report,* Vol. 11, No. 1 (1981).

11. *Ibid.*

12. *Meyer v. Nebraska,* 262 U.S. 390, 399 (1923).

13. *Ibid.*

14. *Cf.,* footnote 7.

Case Study VIII: Structures, Attitudes, Regulations, and the Rights of the Elderly

Leah Curtin

Hattie Brown now resides in a nursing home. For eighty-four years Mrs. Brown was independent and fairly healthy. Two years ago, shortly after her husband's death, she developed diabetes. Since that time she has become forgetful, has developed several leg ulcers and is subject to "dizzy spells." The diabetes could be controlled with insulin and a proper diet, but Mrs. Brown forgot or, perhaps, thought it was too much trouble to cook for herself. In her words, "It didn't seem worthwhile to go to all that bother just for me. I ate a sandwich once in a while or put a T.V. dinner in the oven." Consequently, her neighbors found Hattie Brown in insulin shock twice and in diabetic coma once. She was hospitalized each time and the last time, she almost died.

Her physician was concerned about her eating habits, diabetes, and "forgetfulness." Therefore, he discharged her from the hospital to a nursing home. Because the physician was worried about how Mrs. Brown would adjust to institutional life, he left *prn* prescriptions for Elavil 5 mg. *q4h* and Seconal 100 mg *hs*. She receives no other medications except her insulin.

The nurses caring for Mrs. Brown in the nursing home observed that she seemed unhappy and lonely. She spends most of her time during the day staring out a window or sleeping in a chair. Mrs. Brown is fed regularly and properly, is kept clean and is given her insulin as needed. At night she is restless and disoriented. Several times she climbed over her bed rails and was found wandering about unsteadily in the halls. Once she said she had to put her cat out; another time, she thought the pilot light on her stove was out and, still another time, she thought that she had heard her husband call for help.

For her own safety, the nurses restrained her, but they continued to give her Seconal at bed time. To help combat her depression, they gave her Elavil regularly during the day. Mrs. Brown's behavior did not improve. In fact, she slept even more during the day, and, because she was restrained, she called out often during the night to be free. She was disturbing the other residents. Therefore, the nurses requested and received an order for Librium 10 mg. $q4h$ around the clock and, of course, Seconal 100 mg. at bedtime. Still, her behavior did not improve. If anything, she was more difficult to control.

Hattie Brown's physician visited the nursing home once a month, but he rarely saw her. He generally leafed through her chart and renewed her prescriptions. Her diabetes was under control and, although she seemed to be getting senile, there did not appear to be anything he could do about it. A young nurse, Regina S, was highly critical of the physician because she thought he ought to see Mrs. Brown and be more interested in her progress (or lack of it). She also knew that Medicare paid for his visits and she thought he was cheating the system. Moreover, Regina S was angry because there were other residents whose situations were similar to Mrs. Brown's: their medical conditions were stable but their personalities seemed to be disintegrating. Few of the physicians in charge of the medical regimen of the residents ever actually took the time to see them and yet the government paid them for their "services." On numerous occasions, Regina S was heard to say, "Too much of the money allocated for the care of the elderly by-passes them only to end up in the pockets of physicians!"

What, if anything, can Regina S or other nurses do for Mrs. Brown and other people who share her fate? Where do nurses' professional obligations lie and how can they be identified?

IDENTIFICATION AND CLARIFICATION

Unfortunately, what was a well-intentioned and necessary reform—in this case Medicare legislation—may be distorted and even oppressive when it is translated into the real world of patient care. Situations like those of Hattie Brown raise numerous questions among which are (1) questions of social structure and attitude, (2) questions about appropriate distinctions between medical and nursing care and the duties attached to each type of care, and (3) questions about the formulation and function of appropriate regulations for governmental programs. Although the questions are closely related in real life situations, for the sake of clarity, each will be considered separately.

SOCIAL STRUCTURE AND ATTITUDE

Systems, social attitudes and structures, and institutions shape the context within which professionals practice. To an interesting degree, "health" professionals today perform functions in and for society that, strictly speaking, have little to do with preventing disease, treating disease, curing disease, or even promoting health. Rather many of the functions that have been relegated to health professionals are designed to meet social needs that are of concern to the community.[1] "Hygienic bureaucracy stops the parent in front of the school and the minor in front of the court and takes the old out of the home."[2] Since the early nineteenth century, huge mental institutions, medical centers, and nursing homes have been developed to deliver services to particularly recalcitrant populations.[3] Although such facilities may permit more efficient delivery of care, they also allow "society at large to distance itself from contact with the afflicted."[4] That is, those whose behavior is socially unacceptable or disruptive are put in mental hospitals, those who are dying often are placed in medical centers and those who are old and unable to care for themselves are placed in nursing homes.

Although such institutions may serve useful, necessary, and even charitable purposes in many situations, their inappropriate use or operation may violate the human rights of many of their occupants. If the social function of such institutions is to hide the disconcerting plight of these populations from the general public, or if the operation of such institutions is designed primarily for the convenience of the health professionals who practice in them, their presence is an injustice to those whom, purportedly, they were designed to serve and a sign of moral bankruptcy in a society. Even if society is willing to pay the enormous economic price associated with the upkeep of such facilities solely for the purpose of protecting itself from the misery of some of its members, the sequestering and institutionalized neglect of aged or handi-capped populations is unjustified. The human rights of these individuals are violated as they live and die in a state of not-so-benign neglect: confined in functionally blank environments, kept quiet by drugs, hidden from the eyes of others, and forgotten by the community at large. The lives of these populations are controlled to promote the convenience of professionals and their existences are conveniently concealed from the public's conscience.[5]

The idealistic impulses that originally may have stimulated the development of these institutions often have been perverted. However, institutional life need not be either bleak or dehumanizing and it does not have to be any more expensive than it already is. What it will take to produce a more humane system for the care of those who cannot care for themselves and who have no one who can or will take care of them is twofold: (1) *public demand* for reform, stimulated perhaps by health professionals, and (2) *commitment* on the part of health professionals (principally nurses) to the improvement of the quality of the lives of those who cannot be cured and whose diseases or disorders are "com-plicated" by loneliness, neglect, poverty, and hopelessness.

As long as a majority of the citizens in a society and as long as the members of the health professions are willing to contribute to the neglect of these populations, the human rights of these people will be violated. Even if nurses and other health professionals are faithful to the promises of their profes-sions, they will not be able to effect social change without widespread com-munal support. Institutions are necessary and even vital to the well-being of certain populations; however, their purposes are perverted when they are used as dumping grounds for society or when they are used solely to provide employment, or as a form of undeserved largess for health professionals, or as a form of punishment for those who inconvenience others in society. In short, what is needed is a change in social attitude: a realization that mere allocation of funds is not sufficient to human need if it is unaccompanied by an understanding of the distinctly human needs of people.

DISTINCTIONS BETWEEN MEDICINE AND NURSING

The care given (or not given) to Hattie Brown and others highlights the distinctions that should be made between medicine and nursing. The physician was concerned with Mrs. Brown's medical condition which, in fact, was improved and stable. He also knew that the adjustment to institutional life could be difficult for her and that is why he prescribed the Elavil and Seconal. However, it should be noted that he prescribed both these drugs *prn*, that is, as necessary. One legitimately may ask, "As necessary according to whose judgment?" The physician rarely saw the patient—certainly no more than once a month at best. Therefore, it safely can be assumed that the drugs were to be given when the nurse(s) thought they were necessary.

Although one may wonder why a physician who looked at a patient's chart at least once a month did not connect the drugs (and the frequency of their administration) with the patient's unusual behavior (her sleeping during the day and her restlessness and disorientation at night), was it his responsibility alone? Have nurses no knowledge of pharmacology, the side effects or reverse effects of drugs and the possible reactions that elderly people in particular may have to tranquilizers, mood elevators, and sedatives? The nurses had an opportunity to observe Mrs. Brown daily; the physician did not. Although the physician prescribed the Librium, it was the nurses who requested it. Moreover, the physician did not prescribe that the drugs be given routinely; it was the nurses who decided to give them routinely. In addition, the nurses observed Mrs. Brown's behavior but they did not institute any nursing interventions to try to change it. They relied on medical pharmacologic means only. Not only did the nurses fail to connect the medications with certain physiological reactions, but they also failed to diagnose or treat Mrs. Brown's human responses to institutionalization, disease, and isolation.

The physician is not free from all responsibility but, clearly, the locus (and, thus, the responsibility) of decision making in this particular case rested with the nursing staff, not the physician. It is possible, although unlikely, that these nurses knew too little about pharmacology, physiology, or the effects of institutionalization to take effective action—to formulate hypotheses and to predicate alternative solutions to the problem. More likely, the nurses as well as the patient were victims of an unconscious attitude, an ingrained assumption that elderly people automatically are senile, difficult, and useless.[6] This is precisely the attitude that obstructs the effective and humane care of elderly, institutionalized people.[7]

If nurses accept Kant's imperative that all people are to be treated as persons, and if they take seriously the commitments of nursing, how can nurses (individually or collectively) account for Spetter's observation that "visiting any nursing home and seeing fine men and women nodding as in a coma [from overmedication with tranquilizing drugs] can be a vision of a particular hell in which those condemned to vegetation have been singled out by the socialization of cruelty and rejection."?[8] The fact is that such a hell is more a product of poor nursing care that it is of poor medical care.

Attempts to place the responsibility elsewhere—with the social system or with the physician—simply do not survive close scrutiny. One of nursing's peculiar strengths, a distinguishing characteristic, lies in its capability to improve the quality of people's lives. To misuse or to ignore this capacity—to rely solely on medical, pharmacological, or technical means in the care of people—is to prostitute the profession of nursing. Indeed, it is to reduce the role of nursing solely to that of physician assistant and thus to make the nurse a technological extension of the physician.

The major issue raised in this case study is not the physician's decisions or even his undeserved collection of Medicare funds; it is the nurses' failure to meet the promises and potential of their profession. It was a lack of understanding or respect for the humanity of the patients that led inexorably to poor nursing care—not lack of education or technical expertise. This does not excuse the physician's conduct, but it fixes responsibility where it belongs: squarely on the shoulders of the nurses caring for Mrs. Brown.

THE FORMULATION AND FUNCTION OF APPROPRIATE REGULATIONS

Appropriate governmental regulation of professionals and of programs that include professionals' services is a function of (1) the state's legitimate power and duty to protect the public from fraud or abuse and (2) the accountability of the government to the people for the expenditure of tax monies. However, to make sense, governmental regulation must be rooted in the specific competence of the professions. Competent practitioners are expected to make decisions that are based on their specific education and experience and that are within the boundaries described by statute, by institutional policies, and by governmental regulations. The essential link between appropriate regulation and practice is the regulator's understanding of the functions and services of the professions that are regulated—in this case medicine and nursing.

However well-intentioned and necessary a structural reform, its purposes can be distorted by failures at the bureaucratic level. The result may be that tax monies, if controlled and allocated inappropriately, brusquely by-pass those people whom they were intended to help. What Mrs. Brown and thousands like her really need is good nursing care; however, reimbursement regulations grant access to and control of this necessary resource solely to physicians, who may or may not understand the limits and potential of nursing care. Physicians, quite naturally, are inclined to identify, prescribe for, and treat the medical needs of patients or clients. They are not equipped to recognize or prescribe for the nursing needs of people. It is possible that the physician in this case study failed to see Mrs. Brown because he could perceive no need for him to see her: she was not ill. Mrs. Brown does have diabetes mellitus, but her disorder is under control. However, even though Mrs. Brown is not sick, she does need nursing care to help to maintain her health and possibly even to sustain her life.

Regulations that require that nursing services to the elderly must be certified and supervised by physicians seem to be predicated on several suppositions: (1) that aging is a disease rather than a normal process; (2) that nursing is an extension of, although subordinate to, medicine; (3) that physicians know how to evaluate the nursing care needs of people and prescribe the type of nurses' services to fill those needs; (4) that nurses need physicians to supervise the delivery of nursing services; and (5) that people must be sick to require nursing services.

CONCLUSIONS

In an ideal world, Mrs. Brown could remain in her own home with assistance. However, even in our less than ideal world, her life need not be altered by the administration of tranquilizers, mood elevators or barbiturates.

Residence in a nursing home need not include the assumption of a "sick role" or the surrender of personal dignity and control. To a certain extent, inappropriate formulation, promulgation and enforcement of regulations are the culprits. Because those who write and enforce regulations fail to recognize distinctions between health and illness care and between nursing and medical care, well-intentioned and even well-funded programs fail to meet people's needs. Nurses have an obligation to point out these distinctions and to lobby for necessary changes in regulations, but they also must address the degree of their fidelity to the promises of their profession. In this case study, the physician is less responsible for Mrs. Brown's plight than the bureaucracy and the bureaucracy is less responsible than the nurses. Social attitudes can explain, in part, the reasons for Mrs. Brown's plight, but they do not justify it.

COMMENTARY: CASE STUDY VIII

M. Josephine Flaherty

A number of observations can be made on what was done and not done in Mrs. Brown's situation.

The physician's decision to refer Mrs. Brown to a nursing home was a reasonable one, given the fact that appropriate resources to support her continuing to live at home were not available. What kind of care she received in the nursing home was dependent on the planning and decision making of several individuals and groups, each of which will be treated separately.

Society played a role in the situation through its informal and formal decision making about the care of elderly people, with or without major health problems. Few societies in the world today have made fully satisfactory arrangements for older people whose families are unable to care for them, and increasing attention is being paid today to this issue. Nursing homes have been built in the United States and regulations have been made for state support of some nursing home care. It has been noted that the regulations are not perfect. However, health care professionals, at both personal and professional association levels, do have responsibilities to examine and to evaluate current legislation and to press for changes in it if these are deemed necessary. Can one assume that the health care professionals in this situation were engaged in such activities or that they intended to become so engaged?

Government regulations are made usually after careful study of needs and resources and with advice from appropriate members of the public, including, in this instance, health care professionals and administrators. The efficacy of regulations is monitored by various types of governmental monitoring mechanisms that usually include nursing home inspectors. When such people visit the agencies involved, they should audit types and quality of care through direct observation and through study of a sampling of patient records, as well as through attention to whether the agencies are "following the rules." If the regulations are not adequate to situations, government inspectors should be so informed and should take action to have either the regulations or the situations modified. Hence, there is little or no excuse for the continuing existence of regulations that "everyone knows are not adequate."

Professional staff members in situations such as nursing homes have professional and ethical responsibilities to ensure that high quality and appropriate care is given to patients. In this situation, the physician was responsible for Mrs. Brown, because he had referred her to the nursing home, was still maintaining her as a patient and was collecting fees for his visits. He should have been seeing her regularly and doing periodic physical, social, and emotional evaluations of her condition in cooperation with other members of the health care team. His failure to do this constituted unprofessional and unethical behavior that should have been reported to the chief medical authority of the nursing home, and if necessary, to the statutory body for physicians and to the government funding source. There is a precedent for this in Canada where nurses in a long-term care agency, who were unable to influence physicians to see their patients regularly and to provide adequate care, took the matter to the licensing board for physicians. Action was taken and the situation was resolved. Here the nurses were exercising the patient advocacy role that is within the generally recognized scope of nursing practice. One would wonder why the nurses, particularly Regina S, who had recognized the problem, did not take action. If this nurse was highly critical of the physician, did she confront him with her concern? Perhaps he was not aware of the problem and was relying on the nurses to keep him informed. If the information was on the chart, he should have been aware of it, but maybe he was not reading the chart.

It is obvious that at least some of the nurses were concerned; what is not clear is how much action they took to remedy the situation. It appears that they chose to use *prn* medications without giving thought either to the effects of them on the patient or to alternative methods of care. This action by nurses could constitute statutory incompetence on their part, because they displayed, in their professional care of this patient, a lack of judgment or a disregard for her welfare. This could also be regarded as a breach of their contracts with the employer who hired them to behave as competent health professionals.

One would question whether there had been one or more patient care conferences about Mrs. Brown, for purposes of the evaluation and modification of the nursing care plan of the patient that is part of the nursing process. The nursing supervisors in the institution must have been aware of the problems Mrs. Brown was experiencing and one would wonder how much they had done to encourage the evaluation of the nursing care being given and to counsel nursing staff members about it. There is no mention of occupational therapy or recreology (recreational therapy) departments in the institution and one would wonder if these existed or, if not, why not. The nurses and supervisors also must have shared a concern for the welfare of the other patients who were being disturbed by Mrs. Brown.

The pharmacy in the agency supplied the drugs to the ward and should have been doing periodic evaluations of the amounts used and the effects of these on patients. Conferences between pharmacists and nurses, with appropriate communication with physicians, should take place at appropriate intervals, for discussion and possible solution of problems such as those described in Mrs. Brown's situation.

In summary, the physician, the nurses, the institution, the government, and society shared the responsibility for the failure to deal adequately with Mrs. Brown's difficulties. There is no excuse for any one of these individuals and groups "passing the buck" and leaving the responsibility for action with the others. The whole notion of a health care team puts professional and ethical responsibility for patient care on the shoulders of each and every member of the team. In this situation, they failed to assume and act on this responsibility.

NOTES

1. Bockoven, S. "The Moral Mandate of Community Psychiatry in America," *Psychiatric Opinion,* Vol. 3 (Winter 1966) p. 34.
2. Illich, Ivan. "Excerpts from *Medical Nemesis,*" in Robert Hunt and John Arras, eds. *Ethical Issues in Modern Medicine* (Mayfield Publishing Company, Palo Alto, California, 1977) p. 473.
3. May, William F. "Normative Inquiry and Medical Ethics in Our Colleges and Universities," in David Smith and Linda Bernstein, eds. *No Rush to Judgment* (Indiana University Foundation, Bloomington, Indiana, 1978) p. 352.
4. *Ibid.*
5. *Ibid.,* p. 353.
6. Spetter, Matthew I. "Growing Older in America: Can We Restore the Dignity of Age?" in Elsie Bandman and Bertram Bandman, eds. *Bioethics and Human Rights* (Little, Brown, Boston, 1978) pp. 202–204.
7. Buschmann, M. B. Tank. "The Nurse's Relationship to the Aged," *Nursing Forum,* Vol. XVIII, No. 3 (1979) p. 268.
8. Spetter, *op cit.,* p. 203.

Case Study IX: Nursing Education—The Unethical Conduct of the Role Models

M. Josephine Flaherty

Janet R, a nursing student, approached her instructor, Barbara D, during a period of clinical experience on a medical ward, to say that one of her patients was nauseated and she would like to give him the Gravol that was ordered for him. Barbara D agreed to supervise the preparation of the medication and Janet R brought the chart and medication kardex to the medicine cupboard; the medication was poured. A few minutes later, Janet R returned to Barbara D to tell her that she had given the medication to Mr. McKay, whose chart she had used in its preparation, and that immediately afterward, she had realized that it was Mr. Turner, who was in the next bed, who was nauseated and who needed the Gravol.

Janet R reported the medication error to the head nurse and to the staff nurse, Elizabeth S, who was responsible for the care of both patients involved when the nursing students were not on the ward. Appropriate charting was done by the student on the nurses' notes and the patient, Mr. McKay, was watched closely. Medication error forms were completed and signed by Janet R (the student), her instructor (Barbara D), the staff nurse (Elizabeth S), and the head nurse. According to hospital policy, one copy of the error form was to be sent to the nursing office to be placed in the staff nurse's file and the other copy was to become part of the patient's chart. For the time, both copies were left on the patient's chart. Mr. Turner, the patient who had complained about nausea, received his Gravol and was feeling somewhat better.

Later in the day, when Barbara D was reviewing the incident with her student, she looked for the medication error form on the chart and it was not there. The staff nurse had finished her shift and had gone home. Barbara D asked the head nurse about the error form and she replied that she did not know where it was, but that Barbara should do nothing now, as it "probably would turn up." She noted further that it probably did not matter anyway, because no harm had been done: both Mr. Turner and Mr. McKay had orders for Gravol *prn* for nausea, no side effects of the drug had been observed in Mr. McKay, and it was just as well that the staff nurse (who was ultimately responsible for the patients, but who really should not be chastised for a student's error in the presence of her instructor) would not have a record of this error in her employee file. Both the student and the instructor were surprised and disturbed. It was agreed that the staff nurse would be asked about the missing error form the next day.

On the following day, the staff nurse disclaimed any knowledge of the whereabouts of the error form and was not prepared to pursue the matter or to sign another error form; the head nurse agreed that the matter should be dropped; Barbara D, the instructor, was nonplussed about how to explain the situation to Janet R, the student, who was very confused about the whole affair.

What principles and policies were involved and how appropriate were they? What individuals, actions, rights, and responsibilities were involved? What should the instructor and the student do in such a situation?

ANALYSIS OF THE SITUATION

Essential Data

1. In the hospital cited, nursing students must be supervised for the pouring of medications by a registered nurse, who most often is their instructor.

2. A staff nurse always has ultimate responsibility for patients for whom students are caring; medication errors made by students are charged against the staff nurse and filed in his/her record.

3. The *prn* medication was prepared correctly and given to a patient according to the orders on his chart; however, he was not the patient who needed the medication on that occasion.

4. The instructor supervised the preparation of the medication and accepted the student's word that the chart she used was the chart for the patient who was nauseated. It did not occur to the teacher to verify the correctness of her student's identification of the patient who had complained of nausea.

5. The correct forms were completed and signed and placed on the patient's chart, according to hospital policy and practice, and appropriate nursing personnel were notified and signed the forms.

6. The form disappeared from the chart. Neither the staff nurse nor the head nurse admitted having any knowledge of the whereabouts of the forms and neither was willing to pursue the matter.

7. The instructor discussed the original error in detail with the student and was troubled about what she should do about the missing error forms.

Rights and Responsibilities Involved

A number of rights and responsibilities were involved in this situation, among which were:

1. The rights of both Mr. McKay and Mr. Turner to skilled and safe nursing care

2. The responsibility of the student to provide safe nursing care

3. The responsibility of the instructor to supervise the work of students

4. The responsibility of the staff nurse for the quality of care given to the patients who were assigned to her, including the ones who were assigned temporarily to students, and the responsibility to practice according to the standards for which she is accountable

5. The responsibility of the head nurse to ensure that the nursing care on the ward is given according to the standards of nursing practice, the ethical code for nurses and the policies and practices of the hospital

6. The responsibility of the hospital to ensure that its policies and practices are appropriate and are implemented; and the right to expect integrity from its staff members and "guest practitioners" such as nursing students and instructors from the schools of nursing with which the hospital has practice agreements

7. The responsibility of the school of nursing to ensure that the clinical situations to which students are sent are compatible with the standards of practice that are being taught in the school and that the students and instructors respect and conform with the policies and practices of the agencies according to the hospital-school practice agreements.

1. The Patients

In general, the care provided was appropriate and safe. When the error was made it was reported and recorded and Mr. McKay was observed carefully for side effects. The situation was explained to him and to Mr. Turner who subsequently received his medication. Both patients accepted this situation gracefully, and no negative results were noted for either patient. Hence, it cannot be said that there was a serious denial of rights beyond the human error that was acknowledged and dealt with in what was apparently the best way possible in the situation.

2. The Nursing Student

Janet R made a serious error that could have had a very negative effect on her patient. Fortunately, the medication did not have a harmful effect on Mr. McKay. Janet reported the error immediately to the appropriate sources, discussed the matter in detail with her instructor, and acknowledged her fault and its implications, in writing, on the medication error form. She learned a valuable lesson from her behavior in this incident and will be much more careful in the future regarding accurate identification of her patients.

When the medication error form disappeared, Janet worked with her instructor in an effort to locate it. She did not encourage the "letting the matter drop" that was suggested and was very upset that the situation developed as it did.

3. The Nursing Instructor

Barbara D believed that she could trust Janet R, a senior student, to identify her patients correctly, to bring the appropriate chart for the pouring of the medication, and to administer the medication safely. Her position was understandable, as Janet R was a strong student and Barbara had worked with her for some months. She took pains to ensure that Janet R understood fully the implications of the error and she asked Janet to share the incident with the other members of the class to reinforce the importance of medication policies and practices, the effects of medications on patients, and the significance of safe nursing care.

When the error form disappeared, Barbara put considerable effort into her attempts to locate the missing documents or to have them re-done. When she was rebuffed in these efforts by the staff nurse and the head nurse, she reflected on it and consulted colleagues about whether she should report the incident to the director of nursing of the hospital or to the director of the school of nursing, or both. She realized that such reporting could be considered to be accusations that the head nurse and/or the staff nurse were involved in some way in the disappearance of the documents and hence that they were dishonest. If she pressed the matter of their refusing to complete the forms again or to inquire further into the matter, Barbara could be accused of harassing them, of questioning their judgment, and of trying to make a "big thing" out of a human incident. She believed, however, that if she let the matter drop, she would be failing to practice nursing with integrity and honesty, would not be working within the policies of the agency and would be failing to behave as a worthy role model for her students. She brought the matter to the head nurse's attention again and was told that the forms had never "turned up," that the matter was finished, and that she should do nothing more about it. She considered pursuing the matter with the director of nursing and realized that if she did this, she might engender the hostility of the head nurse and other nurses in the agency and jeopardize her and the school's relationship with the agency and thus threaten the students' future experiences in the agency. She shared her concern with her teacher colleagues and was advised to let the matter drop. The director of the school of nursing agreed with this advice. Barbara explained to the students what had happened, noted that it was an unfortunate situation and said nothing more about it. However, she is worried about it, believes that a similar incident may take place again and is concerned about how it will be handled.

4. The Staff Nurse

The staff nurse knew about the incident and signed the forms. She did not want to be held responsible for the actions of nursing students over whom she had no authority. She could not understand why the student's error had to become part of her record of employment, and why this was a hospital policy. As an employee of the teaching hospital, she had no choice about whether students would care for some of her patients. She did enjoy having their assistance with her patient load but she resented that she had responsibility without authority for them. It is not known whether she ever had discussed this matter with her superiors but she should do so. Whether she had anything to do with the disappearance of the error forms is not known and probably never will be known. It is assumed that nobody asked her directly if she had taken the forms because she said that she had no idea where they were. That she refused to sign another set of forms could indicate that she was not fulfilling the policies of the agency. However, as she said, she already had signed one set of forms and hence had done her duty in this regard. Her conviction that she should not be blamed for something over which she had no control is understandable. It is unfortunate that at least some of the people involved in the situation are suspicious of her, largely because of her refusal to take further action on the issue. Whether or not she was fulfilling her professional responsibilities for record keeping is a moot point, as no staff nurse can be expected to stand guard over patient records when she is not on duty. In addition, it could be argued that the addition of a new medication error form, that has been re-done from memory to replace the original one that had been filled out previously, could constitute interference with or falsification of a record. Only the staff nurse herself could determine with certainty whether or not her behavior was truthful and ethical.

5. The Head Nurse

She, too, was familiar with the incident and had signed the original error forms. Her refusal to delve into the disappearance of the forms from the chart, her advice to the instructor to drop the matter and her comments to the effect that it was "just as well" that the report of the error did not have to be in the staff nurse's file throw some suspicion on her. It is clear that she was responsible for ensuring that hospital policies were carried out and that she was not fulfilling this responsibility in this case. By knowingly allowing a patient record to be inaccurate, through omission of a part of it, she was not practicing according to the standards of practice and of ethics of the jurisdiction in which she was registered, and for this she could have been disciplined. By not reporting the incident to higher authorities in the agency, she was in breach of hospital policy. By not demonstrating a high quality of professional behavior to the instructor and students and to her staff, she was failing to be the positive role model that senior nurses are expected to be in their professional practice. The others who were involved in the situation did not have the same amount of confidence in her that they had had previously and hence the trust relationship between her and them was threatened.

6. The Hospital Administration

The administrative personnel of the hospital had developed and were implementing the policy that placed responsibility without authority for students on staff nurses. This imposition of responsibility is questionable. The hospital believes that it is only by means of a policy like this one that continuity of patient care and responsibility for it can be ensured. However, it does force staff nurses to assume an additional burden for which they may not be well prepared and qualified.

The justice or injustice of the regulation should be examined and evaluated. It should be noted that on at least one occasion in the jurisdiction involved, a staff nurse was reprimanded by the statutory body as a result of a similar instance. Hence, there is a precedent in support of the continuation of a policy like this one where nursing students are involved in clinical practice experience. This may help to assure the hospitals and the schools that patient safety will be increased because the responsibility for it is on the shoulders of the staff nurse. However, unless the staff nurse has the authority to direct and supervise the care given by students, one can question the justice of the responsibility being imposed on the registered nurse. Such a policy could be thought of as incompatible with the hospital's responsibility to provide conditions under which nurses can practice according to accepted standards.

7. The School of Nursing

The whole matter should be examined and discussed by the hospital and the school of nursing. The latter, in agreeing to let the matter drop, was not fulfilling its responsibility to ensure that its staff and students respect and adhere to policies and practices of the agency. Students were not shown the proper methods for handling record keeping in this instance and the school has a responsibility for this. By counselling the instructor to do nothing more in the situation, the director and staff of the school were not supporting their nursing colleague according to the standards of practice. However, it may be that in their professional judgment, given the context and the lack of hard data about the events surrounding the disappearance of the error forms, they believed that this was the best course of action for the instructor.

Conclusion

This is a complex but not unusual situation on which nurses should reflect. How else could it have been handled? Would the problems caused by further investigation of the incident have changed the situation? Is the policy about staff nurse responsibility for students a good one? Why or why not?

COMMENTARY: CASE STUDY IX

Leah Curtin

Nursing students and instructors of nursing, as Flaherty notes, are guest practitioners in the institution who have a responsibility to respect and adhere to policies and practices of the agency. Although the medication error in this case situation does not appear to have been a serious one, the policy involved is significant. Moreover, the disappearance of the report forms and the circumstances in which they disappeared are of great significance. What really is at issue in this case is not a relatively minor medication error, but rather the integrity of the nurses involved. Other significant issues include the institution's responsibility for the safe care of patients, its responsibility to investigate any errors made, and the obligations of health professionals to inform administrative personnel of any errors or untoward incidents that occur on the wards in the care of patients. The institution cannot fulfill its responsibilities to monitor the quality of care patients receive if information about errors is withheld. Barbara D had reason to suspect that information about the error was being suppressed deliberately, probably to keep the error out of the staff nurse's personnel file.

This is unfortunate for several reasons. Nurses have professional collegial obligations to support, guide, and correct one another. A situation such as this one offered an opportunity to the nurses to perform these services for one another. For example, had this situation been handled properly, it would have provided an opportunity for the head nurse, the staff nurse, the nursing instructor, and the nursing student to discuss the propriety of the policy that required staff nurses to assume responsibility for the practice of students over whom they were denied authority. As a result, the policy could have been modified or eliminated. The policy could have been modified to provide that students and/or their instructors consult with the staff nurses responsible for the patients' care prior to the administration of medications, thus granting a measure of control to the staff nurses. The policy also could have been modified by the director of nursing in conjunction with the director of the school in such a manner that a copy of the medication error report would be included in the instructor's personnel file and/or in the student's file rather than in the staff nurses' personnel file, thus relieving the staff nurse of responsibility where she had no authority. It is important to note that legal responsibility for an error in the administration of medications falls primarily on the person who administered the medication, on the person (if any) who directly supervised the administration of the medication and finally on the institution that is accountable for the care patients receive. The chart itself is considered a legal document and those who sign it can be held accountable under the law for any procedure, treatment, medication, or care for which they have signed—whether or not they personally delivered the care, performed the treatment, or gave the medication. There is evidence in the case study that the student charted this occurrence appropriately in the nurses notes; thus, the student is accountable for the error.

There is evidence to support the claim that the nursing instructor used this incident as a learning tool to reinforce to the student the importance of care in the administration of medications and to teach the student what procedures to take in the event of a medication error. However, one well may wonder what else the student learned. She may have "learned" that adherence to agency policies is important only if the people involved place importance on it. She may have "learned" that her instructor's counsel regarding the importance of any medication errors is valid only if the patient suffers significant side effects (a fact, unfortunately, that cannot be known until it is too late to correct it). She may have "learned" that nurses do not support one another as she witnessed the head nurse and the staff nurse undermine the authority of her nursing instructor. She may have "learned" that nurses, rather than seeking to change inappropriate policies, violate them instead of changing them. She may have "learned" that nurses lack integrity. Although there is no hard evidence that someone deliberately destroyed the medication error report forms, there certainly is suspicion that this is what actually occurred. Moreover, she may have "learned" that the director of her school would rather compromise the integrity of nursing instructors, students and the school of nursing than risk the displeasure of the hospital nurses.

Although one can hope that the student did not "learn" such things, it must be noted that the adage "example is the best teacher" is not without foundation. The handling of this situation by the head nurse, staff nurse, and director of the school is reprehensible. In the final analysis, nursing students undoubtedly are affected by the role models they observe and their ideals about the importance of integrity, accountability, and excellence in practice will be formed, or at least affected, by their teachers and the practicing nurses with whom they have contact.

Case Study X: Cardiopulmonary Resuscitation and the Nurse

Leah Curtin

As I walked into Christy's room with a tray full of pills, I heard her ask her mother, "Mommy, what's it like to die?" I stopped—halfway through the door. Her mother answered, "Honey, it's sort of like this. Do you remember when you were at home and you'd fall asleep downstairs? Daddy would pick you up in his arms and carry you upstairs and everything would be all right. Well, dying is something like that, only this time God will pick you up in His arms and then everything will be fine." I entered the room then and Christy's mom and I gave her the medications.

Christy was a three-year-old child, made mature beyond her years by suffering. She was dying of lymphosarcoma. For three months, she had been in and out of the hospital—and this trip was the last one. Everyone knew that she was dying: her physician, her parents, and her nurses. Christy's mom stayed with her all day, every day, and her dad usually spent the nights with her.

One night about 12:30 a.m., I went into her room. She was resting quietly, but her mother had had about all she could take. Tears of exhaustion, pain and grief were sliding silently down her cheeks. I sat down next to her and we stayed together for a few minutes until her husband arrived. The floor was fairly quiet that night, so I suggested that both of them go down to the automat for a cup of coffee and a little time together. I promised that I would not leave Christy's room until they returned.

Perhaps ten minutes after they left, Christy awoke. She was much worse and appeared to be very frightened. I called the practical nurse and told her to call the doctor, the supervisor, and the chaplain and to send an aide down to the automat *stat* to get her parents. Christy was struggling to breathe and there was fear in her eyes. Suddenly, I remembered what her mother had told her.

293

Gently, I leaned over and picked her up and held her in my arms. She seemed to relax as she laid her head against my shoulder. She died like that—quietly in my arms. I do not know how long I stood there holding Christy. It seemed like an eternity but it could not have been more than a few minutes.

Her parents rushed into the room, I looked at them—and they knew Christy was dead. As we were tucking her into bed, a young resident physician entered the room. He took one look at Christy and said, "My God, why didn't you call a code?" He started to pound on Christy's chest, but her father stopped him. I turned to Christy's mom and said, "I'm so sorry." She started to cry and so did I. I held her in my arms and she held me. In a few minutes I was able to tell her how Christy died, how I held her in my arms and how she wasn't afraid anymore. The chaplain arrived about that time and we all went to the lounge. As he talked to them, I left to get coffee from the nurse's locker room.

The priest was talking with the parents, and other children on the floor needed my attention, so I did not stay long. I made rounds and then helped to prepare Christy's body for the morgue. I thought the incident was ended—although I knew I would never forget Christy or her parents. However, the incident was far from over. The next morning I was called to the nursing office. Why hadn't I called a code on Christy? Hospital policy required that a code be called on all patients unless there was a written no code order. Her pediatrician had not written a no code order; who was I to make such a decision?

In all honesty, I could only respond by saying, "It never occurrred to me to call a code. Everyone knew Christy was dying; no one disagreed. Even if I had called a code, it probably wouldn't have been successful. If it had been, the only result would have been that Christy would have suffered longer before she died." Fortunately for me, the chaplain had heard (through the super-efficient hospital grapevine?) that I was in trouble. He made an impassioned plea in my behalf and I was "let off" with a severe reprimand. I feel no guilt about my care of Christy—only sorrow for her suffering and her death at so young an age. I also feel privileged to have known Christy's parents: gentle people of courage and strength. However, there are other children like Christy; doctors still won't write no code orders (no matter what they may say) and the hospital policy remains the same. If I fail to resuscitate some other dying child, I don't know what will happen. What will (or should) I do when faced with similar situations in the future?

IDENTIFICATION OF THE ISSUES

Quite frequently, staff nurses are placed in the position of either resuscitating a patient or acquiescing to the person's death simply because no one else is there. Moreover, nurses often are placed in paradoxical positions by conflicting written and verbal instructions from physicians; by physician directives that conflict with hospital policies; by conflicting statements from patients, family members, and physicians; by their own conflicting perceptions and values; and, finally, by the absence of a clear, rational, and humane policy regarding cardiopulmonary resuscitation. It is not uncommon for nurses to be asked to employ such subterfuges as the "Slow Code" (otherwise known as "walk, do not run, to the phone"). These so-called slow codes not only are dishonest, they may cause untold anguish and do cost a great deal of money—to no avail. The health professionals are not trying to succeed. Either one codes or one does not: there is no such thing as a "slow code."

Today, hospitals no longer are seen as places people go to die, but rather as places people go so that they may live or live more fully. A technological advance as dramatic as CPR inevitably stimulates the imagination of health care professionals and the general public alike. Yesterday's extraordinary achievement becomes today's demanded result.

Cardiopulmonary resuscitation was developed primarily to assist heart patients and those whose hearts were affected temporarily by trauma or disease. The use of this technique might buy enough time for either surgical intervention or natural healing to occur. It is not a cure for any known disease; it can prevent death from occurring but it cannot re-create life or reverse the ravages of disease. Should this technique be used when the only projected outcome will be to prolong the dying process? Should it be used when the only projected outcome will be the maintenance of life in a state of profound disability? What constitutes the use and misuse of this technology? Who decides?

When a patient experiences a cardiac arrest, there is no time for reflection or weighing of values. This is all the more reason why the decision to use or not to use CPR demands participatory preparation: prior consultation, communication, and deliberate thought among all people involved. Adequate preparation should help to eliminate indecision, to moderate stress, to assure compliance and to increase effectiveness. Decisions about the use of cardiopulmonary resuscitation should not be made impersonally nor should they be made in an under-the-table manner. The issues involved demand careful consideration, clear communication, and individual application. Conscious and rational decision making in these areas must not be avoided. Some professionals try to buy time and distance from disappointment or blame by appeals to tradition, to rules and to regulations—to any external restraints that come to mind. Others try to measure the value of a technological advance by the degree of its predictability. The successes of CPR still urge one to act affirmatively: its failures still encourage one to refrain. How can health professionals be sure that those who can benefit from resuscitation will receive it, while those who cannot, will not receive it? Blanket policies (*e.g.,* always resuscitate every patient) produce nothing but frustration;

they stifle humane tendencies, lead to decisions made by default or, worse still, to decisions made and carried out *sub rosa*.

By and large, physicians, hospitals, and nurses do not want to prolong people's suffering or to mechanize their dying. The real obstruction to their ability to deal openly with these problems is fear—not so much fear of death or even the responsibility for decision making (although it *is* onerous), but rather the mundane, materialistic, and realistic fear of malpractice suits. As a result, the physician will not write a "no code" directive, the hospital establishes a blanket policy, nurses are caught in a painful dilemma—and patients may suffer a prolonged and mechanized death.

TOWARD A RESOLUTION*

Since the 16th century scientific endeavor has built a shelter of confidence on the dramatic successes arising from rational application of technologically improved tools. Solutions were positive, life-expanding, *automatic,* and tangible. The human mind was extolled and human emotions were deprecated. Indeed, mind was set against emotion. Problems, failures, and side-effects were ignored by the general public—to be examined only by a very small elite of professionals. Today, with the rapid diffusion of knowledge to a public in highly diverse states of intellectual and psychological development, this era has passed.

INSTITUTIONAL WILL

In the past, decisions about CPR supposedly were left to the discretion of the physician alone. In the final analysis, however, nurses often were left to make such decisions alone—without support or guidance. Largely as a reaction to a perceived malpractice crisis, hospitals established blanket CPR policies requiring resuscitation of all patients, and physicians refused to write no code orders. Nurses were commanded by institutions and by physicians to resuscitate. The wishes or needs of patients and families, while often communicated to the nurses, seemed to be ignored by physicians and institutions—as was the likelihood of success.

In eras of few options, man-powered techniques, short time spans, immobile capital resources and limited access to knowledge, command ethics may have been appropriate. However, that epoch is gone. Burgeoning technology, multiple options, and diffusion of knowledge have rendered the command ethic obsolete. Because many people are involved in decisions such

---

*This section is a revised version of "CPR: Optimal Care vs. Maximal Treatment." It appeared in the August 1979 issue of *Supervisor Nurse* and is reprinted here with the permission of S-N Publications, Inc.

as those related to CPR—patients, families, health professionals, institutions—the notion of institutional will (*i.e.,* guidance, support, and shared decision making) is taking the place of command ethics.

However, the method of implementation of institutional will must be clear. To make *ad hoc* pleas for rational and compassionate behavior is very nice, but hardly helpful in situations like the ones where CPR is considered. It is far more useful to provide a clear, written statement of what is considered rational and humane in specific circumstances. Articulation and dissemination of policy helps to focus attention on what is being done, by whom and for what reasons. It helps to ensure that those who should make decisions actually do so—and hence, decisions are not avoided, made by default, or handled *sub rosa.* Thus, potentially tragic errors in judgment—or misplaced compassion—will be minimized.

Another value of the development of a flexible CPR policy is that it focuses institutional attention on the problem of life-prolongation. The guidelines that are developed can be applied to other techniques in similar situations. They can begin to lay the groundwork for the compassionate application of technology throughout the institution. Moreover, CPR policies can provide a recognizable basis for the development of accepted community standards of practice. Once such standards are developed, the threat of resuscitation-related malpractice suits will be reduced.

ELEMENTS OF A SOUND CPR POLICY

The primary goal of any hospital or health professional is to provide optimal care to all patients. However, optimal care often is confused with maximal treatment.[1] "The right medical practice will provide those who may get well with the assistance they need, and it will provide those who are dying with the care and assistance they need in their final passage. To fail to distinguish between these two sorts of medical practice would be to fail to act in accordance with the facts."[2] However, the care and treatment of the terminally ill in North America has been gradually shifting from optimal care to maximal treatment[3] partly because of an increased reliance on technology,[4] partly because of legal bias for maximal treatment,[5] and partly because of poor clinical judgment.[6] Moreover, reliance on the traditional distinction between ordinary and heroic measures of prolonging life has reinforced this trend.[7] Attention is directed toward pieces of equipment or techniques (is it heroic or ordinary?) rather than the condition and wishes of the patient. To correct this situation, *any rational general policy includes a method of distinguishing between those who enter the hospital to die and those who enter the hospital to recover.*[8] Although a short-term acute care facility is no place for dying human beings, they *are* there. Their need is for intensive caring, not intensive technological care. If they are conscious at all, they need their families and loved ones around them.

The modern intensive care unit is a technological marvel: it epitomizes maximal treatment, but, for dying patients, that does not represent optimal care. Therefore, hospital policy *should provide for the placement of irreversibly dying patients in other, more appropriate areas of the hospital.*

Provision also must be made for those individuals who enter the hospital to recover, but whose conditions cannot be treated successfully and who subsequently become irreversibly terminally ill. General hospital policy *should distinguish between those already admitted to the hospital whose conditions have become irreversibly terminal, and those whose conditions may respond to treatment.* A patient classification system similar to that outlined by the Critical Care Committee of the Massachusetts General Hospital may prove most helpful.[9] According to such a policy, critically ill patients are classified as follows: "*Class A*—maximal therapeutic effort without reservation; *Class B*—maximal therapeutic effort without reservation, but with daily evaluation because probability of survival is questionable; *Class C*—selective limitation of therapeutic measures. The criterion which determines every aspect of the therapeutic regimen continues to be the overall welfare of the patient. At this time certain procedures may cease to be justifiable and become contraindicated . . .".[10]

Far too often health professionals and hospital administrators act as though resuscitation problems are their private preserve. They are not. A humane policy should include a method whereby patients or their families can express their wishes or expectations in the event that cardiopulmonary resuscitation does not offer hope of benefit to the patient. The Beth Israel Hospital of Boston demonstrates a scrupulous respect for patients in its document, "Orders Not to Resuscitate."[11]

The contemporary modern realizes that success lies in reconciliation of the claims of intelligence and of emotion. Today's health professional knows that stress must be managed by proper channeling of persons, resources, and controls. Any systematized group (institution) increases the number of options that are available to support persons against their personal limits of knowledge and of psychological strength. Justifiable institutions moderate the stresses of conflicting claims on the persons they serve—and who serve in them. Institutions demonstrate these activities through the policies they proclaim and practice and through the behavior of their leaders. To offer viable options, institutions must provide a continuous flow of education, support, and correction. They also must convey a sense of reliability: of honesty to the tasks they claim.

The development of a rational and humane policy regarding the use of cardiopulmonary resuscitation represents one option that is open to institutions to help reduce stress and to increase accountability to the public. It is not an easy task and certainly not an agreeable one—difficult distinctions must be made and lines drawn. Many values are involved, and sometimes they conflict.

While declaring that the hospital's general policy is "to act affirmatively to preserve the lives of all patients," the Beth Israel document establishes procedures by which a patient (or family in the case of an incompetent patient) can collaborate in a standing order not to resuscitate.[12] Such collaboration depends on certain provisos—specifically that the patient's condition is irreversible and irreparable and that death is imminent. Although this practice relinquishes only a small degree of control to patients or their families, it could help to alleviate fears of under- or over-treatment. *Any humane general policy should establish procedures by which patients (or their families) can express their wishes when the patient's condition is irreversible and irreparable and when death is imminent.*

To facilitate communication, ensure accuracy and secure compliance, *a hospital policy should require "do not resuscitate" orders to be written in an appropriate place on the patient's chart.*

A body of consultation or appeal should be provided for difficult cases. *The hospital's policy should designate a standing committee for consultation or appeal,* for example, an Optimum Care Committee or an Ethics Committee.

Because of the sensitive nature of this issue, it is advisable to permit flexibility and discretionary judgment in the implementation of a CPR policy. The hospital is not determining arbitrarily who shall live and who shall die but rather is attempting to ensure that no one dies unnecessarily, and that those who must die will do so without discomfort or indignity.

To establish CPR policy is one thing; to achieve compliance is quite another. If major departments of the hospital are included in the development of the policy (medicine and nursing should be represented heavily), eventual success is more likely. The hospital's legal counsel can be of assistance in at least three ways: (1) in the research regarding the laws of the state or province and other jurisdictions to assure that the policy does not violate law; (2) in the collection of written statements of such national bodies as the American Hospital Association, the Catholic Health Association, the American Nurses' Association, the American Medical Association, the American Heart Association, and the American Bar Association; and (3) to peruse a draft of the policy to advise the committee regarding the possibility of liability. A lawyer, however, should not determine policy with regard to patient care; he or she should be a member of the committee and not a committee of one!

Hospitals and health professionals within a geographic community should protect themselves by cooperating with each other in the development of CPR policy. In such manner, accepted community standards of practice can be developed.

Health care institutions must reconcile human needs and technological demands, combat fruitless skepticism, and calm fears (their own and others'). Technological skills are great and growing, and this knowledge will continue to grow. To moderate the stress of expanded choice, human beings must take the time to determine together how best to apply knowledge and technology to the greatest benefit of patients, health professionals, and society.

PRAGMATIC CONSIDERATIONS

Until such time as flexible, rational policies regarding the use of CPR are developed, disseminated and in practice, nurses will continue to be placed in untenable positions. The decision not to resuscitate should not be uni-lateral—whether the person making that decision is a nurse, a physician or a family member. The only person who has a perfect right to make that decision is the competent patient. However, for many reasons, this "easy way out" often is not available. As a rule, irreversibly dying individuals should not be subjected to cardiopulmonary resuscitation. Pragmatically speaking, it achieves nothing. All that results is more agony for the dying and lasting scars for the living. It is a degrading and unnecessary interruption of a person's dying.

In cases where there is some hope for recovery, CPR should be employed unless it is prohibited specifically by the competent, adult patient with particular attention directed to the consent process. However, such an approach is difficult to implement in the face of institutional or legal opposition.

In this particular case study situation, the nurse acted appropriately—she calmed the fears of a dying child and made her death more comfortable and, yes, dignified. One hopes that her fear of legal, institutional, or professional censure will not induce her indiscriminately to resuscitate irreversibly dying individuals. A nurse's first obligation is to her own integrity and to the overall welfare of the patient. Both would be violated if she followed this course of action. However, to proceed on her own, without input or support from others, arbitrarily to determine whom she will or will not resuscitate poses problems of its own.

This latter course of action is fraught with danger for both patient and nurse: the possibilities for abuse are enormous. Given a respect for human rights and a consideration for the fact that many people are involved in such decisions, it is not permissible for one person to make a unilateral decision for death for another person. One individual's understanding of the facts may be imperfect, or his or her compassion may be misplaced. The possibilities for errors or injustice are so great that shared decision making is required. Moreover, the burden is too onerous for one person to bear alone. Nurses and other health professionals may have to force the issue if hospitals and physicians refuse to face it. For the patients' sake and for their own protection, nurses must not act precipitously on a shaky data base or only according to their personal values. Another individual's life is at stake and that is not a small matter.

COMMENTARY: CASE STUDY X

M. Josephine Flaherty

This case study situation brings to light a number of areas of responsibility, on some of which Curtin has commented. The benefits and risks of technological approaches to health care, such as cardiopulmonary resuscitation, have been pointed out and the conflicting views and behaviors of various members of the health care team have been highlighted.

One cannot help but wonder how familiar the young resident physician was with the patient's condition and with her family's point of view. One could ask whether he knew how long the child had been dead and whether his decision to try to resuscitate her was based on reason or simply on an almost reflex reaction. It has been noted in some situations that attempts should be made to resuscitate all patients, because it is "good experience" for the staff. The inhumanity of such a statement is astounding, but it probably is the result of the devotion of some health care professionals to technology rather than to the care of human beings.

In view of the father's reaction to the physician's attempts to resuscitate the child, it is even more astounding that the nursing administration personnel would reprimand the nurse for what was the only possible ethical and professional choice of action that she could have taken. Why was it only the chaplain who came to the nurse's defense? Chaplains do not have a monopoly on humanitarian behavior. The nursing profession alleges that its hallmark is the caring quality of its members' behavior, and yet it was that profession that censured the caring behavior of one of its own members. The policy of the institution to resuscitate all patients and the behavior of its nursing leaders were both in conflict with the caring behavior that was required in the case study situation.

Curtin has suggested that agency policies about cardiopulmonary resuscitation should be developed by committees in the agencies, with heavy representation from nursing and from medicine. If nursing had been represented in the development of policy in this agency, it must have been either not willing or not able to focus attention on the human aspect of the policy. The responsibility of nurse administrators to demonstrate accepted standards of practice and to be faithful to the promises of the nursing profession extends beyond their own behavior to include responsibility for the behavior of those who are part of the nursing department. The reprimand should not have been registered against the nurse. It should be removed from her record, unless it can be proven that her failing to observe the blanket rule to resuscitate in the hospital was demonstration of incompetence or professional misconduct, that is, failure by her to exercise appropriate and sound judgment in the application, or lack of it, of hospital policy. The nurse in this situation would be wise to seek the advice of her registering body on this incident.

A nurse administrator who supports the reprimand in this type of situation could be accused of poor judgment and of failure to implement an acceptable nurse–nurse relationship. The behavior of the resident physician should be investigated and appropriate action taken to clarify and/or modify the policy of the institution. A hospital that continues to implement an uncompromising policy such as this one should examine its purposes and its policies and practices to determine whether these are compatible. It is only through actions like these, as Curtin has suggested, that the obligations of hospitals and professionals to care for patients can be realized and that the use of high technology can be kept within the boundaries of humane care.

NOTES

1. May, William F. "The Right to Die and the Obligation to Care: Allowing to Die, Killing for Mercy, and Suicide," in David H. Smith, ed. *No Rush to Judgment* (Poynter Center, Bloomington, Indiana, 1977) p. 74.

2. Ramsey, Paul. *The Patient as Person* (New Haven, Yale University Press, 1970) p. 133.

3. Cassell, Eric J. "Dying in a Technological Society," *The Hastings Center Studies,* Vol. 2, No. 2 (May 1974) p. 31.

4. *Ibid.*

5. *Cf.,* Silving, C. "Euthanasia: A Study of Comparative Criminal Law," *Pennsylvania Law Review,* Vol. 103 (1954) pp. 350–356.

6. Crone, Diana. *The Sanctity of Social Life: Physicians' Treatment of Critically Ill Patients* (Russell Sage Foundation, New York, 1975).

7. Ramsey, *op. cit.,* p. 133.

8. "Optimum Care for Hopelessly Ill Patients: A Report of the Critical Care Committee of the Massachusetts General Hospital," *The New England Journal of Medicine* 295:7 (August 12, 1976) pp. 362–364.

9. *Ibid.,* p. 362.

10. *Ibid.*

11. Rabkin, Mitchell, George Gillerman, and Nancy Rice. "Orders Not to Resuscitate," *The New England Journal of Medicine* 295:7 (August 12, 1976) pp. 364–366.

12. *Ibid.,* p. 366.

Case Studies XI and XII: Hyperalimentation—The Distribution of a Scarce Resource

Leah Curtin

CASE STUDY XI

Jaime was born of illegal immigrant parents in a South Texas hospital. His mother left the hospital three days after his birth and has not been heard from since that time. Jaime has short bowel syndrome and he was started on hyperalimentation several days after his birth. That was 11 months ago. Jaime is not considered adoptable and the cost of his care is not covered by any existing plan. The hospital has tried to get Medicaid to cover the cost of his treatment and to transfer Jaime to an orphanage—without success.

Jaime is doing well—in fact, thriving—but hospital authorities are threatening to discontinue his care because of its cost. One physician suggested that rather than let Jaime die of starvation and dehydration, it would be safer to let him die of septic shock. Presently, Jaime does not have an infection, but "sloppy" technique would provide one quickly enough. In short, he suggested that "someone" should inject a contaminated solution into the hyperalimentation catheter (and thus directly into Jaime's blood stream via the superior vena cava). He left verbal directions to this effect with the nurses.

The social worker agrees with the physician. She has tried unsuccessfully to get social agencies to pay for Jaime's care and none will do so. Moreover, she sees no reason why society should be burdened with the cost of caring for him.

Many of the nurses are outraged about the physician's verbal instructions. Moreover, they are angry about the social worker's attitude. In addition, an element of mutual mistrust has entered relationships among the nurses and between the nurses and the physician. The nurses have been caring for Jaime for eleven months. They have seen him through critical times and have rejoiced as he gained in strength and started to develop normally. They know that Jaime will need hyperalimentation as long as he lives—and they also know that, barring infection, he could live out a normal life span. Some of the nurses think that Jaime should have been permitted to die of his birth defect quickly without intervention. Others think that it would be merciful if Jaime did get an infection naturally (not induced) and die rather than to have to depend on hyperalimentation for the rest of his life. Some of the nurses think that if the doctor injects a contaminated solution, that is his business but they will not do it. Others guard Jaime closely and monitor his care carefully to assure that *no one* uses "sloppy" technique. The nurses do not think that Jaime should be starved to death—at least not if they are involved in any way. What can or should be done in this situation? What, if anything, can or should the nurses do?

CASE STUDY XII

Jeremy Jones is a 47-year-old cancer victim. He is married and the father of three pre-adolescent children. He is an expert auto mechanic and owns his own small service station. He has medical insurance, although his private policy does not provide extensive coverage. His abdominal cancer was extensive and both an ileectomy and a colectomy were performed. There was no immediate evidence of further metastasis, but the probability of it is quite high. His postoperative period was uncomplicated; he progressed well and was released three weeks after surgery. Because his intestines were removed, his nutritional status must be maintained through the administration of hyperalimentation. Mr. Jones was fitted with an ambulatory vest* and he was referred to the hospital's home hyperalimentation team for follow-up care.

Through the use of this vest and the follow-up care offered by the team, Mr. Jones was able to live a nearly normal life at home and even returned to work. However, Mr. Jones' insurance does not cover hyperalimentation and there are no social programs to help him. (Hyperalimentation usually is not covered by Medicaid.)

Sheila J is a registered nurse who works with the home hyperalimentation team. She is caring for Mr. Jones and his family. Unfortunately, Mr. Jones is unable to meet the cost of his treatment and has not paid his bill in over six months. Despite the intervention of various persons, from social workers to bill collectors, Mr. Jones does not pay simply because he cannot pay. Therefore, he was informed that his treatment was to be discontinued. He told Sheila that he will pay what he can, but he simply does not have enough money. He wants to live as long as he can. "How can you take my food away? You'll be killing me. What right do you doctors and nurses have to take out my intestines so I can't eat and then starve me to death?"

Sheila explained to him that if he stopped working, they probably could qualify him for total disability. In all fairness to the hospital and health team,

---

*A polyester mesh vest fitted with two 500 ml. bags of hyperalimentation fluid and a small volumetric infusion pump to control volume to an implanted catheter that goes directly into the superior vena cava.

they tried to have Mr. Jones' treatment covered by Medicaid but the case workers refused the petition: Mr. Jones is not destitute. He owns his own home (at least, he is making payments on the mortgage), a three-year-old car and his own business.

These facts were laid before Mr. Jones and he responded, "My family needs a place to live; where can we live more cheaply than we do? My house payments are only $175 a month and that includes insurance and taxes. If I sell my car, neither my wife nor I will be able to get to work or even to the grocery. I work, I pay my taxes, I don't owe anything to anybody except for these darn treatments. Sure, we could become beggars, but why should we when we only need help in this one area?" Mr. Jones does not understand why he must quit working, sell everything he has, give it to the hospital, and become totally dependent on society just because his "food" costs three times as much money as he makes in a year. He is a proud man who "takes care of his own." He pays his taxes, he works as hard as he can, he wants his wife and his children to have pride and to earn their own way. He refuses to make paupers of them so that he can live. He asked Sheila please to help him, but not to demand that he beg.

What can or should Sheila do to help him? Should she point out that it is his choice: he can die of starvation or he can "qualify" for help. What other options, if any, are open to Sheila?

GENERAL DISCUSSION AND SOCIAL CONSIDERATIONS

Both of these seemingly exotic case situations capture and poignantly illustrate a modern day dilemma: the prolongation of life (not death) through the use of technological advances. Neither Jaime nor Mr. Jones could have survived even a decade ago. Today, their lives can be prolonged, but in the process, they have become dependent on artificial, expensive and relatively scarce resources. To a certain extent, parallels can be drawn between these cases and some of the problems that have occurred in the past. For example, when insulin was discovered for the treatment of diabetics it, too, presented similar problems. When urinary dialysis and kidney transplants first were developed, they also presented similar difficulties. In the former case, the problem was solved by another technological advance—the development of a relatively inexpensive way to produce insulin. In the latter case, the United States Congress passed an amendment to the Medicare–Medicaid legislation that provides coverage for dialysis and kidney transplant patients even though the individuals involved do not meet the other economic or age requirements. A natural lottery singled out those individuals who, through no fault of their own, could not meet a fundamental need. The Congress recognized that average citizens simply cannot afford certain treatments that are necessary to prolong their lives and it made limited provisions for such care. In such a manner, the demands of social justice were met. A just society provides for each according to his need.[2]

Jaime and Mr. Jones are not irreversibly dying. They are not suffering significantly from anything other than society's inability or unwillingness to come to grips with the type of problem they represent. Although both of them will die without treatment and, although both cases are examples of involuntary withdrawal of treatment, neither case can fall under the broad umbrella of euthanasia. Dying of dehydration and starvation is not merciful by anyone's criteria, nor is there any physical necessity for such a death. The conditions involved are incurable, but with treatment they are not terminal. Perhaps some might consider the deaths of these patients to be an economic necessity, but few would be dishonest enough to call this merciful.

A good case could be made for the inclusion of hyperalimentation in the Medicaid program and an amendment has been introduced to this effect;[3] however, the fact remains that at this time, no such provisions have been made. Approximately 1,500 persons across the nation currently require sustained or long-term hyperalimentation and it is anticipated that this number will increase by about 1,000 per year if financial assistance is made available. Moreover, barring unforeseen circumstances, many of these individuals could have a normal life span.[4] The cost for the hyperalimentation fluids and administration alone (not including hospitalizations and so forth) is about $150 per day per person in 1980 dollars[5] —approximately 53 million dollars per year in total. However, the cost in 50 years' time (excluding both inflation and the possible breakthrough of new, cheaper means of providing hyperalimentation) conceivably could be two billion, six hundred and fifty-five million dollars per year.

As medical technology advances and new ways of treating formerly fatal diseases and disorders are developed, thousands—perhaps millions—of people will be offered a second chance at life.[6] However, until or unless the technology is made both affordable and available, distressingly practical decisions will have to be made. In the late 1950s and early 1960s, when kidney dialysis patients and the health professionals who cared for them faced similar problems, special committees of laymen and women were organized to decide who among the candidates actually would receive the treatment.[7] Among the selection criteria they used were the following:[8] (1) *The relative likelihood of success* (*e.g.*, were there any other complications that could interfere with the success of the dialysis?). For example, a person suffering from renal shutdown secondary to polycystic kidney disease would have precedence over a person suffering from the same condition plus, let us say, a congenital heart anomaly. Psychological factors also were considered—for example, a person's will to live and his willingness to comply with the necessary dietary and physical restrictions. A person's attitude toward the treatment could make the difference between success and failure. (2) Among those who had a good chance for success and whose attitudes were positive, a second criterion was employed: *the future life expectancy of the applicant.* In this category, the age and general condition of one patient were weighed and balanced against those of another. All things being equal, a younger person generally would be preferred over an older person. However, this criterion was modified by consideration of the potential recipients' family roles—what responsibilities, if any, do the applicants have for other family members? In this vein, a middle-aged mother of teenage children might be considered more eligible for treatment than a younger bachelor. On the other hand, these last two criteria could be modified by consideration of two other factors: a person's past contributions to society and the potential future contributions that an individual (if successfully treated) could make to society.

Moreover, a specific set of procedures had to be developed for systematic weighing and ranking of each of the criteria. There had to be rules to assure equity. The likelihood of success and the future life expectancy of an applicant generally were assigned greater weight than were family responsibilities. In other words, a young man with multiple complications would not be given precedence over an older man without complications, even if the younger man had a wife and several small children for whom he was responsible and the older man was a bachelor with no obligations. However, the inclusion of such factors as family role and past and future contributions created controversy. Many ethicists have suggested that the only way to choose equitably among those who have a good chance of benefiting from the treatment is random selection. Given that all human beings have an equal right to life, and that all of the candidates are in equal need of the procedure, and that all have an equal chance of success, there is no persuasive reason why one should be preferred consciously over another merely because he is married, a parent, well educated, morally upright and so forth.[9] The best principle to be applied is random choice among equals.[10] Random selection could be implemented either through a lottery or on a first-come-first-served basis.[11]

Such approaches, however, can help only to select patients for treatment. The problem presented by both Jaime and Mr. Jones involves a choice between continuation of treatment or withdrawal of it. Certainly, no persuasive argument can be put forth that Jaime certainly would want to die if given the choice and Mr. Jones already has voiced his desire to live. Both of them need the treatment to live and in both cases treatment already has been initiated. Thus, both Mr. Jones and Jaime, by choice or by chance, already have been "selected" for treatment. How can one justifiably remove from them what they need to live?

CHARACTERISTICS OF THE PROBLEM

Although the prolongation of life through the use of artificial means of feeding is part of a larger problem involving social justice in the distribution of scarce resources, there are some aspects that are unique to discussions involving the termination of parenteral and enteral therapy—problems that make such discussions perhaps even more trying than are decisions not to resuscitate or to discontinue a respirator or even to withdraw an artificial kidney. Quite specifically, these aspects include the following considerations:

1. Adequate nourishment often is regarded as a basic human right; certainly it is more commonly agreed upon than is a right to medical treatment. Although an artificial kidney is just as essential to persons who are in kidney failure as adequate nourishment is to those persons whose intestines are non-functional, there is a subtle shade of difference. The filtering out and disposal of wastes is an internal body function while the providing of nourishment is an external function. To be sure, the digestion of nutrients is an internal function but the provision of them is an external function. Although both the dialysis patient and the hyperalimentation patient need to have certain of their internal bodily functions performed artificially, the withdrawal of treatment from the hyperalimentation patient also involves a refusal to supply the external aspect of the need. The withdrawal of treatment from the dialysis patient does not represent the same thing. It seems to be more acceptable for a person to die from internally produced toxins than from externally induced dehydration and starvation. This is not to claim that it is, nor is it necessarily just to try to balance the rights of one person against the rights of the other. However, this additional factor seems to be morally significant.

2. The use of kidney dialysis, respirators and so forth clearly falls within the purview of medicine, while the provision of adequate nourishment does not. However, as means of providing nourishment artificially have become more sophisticated and effective, the line between what is medical treatment and what is ordinary feeding is blurred. Would any among us consider bottle feeding an infant or spoon feeding a debilitated adult to be a medical treatment? Yet both are artificial means of feeding. To take this argument a step farther, a premature infant may need a "ducky" nipple because his sucking reflex is not developed adequately. Perhaps an adult has no teeth and needs his food mashed. Are these now medical treatments or merely minor adjustments in the feeding process? From here, it is a short step to the use of tube feedings for infants who are so premature that they have no sucking reflex and adults who are so debilitated (either temporarily or permanently) that they are unable to swallow. When digestion is permanently or temporarily impaired, the most efficient and effective way to provide nourishment is the use of hyperalimentation. At what, if any, point in this progression does feeding become a medical intervention? This point is important or it becomes important when physicians order the discontinuance of artificial means of feeding. Is providing food by whatever means legitimately within the medical prerogative? Do the rights of persons to adequate nutrition depend on their age or their degree of debility or dependency? Do physicians have the moral and legal authority to withhold nutrients?

3. The thought of dying of starvation and dehydration is abhorrent—particularly when food and water are available. It seems far less justifiable to die of dehydration and starvation than to die of a birth defect, cancer, renal failure, or cardiac and respiratory arrest. Why? Probably because every human being needs food and water to sustain life, while very few need dialysis, respirators, cardiopulmonary resuscitation, and so forth.

Some people have suggested that the best course of action is to withhold the information that this option (hyperalimentation) is available and, thus, people will die of their disorders. However, this course of action is dishonest. Individuals can lie by denying or distorting a fact or they can lie by deliberately withholding the truth. To espouse this course of action is to place absolute authority over another's life and death in the hands of one person—a health professional—who will use whatever arbitrary criteria he chooses to determine who will or will not be made aware of options. It totally excludes patient, family, and community from decision making. In short, it is a giant step backward in the development of a just relationship between the health provider and the health consumer.

4. It is very difficult, if not impossible, to provide a good argument from the standpoint of mercy for withdrawal of withholding of nutritional life support systems. Every person must die, but how people die is not without significance. Certainly, if people still can feel anything at all, dying of starvation and dehydration must rank among the most agonizing ways to die.

TO KILL OR TO LET DIE

It is one thing to fail to resuscitate an irreversibly terminally ill patient; it is quite another to starve to death a person who has some hope of survival. For one thing, there is the distinction between allowing to die and killing. Deliberately to allow a person to die is morally justifiable only if the person has no significant chance to live or if it is in keeping with a competent person's fully informed decision.[12]

James Rachels, in an article entitled, "Active and Passive Euthanasia," presented what is considered one of the strongest arguments for elimination of the distinction between allowing to die and killing (commonly known as the distinction between active and passive euthanasia).[13] To make his most telling point, Rachels uses two examples. In the first instance, a Mr. Smith drowns his cousin in a bathtub and arranges to make it look like an accident. In this manner, he gains a large inheritance. In the second example, Mr. Jones also covets his cousin's money and plans to drown him in his bath. However, when Jones enters the bathroom an accident already has occurred and his cousin is in the process of drowning all by himself. Jones merely stands there and allows his cousin to drown. Rachels concludes that if there were any intrinsic moral relevance to the difference between killing and letting die, then there should be a difference in the assessment of Smith's and Jones' conduct.

Actually, Smith's and Jones' behaviors are both morally reprehensible because both constitute killing—one by an act of commission and the other by an act of omission. Moreover, this analogy's relevance for euthanasia is inept. For one thing, neither Smith's nor Jones' cousins consented to their deaths. For another, neither of them was suffering from a terminal disease. Their lives were endangered, but this danger was easily reversible. For a third, the intentions of both Smith and Jones could not be described as either benign or merciful.

The conclusion that can be reached from Rachels' argument is that withholding or withdrawing life saving help without consent from those who could benefit from it, and taking direct action to end a life, both constitute killing. On the other hand, allowing to die presupposes that an individual either is beyond assistance or knowingly has refused assistance. Perhaps the distinction could be made more appropriately by substitution of the words "acquiescing to a person's inevitable death" for the phrase "allowing to or letting die."

A RIGHT TO AID

If individuals have any rights at all, they must have a right to life—a precondition for all other rights. If the right to life means anything at all, it must entail a right *not* to be killed. The right not to be killed logically must include a right to aid "when one is in serious need or jeopardy provided that such aid can be rendered without excessive risk or loss to another."[14] According to Rawls, a limited duty of mutual aid is a necessary correlative of the right not to be killed.[15] Not only does the formulation of a limited right to aid recognize our mutual vulnerability and dependence, but it also greatly adds to a person's sense of security and thus to the quality of life in a given society. "The primary value of the principle is not measured by the help we actually receive but rather by the sense of confidence and trust in other men's good intentions and the knowledge that they are there if we need them."[16]

Moreover, the patient–professional relationship includes a contractual duty to render assistance. Thus, an individual's claim on a health professional for aid certainly is stronger than is his claim on members of the general public.[17] Therefore, for health professionals to withhold or withdraw life-saving or life-sustaining aid, where it is necessary, desired, and of possible benefit to a patient, can be viewed as killing. However, to claim that withholding or withdrawing aid is killing in any form, when it is unnecessary or ineffective, undesired, and/or offers no hope of benefit to the patient, is both inappropriate and unjust. To recognize when death is inevitable and to withdraw treatments that add pain or indignity is not killing. Rather it demands a sense for what the stoics called "the fitting"—it is a mature recognition of the Biblical imperative, "To every thing there is a season, and a time to every purpose under the heaven; a time to be born, and a time to die; a time to plant, and a time to pluck up what is planted . . . " (Ecclesiastes 3:1–2).

DENOUEMENT

Given these general reflections, and in acknowledgement of the fact that hyperalimentation already has been started on both Jaime and Mr. Jones, it can be concluded that to withdraw this treatment in either case constitutes killing. The act is not morally justifiable and may not be legally justifiable.

The nurses are faced with a number of problems. In Jaime's case, the physician's verbal request for "someone" to inject a contaminated solution into the baby's bloodstream is both immoral and illegal. The nurses have both a right and a duty to refuse to comply. Starving Jaime to death may not be illegal, but it is immoral. If the physician discontinues hyperalimentation, the nurses should take definitive steps to protect Jaime—steps that other professionals have taken in the past when faced with similar problems. To handle the immediate problems, the nurses can: (1) contact the various corporations that supply hyperalimentation fluid to the hospital and ask them to donate a supply for Jaime (this has worked in the past and, although there are limits, the corporations usually are most generous—particularly if they are assured favorable publicity); (2) make a direct appeal for help to the public through newspapers, radio or television; (3) contact personally various child welfare groups (public and private) and ask for help for Jaime; and (4) contact the local Child Protective Association or the county prosecutor's office if all else fails.

Such actions generally will produce results on a short-term basis for one case. However, to effectuate on-going aid, health professionals must band together with interested lay persons (1) to lobby Congress to have hyperalimentation included among medicaid benefits; (2) to establish a private foundation to collect donations from the general public to aid those in need of hyperalimentation; and (3) to provide for citizen participation in committees, the purpose of which shall be to limit access to this resource if there is no other alternative. Although limited access to scarce resources is not necessarily unjust, the issues involved are too important to be the sole decision of one health professional—or even a group of health professionals.[18]

In Mr. Jones' case, the professionals must find some way to help him without reducing him to penury. As Feinberg put it so well, "having rights enables us 'to stand up like men,' to look others in the eye and feel in some fundamental way the equal of everyone."[19] These are the rights that Mr. Jones claims and it is a cruel, quixotic, and unjust society that would deny them. Until such time as a social program is developed to handle these problems on a broad scale, the same steps can be taken, with Mr. Jones' permission, for him as were suggested in Jaime's case.

The actual outcomes in these cases are as follows. Jaime died of septic shock secondary to an overwhelming infection. No one really knows if the infection had been induced. However, mistrust, doubt and suspicion have damaged, substantially and perhaps permanently, the relationships among the health professionals. Sheila J made a personal plea to the corporation that supplies

Mr. Jones' hyperalimentation fluid and the company donated a year's supply to him. At the end of this period, Mr. Jones and Sheila will be faced with the problem again unless either his cancer has metastasized and he dies, or some more permanent way of funding care for people like Mr. Jones has developed.

COMMENTARY: CASE STUDIES XI AND XII

M. Josephine Flaherty

As Curtin has pointed out, the situations described here have far-reaching implications for health care professionals, for institutions, for society and, of course, for patients who are in need of parenteral therapy. As she has noted, these situations may be only the beginning—as equally far-reaching scientific advances within the next few years probably will open the door to other possibilities that may make radical differences in the probabilities that many people with major health problems will live long and productive lives, provided that they have access to complex and expensive technical assistance. These situations will place major stresses of various kinds on a number of people, including nurses, in relation to decision making about when, where and how the technological mechanisms will be used.

In the instances described, the nurses used creativity and persistence to fulfill their responsibilities for the care of their patients—sometimes at considerable personal and professional cost. The nurses who cared for Jaime were put in an untenable position by a physician who suggested that someone "kill" the patient by injecting a contaminated solution. It is clear that the nurses were justified in their refusal to comply with this suggestion. However, one would wonder what action the nurses took to report this incident to the appropriate authorities and what was the result of such reporting, if it did take place. The physician in question was practicing in an unprofessional, illegal, and unethical manner and was not faithful to the promises of his profession. It is interesting that he suggested that someone else do the deed that, obviously, he was not prepared to perform himself. Perhaps he remembered something about his profession's Hippocratic Oath and its Code of Ethics, but not enough to prevent his making the incredible suggestion that someone take the action.

It is interesting to note that there was not complete agreement among the nurses about what should be done. This, of course, led to mistrust among the nurses that was added to their lack of trust and confidence in the physician and in the social worker. It appears that, as a result, there was little collegiality remaining in the situation and one would wonder how a collaborative and cooperative health care team could function there. It is hoped that action was taken to correct this situation as it could have serious negative implications for the future of care in the institution and for the future performance of the health professionals involved.

The action of the nurses to obtain outside help for both patients was commendable and is part of the advocacy role of the nurse. Their action to lobby government to make statutory provision for situations like this one demonstrates their commitment to go beyond direct patient care to consider and act on the nature and shape of the health care system and to sensitize members of the public about problems and possibilities in society that have implications for health. It also demonstrates that they are prepared to examine their own values and positions and to articulate and act on them in the face of difficulties and to modify them in the face of convincing information. Thus the nurses are living Socrates' "examined life" and are demonstrating a genuine professional concern for the needs and resources of society as a whole, and not just for their own small part of it.

NOTES

1. Outka, Gene. "Social Justice and Equal Access to Health Care," in Thomas Shannon, ed. *Bioethics* (Paulist Press, Ramsey, New Jersey, 1976) p. 380.
2. *Ibid.*, p. 385.
3. S. B. 7789 would place hyperalimentation under the Medicaid provisions of the Social Security Act just as kidney dialysis is placed there.
4. Private conversation with Deanne Englert of the American Society for Parenteral and Enteral Nutrition, August 10, 1980.
5. *Ibid.*
6. Alexander, Shana. "They Decide Who Lives, Who Dies," a *Life Magazine* reprint (Time, Inc., New York, 1962) p. 2.
7. *Ibid.*
8. Rescher, Nicholas. "The Allocation of Exotic Medical Lifesaving Therapy" in Robert Hunt and John Arras, eds., *Ethical Issues in Modern Medicine* (Mayfield Publishing Company, Palo Alto, California, 1977) pp. 422 and 437.
9. Ramsey, Paul. "A Human Lottery?" in Robert Hunt and John Arras, eds. *Ethical Issues in Modern Medicine* (Mayfield Publishing Company, Palo Alto, California, 1977) p. 447.
10. *Ibid.*
11. Childress, James. "Who Shall Live When Not All Can Live?" *Soundings,* Vol. LIII (Winter 1970), pp. 339–62.
12. Fletcher, George. "Prolonging Life: Some Legal Considerations," in Samuel Gorovitz, *et al.,* eds. *Moral Problems in Medicine* (Prentice-Hall, Englewood Cliffs, New Jersey, 1976) pp. 263–264.
13. Rachels, James. "Active and Passive Euthanasia," *New England Journal of Medicine,* Vol. 292 (1975) pp. 78–80.
14. O'Neil, Richard. "The Moral Relevance of the Active/Passive Euthanasia Distinction," in David Smith and Linda Bernstein, eds. *No Rush to Judgment* (The Indiana University Foundation, Bloomington, 1978) pp. 188–189.
15. Rawls, John. *A Theory of Justice* (Harvard University Press, Cambridge, Massachusetts, 1971) p. 114.
16. *Ibid.*, p. 339.
17. Foot, Phillippa. "Euthanasia," *Philosophy and Public Affairs,* Vol. 6 (1977) p. 101.
18. Nabarro, J.D.N. "Selection of Patients for Hemodialysis," *British Medical Journal* (March 11, 1967) p. 622.
19. Feinberg, Joel. "The Nature and Value of Rights," *The Journal of Value Inquiry,* Vol. 4 (1970) p. 244.

Case Study XIII: Confidentiality of Patients' Records

M. Josephine Flaherty

Jane S was the occupational health nurse in a federal hospital. Among her responsibilities was the completion of the health status section of the form, which included both personal and health history, for the periodic health examination that was done for each of her clients—that is, persons who were employees of the federal government in the region in which the hospital was located. The occupational health physician completed the medical portion of the health report, recorded a decision about the employee's fitness for work and returned the report to Jane S, who also maintained a confidential file for employees' health reports and records. Employees were asked to sign a statement on the health report to the effect that information in the report, that had implications for the employees' fitness for the job, could be shared with the employer, that is, the supervisor in charge of the immediate work situation, as necessary.

One day, Jane S received a memorandum directing her to send a copy of Mr. Collins' (he was an employee on whom the health report had just been completed) health report to the federal capital city for filing in a centralized data bank. Jane questioned the request and asked for an explanation of the purpose of the central file. She was told simply that it was a directive from national headquarters and that she should comply. She pointed out that Mr. Collins had given permission for sharing of information only in the immediate situation and that she would get in touch with him and ask him to come in to sign an addendum granting permission for sending of the record to the central file. She could foresee no problems with obtaining this permission. She was told that this was not necessary and she was ordered to send the file immediately. She insisted that such action was contrary to the standards of nursing practice and the code of ethics for which she was accountable; these required that she exercise discretion in the sharing of information about patients and that she maintain records in accordance with the policies of the employing agency. She noted that if she complied with the order without the patient's consent, the statutory or registering body could charge her with professional misconduct. She was told by the senior officers in the hospital, including the hospital administrator, the occupational health physician and her nursing supervisors, that she must obey now and that if she had a problem with the order, she should grieve later under the terms of the collective agreement between the nurses and the federal government (her employer). She complied.

Later that day, Jane filed a grievance that was based on her being required to act in a manner that was contrary to standards of professional practice and that was in conflict with the hospital's policy as outlined on the employees' health record form. The grievance was denied at all levels, including the top level of the department involved, that was located in the national capital head-quarters.

Jane reported the matter to the statutory body with which she was registered. That body referred the matter to the Chief Nurse in the federal government, who although she had no line relationship with the section and the nurse involved, agreed to investigate it. Her inquiry revealed that the most senior officer in charge of the health division involved had denied the grievance on the advice of his senior advisors, without studying the case in detail. At the urging of the Chief Nurse, who was playing an ombudsman role in the matter, the question was re-opened, the decision on the grievance was reversed, and the grievance was upheld; the rationale for the central data bank was re-examined and re-confirmed, but the employees' health record form was revised to include obtaining the employees' permissions for including their health record forms in the central data bank.

Were the various actions that were taken appropriate and correct? Why or why not? What are the implications of these actions for nursing?

ANALYSIS OF THE SITUATION

Essential Data

1. Jane was aware of the standards of practice for which she was accountable and of the policies and practices of the agency.

2. A directive was given that represented a change in policy and practice related to health records and for which a rationale was not provided.

3. Jane attempted to take action to remedy the conflict caused by the directive and was forbidden to carry out her plan of action.

4. In accordance with the collective agreement, Jane obeyed and grieved later.

5. The grievance was denied at all levels, apparently without full consid-eration of it at at least one level (the highest one).

6. Jane referred the matter to the statutory body for nurses that, in turn, referred it to a senior government nurse who assumed an ombudsman role in the situation.

7. Although the specific situation regarding the particular patient, Mr. Collins, was not resolved, as a result of the incident, the nurse's grievance was upheld and the employees' record form was revised.

THE PEOPLE, RIGHTS, AND RESPONSIBILITIES INVOLVED

1. The Patient

In good faith, Mr. Collins cooperated in the health examination process and signed the consent for sharing of information. He had the right to expect that the other party to the consent agreement would honor it, but this did not occur and the patient's right to privacy was violated.

2. The Nurse

Jane was practicing according to the standards of her profession and the policies of the employing agency. She recognized her responsibility, at the statutory and agency levels, for the privacy of patients' records, for the maintenance of the patient–professional trust relationship, for the advocacy role of the nurse, and for her honoring of the terms of the nurses' collective agreement in relation to administrative authority in the agency.

Her concern for these issues led her to question the original order. When the response to her question was not satisfactory, she used initiative and creativity to resolve the situation, by suggesting that she elicit the patient's cooperation in the signing of a new consent form. When she was denied permission to do this, she offered strong arguments (on professional, statutory, and ethical grounds) in defense of the position that she was taking on the matter. When this was to no avail, she obeyed the order and grieved. When even this was not successful, she took the matter to the statutory body.

In her actions, Jane displayed persistence and courage. Many people might believe that it would have been much easier for her to compromise her standards and "go along with" her superiors on the issue. Because she was essentially in a "one nurse in the (occupational health) section" situation, she was virtually alone in her battle, without the support of either peers or supervisors. In spite of this, because of her commitment to the promises of her profession, she stood firm in her position, and when she was coerced into doing something she believed was wrong, she took the matter to higher authorities. When she failed to get support there, she went to the statutory body with the issue. Her behavior is an example of professional integrity—of doing what she believed to be right, regardless of the cost. This action involved considerable risk on her part, as her employer was the only one for nurses in the small and isolated community in which she lived. Hence, she was not free simply to change jobs, because there was none for nurses elsewhere in that community. She also was not free simply to move out of the community, because her husband was employed there.

This nurse, in her persistent efforts to resolve the situation, was demonstrating proactive nursing care, as she was anticipating a repetition of the situation in the future, and she wanted to ensure that appropriate mechanisms were in place to deal appropriately with future occurrences. In agreeing to share her concerns and the details of the situation with the statutory body and with the senior nurse in government, Jane was, in effect, taking the matter to "the highest courts in the land in nursing"; hence, she was subjecting her behavior to the scrutiny of the highest level of decision making in the nursing profession. This demonstrates the risk taking and the courage of one's convictions that are the mark of a true professional nurse. Her actions had far-reaching effects on the policies of the agency and on the practice of other nurses there, who heard about the incident and renewed their faith in the power of a committed individual to affect policy.

3. The Physician

The physician was aware of the statement on the patient record form and must have realized that the new regulation about the central data file involved a conflict with the form and an infringement of the rights of the patients. His failure to question this and to support his colleague, the nurse, in her actions is disturbing. One would wonder whether he, as a professional, had given thought to his own responsibilities for the maintenance of confidentiality and whether he had considered his responsibility to act collaboratively and cooperatively as a member of the health care team.

4. The Administrative Personnel of the Hospital

The administrators, including the senior nurses, must have known about the conflict between the patient record form and the new policy related to the central data file. It is surprising that the hospital administrative personnel were willing to implement conflicting policies and practices and that they refused to support the grievance of an employee who had pointed out the conflict. It is astounding that the nursing administrative personnel were in agreement with the other administrators, particularly when the conflict represented action that, for nurses, including the nurse administrators, was, in essence, professional misconduct according to the statutory regulations for nurses of the jurisdiction. It is rather sad that the supervisory nurses were not prepared to support the obviously correct behavior of their staff member or to question the appropriateness of the order from Headquarters to send records to a central data bank. The senior nurses could have been charged and disciplined by the statutory body for their behavior. They and the other administrators could and should have been reprimanded by the central government agency for failure to exercise judgment in the receipt and implementation of policies and for failure to recognize the correctness of their employee's actions and to uphold her grievance.

5. The Central Government Authority

This authority was negligent in its dissemination of a directive that apparently was not supported by a rationale and was negligent in its imposition of a policy that had not been monitored adequately for its compatibility with current practice. The senior advisors (one of whom was a senior nurse) to the chief executive officer of the central agency, who advised him to deny the nurse's grievance, either failed to investigate the situation fully or were unable or unwilling to admit that the employee was right and that the policy was wrong; thus, they were not exercising their responsibilities to provide sound advice to their supervisor. Hence, they denied the rights of the nurse employee and put the employer (the government) in the position of acting in conflict with its own policies and in conflict with its ethical commitment to serve the public faithfully.

The chief officer of the central agency believed that the advice given to him was sound, but he should not have signed the denial of any grievance, particularly one that had gone through many channels before it reached him, and hence must have been of great import to the grievor who had persisted in it for a long time, without full knowledge of the situation. As a result of clarification of the issue by the chief government nurse (in her ombudsman role), the chief officer did take action to have the employee form changed; in addition, he wrote to the nurse involved to notify her about the action that had been taken on her grievance (the reversal of the original decision) and the action that resulted from her pursuit of a solution to the problem (examination of the situation and modification of the patient health record form). One would hope that he also commended her for her behavior and apologized to her for the difficult situation to which she had been subjected.

6. The Statutory Body

By taking the matter to the senior nurse official, the statutory body chose a course of action through which the situation might be resolved without a charge against the nurse and a formal hearing into her behavior. The statutory body can regulate the practice of nursing but not the policies and practices of hospitals, except through lobbying about policies that infringe on the practice of registered nurses and registered nursing assistants. The statutory body's action was evidence of its support of its nurse members and its willingness to attempt to influence the behavior of employers, as part of the statutory body's mandate to protect the public by ensuring that nursing is practiced according to generally accepted standards of practice and of ethics.

7. The Chief Nurse (Ombudsman)

The action taken by this nurse was not an *explicit* part of her job description, but she believed that promotion of high standards of nursing practice and an ombudsman role in relation to nurses in the country were *implicit* in her responsibility to promote the health and well-being of all citizens of the country. Hence, as a public servant, she felt an ethical, professional and legal responsibility to take action at as high a level as was necessary. This was possible because the nurse involved and the statutory body had trust relationships with her and she had the respect of the senior officers of the government department, who listened to her and took action accordingly.

CONCLUSION

This case illustrates the willingness of an ethical professional to act correctly, even in the presence of coercion from powerful individuals and groups, to persist in her efforts, and to take risks to ensure that the matter would be resolved in a satisfactory manner. Jane S is a professional nurse who examined and clarified her beliefs and values, articulated them clearly, had the courage of her convictions that enabled her to take action, and was prepared to submit her actions to the scrutiny of her peers and superiors. In doing all these things, this young nurse made a significant contribution to the honor, growth, and development of the nursing profession, to the growth and sensitivity of the other professionals who were involved, and to the well-being of patients who will be cared for in federal hospitals.

Case Study XIV: A Patient's Right to Know— A Nurse's Right to Tell

Leah Curtin

William R, a recently widowed man in his late sixties, was admitted to the hospital through the emergency room with a provisional diagnosis of intestinal blockage, probably resulting from a tumor. He had no personal physician, so he was assigned to a house surgeon for care. On admission to the hospital, he was sent to a surgical oncology unit where primary nursing is practiced. Jean S, a staff nurse with 10 years of experience in oncology, was assigned to care for Mr. R. She cared for him for five days prior to surgery and a good rapport developed between them.

She was scheduled for three days off starting on the day of Mr. R's surgery and did not see him again until two days after surgery. She read the surgical reports and checked with her associate nurse to determine both Mr. R's reaction to the surgery and what he had been told about his condition. Mr. R's tumor was malignant and there was evidence of wide-spread metastasis. The physician performed only a simple colostomy to relieve Mr. R's pain and closed him up. The associate nurse reported that Mr. R had asked no questions about his condition and she had not volunteered any information. There was no indication in the physician's note of what, if anything, the physician had told the patient.

Jean entered Mr. R's room not knowing what he had been told. His first few comments indicated that he did not know that his tumor was cancerous, that he did not know that the cancer was metastasized, and that he thought that the colostomy was temporary and would be closed before he left the hospital. He did not know the seriousness of his condition, but he did ask questions that indicated he was concerned. He asked for information regarding the results of his biopsy. He asked Jean directly if the colostomy really was temporary; the physician had not been very clear about this matter. Mr. R also asked if Jean thought it was necessary for him to contact his son and daughter, both of whom were married and lived out of state. He did not want to worry them so he had not told them he was in the hospital. However, if he was really sick, he thought they should be called. What did she think he ought to do?

Jean tried to keep the conversation general and to divert his attention to other things—without success. However, as she listened to Mr. R her concern and consternation grew. A group of surgical residents, led by Mr. R's house surgeon, entered Mr. R's room, asked him how he felt, and examined him. Mr. R said he felt "pretty good all things considered," but he did not ask the physicians any questions. They left the room, telling Mr. R that he looked fine and was doing "great."

Shortly afterward, Jean cornered the house surgeon assigned to Mr. R. She told him she was Mr. R's nurse and that he was asking her a great many very pertinent questions. She asked him how much he had told Mr. R because she needed this information so she could be more open and supportive with him. The physician said that he had not told Mr. R anything about his cancer. When Jean asked why, he responded, "There's nothing we can do for him. He's going to die and knowing it will only increase his anxiety." Jean said, "But what about his children? He wants to call them if it's anything serious. Have you talked with them? What are you going to tell his family?" The physician assured her that he would talk to Mr. R's family but, in the meantime, she was not to answer any of the patient's questions. The physician claimed that giving information to a patient is a physician's prerogative and any act of disclosure on her part would be considered and treated as insubordination.

Ms. S retreated in order to consult the head nurse. The head nurse assured her that the questions she had asked the resident were not inappropriate, but she really was not quite sure how to handle the problem. As the days passed, the relationship between Ms. S and Mr. R became strained. He could not understand why she would not answer his questions and he resented her evasive tactics. When she tried to teach him colostomy care, he paid little attention. Why should he? After all, the colostomy was temporary, wasn't it?

Mr. R was not recuperating rapidly. In fact, he felt terrible. He did call his son and daughter and they both came to the city to see him. They were concerned about his care and how long he would live. They knew he had cancer and they had read about the hospice concept of care for the dying. They asked Jean if there was a hospice in this city. Jean knew there was and told them about it. She again ran into trouble with the physician who told her that he would make whatever referrals he thought necessary.

Jean asked him what arrangements he thought would be necessary for Mr. R's discharge. He did not think that a hospice was a good idea because then Mr. R would know he was dying. He expressed the thought that it is very cruel to take away a person's hope. He told the same thing to Mr. R's family. In his opinion, Mr. R needed skilled care and should be discharged to a nursing home. That way his children would not have to worry about his care and he would not be alone.

When the doctor told Mr. R that he was going to discharge him to a nursing home, he was quite upset. Among other things, he asked why his colostomy was not closed and why he could not go home and take care of himself. The physician said he needed more care than he could give himself at home and that he would close his colostomy when he got stronger. Mr. R. remarked, "I'm not getting stronger. I seem to be getting weaker." The doctor responded, "You'll be as good as new in no time." and walked out. Mr. R turned to Jean and said, "What's going on here? Isn't it about time someone levelled with me? What's wrong? Am I dying? Can't you say *anything*?"

What can or should Jean S do in this situation? Should she follow the physician's lead and assure Mr. R that he is fine? If so, why? If not, why not?

IDENTIFICATION OF ISSUES

This case presents a number of problems and questions. The most significant moral question is: Does a patient have a legal and moral right to information about his own physical condition? Should health professionals lie to people when they think it is in the individual's best interests to do so, that is, is there such a thing as a therapeutic lie? Closely related to these questions is whether the scope of nursing practice includes answering patients' questions about their physical conditions. Put another way, this question involves whether a physician is morally justified in withholding information from patients and in demanding that nurses do the same. Do physicians have the moral, legal, and professional authority to interfere in the nurse–patient relationship? If so, to what extent and why? The multiple issues raised in this case require individual exploration and analysis.

LEGAL AND MORAL RIGHTS OF HOSPITALIZED PATIENTS

Do patients have a legal right to information about their physical conditions? The answer to this question is ambiguous. The courts uniformly have upheld the right of all competent persons to make major decisions involving their own bodies. For example, in *Schoendorf v. Society of New York Hospital,* the Supreme Court of New York stated: "Every human being of adult years and sound mind has a right to determine what shall be done with his own body . . .".[1] In a Kansas case, the court held that "a man is master of his own body and he may expressly prohibit the performance of life-saving surgery or other medical treatment. A doctor may well believe that an operation or other form of treatment is desirable and necessary, but the law does not permit him to substitute his own judgment for that of the patient by any form of artifice or deception."[2] Moreover, a California court said: "A physician violates his duty to his patient and subjects himself to liability if he withholds any facts which are necessary to form the basis of an intelligent consent by the patient to the proposed treatment."[3] In addition, in the case of *Jones v. Regents of University of California,* a jury refused to accept a "defense argument that a physician may withhold some warnings of risk when the emotional condition of the patient might have resulted in intense anxiety that would interfere with his ability to decide rationally on the advisability of accepting the proposed surgery."[4] Therefore, it can be concluded that patients have a legally defined right to information in situations in which medical or surgical interventions are proposed.

However, the disclosure of information to patients *when no medical or surgical treatment is contemplated* may not be required by law. For example, only nine states in the United States have laws that allow patients even limited access to their medical records.[5] At any rate, it can be stated confidently that patients for whom no surgical or medical intervention is planned have no *clearly defined* legal right to information about their conditions.[6]

On the other hand, there certainly is no law requiring physicians or nurses to withhold information from patients. Moreover, the absence of a clear legal imperative to share information cannot be assumed to legitimatize deliberate lying. Why, then, do some health professionals withhold information from patients or even deliberately lie to them?

THE THERAPEUTIC LIE

Differences of opinion on the benefits (or lack of them) of telling the truth to patients are ancient and generally involve considerations of benevolence, that is, doing what is in the patient's best interests. Often, another significant, underlying issue is the attitude of the professional toward the nature of the therapeutic relationship: Does the professional view patients as individuals who are acted upon or does he (or she) view patients as active participants or partners in their care?[7]

Those who argue for the therapeutic lie (whether it would be withholding the truth or outright lying) generally hold that telling the truth in a particular instance will be psychologically damaging for the patient. Those who hold that patients have a right to have their questions answered truthfully, regardless of the consequences, base their arguments on three premises: (1) the duty to respect patients' rights to self-determination, bodily integrity, and personal decision making (autonomy); (2) the desirability of truthfulness in general; and (3) the belief that knowing the truth is in the best interests of individuals in the long run.

However, to present the controversy so simplistically is deceptive. Certainly, there are instances in which the detailed recital of a patient's condition and eventual death could create an emotional state contrary to the person's feelings of well being. In fact, there are few people whose sense of well-being would be enhanced by such a discussion. Moreover, at different times, people are more and less able to cope with the whole truth. Perhaps the best person to determine the time of disclosure as well as the amount of the disclosure is the patient himself. The most obvious indication of a person's readiness to know is the asking of questions. Although some people may not want their questions answered, most do—that is why they ask them.

What should be recognized is that either approach can be less than benevolent. If patients are subjected to a pitiless discourse on all the details of their conditions and their dying, they surely will suffer a shock, probably will be frightened and, quite possibly, will be depressed. However, if all information about a patient's condition and impending death is withheld, he may experience greater anxiety, depression and loneliness than he would if confronted with the truth. In such instances, the individual "is subjected to a kind of premature burial in that everyone—his loved ones included— eliminates him from discussions of the future."[8] Neither approach seems ethically justifiable.

In the first instance, the disclosure of information should never be done in a pitiless manner. Details, to the extent that they are known, should be provided only as they are requested and outcomes only as they can be predicted accurately. Information should not be forced on a person; it should be presented as gently and honestly as possible. There are very few nice ways to present devastating information, but there are some ways that are less brutal than others. In the second instance, to surround an inquiring patient with silence may engender anger, frustration, and fears of a fate worse than death. Frequently, what can be imagined is more devastating than what is. Moreover, lying or withholding the truth robs individuals of their ability to make decisions regarding the disposition of their final days.

A RIGHT NOT TO KNOW

Of course, there are people who really do not want to know what is wrong with them, and who could not bear the finality of a terminal prognosis. Generally, such individuals either may not ask questions or may refuse directly any offers to share information with them. There certainly is no legal duty to provide information in such circumstances and, usually, there is no moral duty to do so. Rights (moral or legal) generally are permissive for the holder of the rights but not for others. That is, the patient himself can refuse to hear information but others have no right to refuse it to him. However, there may be situations in which the patient has an overriding duty that necessitates disclosure of information to him even though he does not want to have it. For example, a twenty-six-year-old father of two preschoolers was diagnosed as having primary cancer of the liver. He asked no questions and persistently resisted all efforts to provide him with information. Meanwhile, he intended to complete several major changes in his and his family's life. He recently had been transferred to a distant city and was in the process of purchasing a new home in that city. The move would uproot his wife and children and place them far from family and friends. Moreover, although his estate was modest, he had not made a will, apprised his wife of their financial circumstances, or made any preparations for the care of his family in the event of his death. The health professionals caring for him, in concert with his wife, gently and as compassionately as possible, finally were able to help him to recognize his condition and to make the necessary preparations. In the end, he transferred all bank accounts, stocks, and ownership of their home to his wife. He made a will and, naturally, informed his employer that he could not accept the transfer. Fortunately, his company had a number of survivors' benefits of which he had been unaware and appropriate action was taken to make the claims; thus, when he died the burdens on his wife were decreased greatly.

In general, patients do not have obligations to know their conditions; that is, they are free to request information or to refrain from requesting it—except in the presence of an overriding obligation to others.

IS THERE A MORAL RIGHT TO THE TRUTH?

In *The Republic,* Plato argued that beneficent lying is justifiable for physicians if their patients are served better by it.[9] However, in his *Nichomachean Ethics,* Aristotle held that truthfulness is indispensible to trust among humans and thus, any deliberate attempt to deceive is wrong in itself.[10] Philosophers and theologians have argued the points of the "beneficent lie" at least since that time. Both Thomas Aquinas[11] and Augustine[12] held that all lying is morally wrong, but that lies told for beneficent reasons do not constitute as serious a transgression as those told in malice. Immanuel Kant taught that any lie is a breach of the duty of veracity required of all men,[13] while Jeremy Bentham held that lies are wrong only if they have evil consequences.[14]

Some distinction should be made between telling an untruth and withholding the truth. Uttering a deliberate lie always is deceptive. Maintaining silence in the face of questions may or may not be deceptive depending on the circumstances, that is, the relationship between the people, the importance of what is not said and the relevance for the listener of the information withheld.[15] Moreover, even if no questions are asked, maintaining silence in the face of important and relevant information may be the equivalent of lying.

What must be understood is that deception by whatever method can succeed only when individuals trust the deceiver—when they believe the individual to be honest and forthright. "Lying, whatever the motive, trades on trust and truth. It can succeed only where truth is the norm. Only when the person who is speaking is regarded as trustworthy can he succeed in lying. Each lie trades on and diminishes the credibility of every truth. Consequently, the practice of lying to terminal patients has made even the truth suspect."[16] Thus, today, the practice of lying to patients has increased mistrust and made even the truth not credible. Therefore, people are not reassured when told "Everything is fine." or "The tumor was benign." because they know we could be lying: health professionals no longer are thought to tell the truth.

To tell deliberate lies to a patient not only robs him of reality, but it can serve to destroy the human relationship between patient and professional. Full disclosure, however, may not be required. The amount of the disclosure depends on a number of factors, including the type and number of questions the patient asks. It also may be that a little information at a time is sufficient. What is necessary is direction, understanding and some knowledge of the person as an individual.

Arguments for truth telling and for sharing information can take several forms. For example, one can consider the requirements of personal privacy. According to Charles Fried, "Privacy is not simply an absence of information about us in the minds of others; rather it is the control we have over information about ourselves."[17] The more information others have about us, the more control they can exercise over us. The more vital the information—particularly if we ourselves are ignorant of it—the greater our helplessness and vulnerability. This is why Fried holds that our personal control of information about ourselves is necessary for liberty. How people behave toward us is, in part, a function of what they know about us. "Acts derive their meaning partly from their social context—from how many people know about them and what the knowledge consists of."[18] In an environment (such as a hospital) that is controlled largely by others, knowledge of who you are *and* what are your problems is central to even a limited exercise of freedom or autonomy. Unfortunately, people—even health professionals—do act differently toward a dying patient than they do toward other patients. If the person is deprived of the knowledge that he is dying, he will not understand the change in attitude or the isolation that inevitably results. People are uncomfortable around a dying person, particularly if they are trying to deceive him. Thus, the individual not only is an unwilling victim of his circumstances but also is an unknowing one.

Just as important is Fried's argument that the control and sharing of information about ourselves is a necessary pre-condition for loving or intimate relationships. People choose to share themselves and information about themselves with certain other people for specific reasons. The willingness to share intimate information with others is one of the foundations of close, trusting human relationships. Therefore, to provide private and vital information to family and friends while withholding it from the patient may "destroy the limited degree of intimacy . . . achieved . . . ."[19] over a lifetime. Moreover, it deprives an individual of choosing those persons with whom he wants to share this information, his thoughts, or his fears. Human beings, rational creatures, are treated as objects when they are deprived of information. For example, dying patients not only are rendered incapable of making sound judgments, but they are deprived of their own dying—of saying good-by, of concluding their affairs, possibly of providing for their loved ones and, finally, of choosing their own attitude toward their impending deaths. Put quite simply, truth telling and sharing of information demonstrate respect for human rights, lying does not. Patients have a moral right to information about themselves and, when they ask questions, they have a right to truthful answers.

ARE THERE LIMITS TO THE RIGHT TO INFORMATION?

Those who believe that withholding information sometimes is justified usually offer several reasons for it. One such reason is to save someone from clear and imminent danger.[20] Another argument put forth is that withholding information really is not a lie. The reasoning is as follows:

(a) All knowledge necessarily is incomplete, that is, no one ever has all knowledge of any one subject.

(b) Because all knowledge is incomplete, one cannot know with certitude what is true and false information.

(c) Therefore, health professionals are justified in withholding incomplete information—and in continuing to withhold all information because the data never will be complete.[21]

Although to some extent this syllogism is logically defensible, it is inept. Its proponents fail to make the critical distinction between complete information and accurate information. Short of putting the patient through medical school and possibly some advanced training, there is no way in which this individual can have even as incomplete a knowledge of his condition as the physician has. However, enough of what is known can be transmitted to the patient to enable him to understand what *is* known of his condition. As imperfect as our knowledge is, it cannot be used to justify withholding as accurate a description of reality as possible. It is absurd to claim that because our knowledge is incomplete (as it is in all areas of human endeavor), distorting, withholding, and falsifying available data are justified.

Another argument put forth to justify the "no lie at all" approach is the notion of mental reservation.[22] According to this approach, a health professional is perfectly justified in responding thus to a patient's question:

Patient: "What is my blood pressure?"

Nurse: "It's normal (while she thinks but does not say, '190/110 is normal for a person with hypertension')."

or

Patient: "Am I dying?"

Nurse: "You're doing remarkably well (while she thinks but does not say, 'for a person in the terminal stages of bone cancer')."

Proponents of mental reservation claim that the speaker is not deceptive; rather the questioner is hasty in interpreting the answer. Such sophistry, of course, could be used to justify all lies. In summary, the term "mental reservation" can be used to replace the term "lie" to designate an intentional deception: the intent is the same, the action is the same, and the result is the same.

Still another argument is advanced on behalf of the "no lie at all" approach to therapeutic deception. In essence, it merely is a variation of the "imperfect knowledge" approach. One need not tell a person that he is dying because it may not be true, that is, unexplained cures and spontaneous remissions have occurred in rare instances in the past and it is at least remotely possible that this person could experience a miraculous cure. A slight variation of this theme is that someone may discover a cure for this disease before the patient dies; therefore, it is inappropriate to tell anyone that his condition is irreversibly terminal. Such an approach begs the question: it places a remote possibility in a superior position to a known probability. Moreover, it cannot be used legitimately to withhold truthful answers to a patient's questions. A health professional need not be brutal in his or her response or take all hope from a patient. However, it is deceptive to say that medicine can cure what it cannot cure. Creating false hopes for desperate people is at least as cruel as denying all hope.

Perhaps the most powerful argument put forth for distortion of the truth (at least with regard to terminal patients) is that one must balance the benefits of truth telling against the risks imposed by that knowledge. For example, a person with a history of cardiac problems might experience a cardiac arrest if told that she has cancer; an individual with a history of emotional instability might attempt suicide if told that he is dying. This approach has been institutionalized in law as "the principle of therapeutic privilege," that is, a physician may withhold information from patients when, in his judgment, such knowledge clearly constitutes a danger to the health of the patients. However, an individual physician is required to meet the standards of truthfulness of other reasonable physicians in his community and in his particular specialty.[23] Such institutionalization of paternalism has been criticized severely by recent commentators[24] and limited sharply by the courts in recent years.[25]

With all due respect for the law, what is legally permissible and what is morally defensible are not necessarily equatable. Moreover, even under the law, the principle of therapeutic privilege cannot be interpreted broadly enough to permit the routine deception of whole classes of patients (*e.g.,* dying patients). Increasingly, justification for deliberate deception of any patient "for his own good," will have to be defended legally.

WHO SHOULD PROVIDE INFORMATION TO PATIENTS?

Clearly, if patients have a legal right to information in at least some sets of circumstances, and they do, and if patients have a moral right to accurate information if they request it, and they do, someone must have a legal or a moral duty to provide information.

In cases where any medical or surgical intervention is proposed, patients have a legal right to at least enough information to make an informed decision. The legal duty to provide this information rests squarely on the shoulders of the physician proposing the course of action and he can be held liable if he fails to present an adequate amount of truthful information. A nurse may deliver a consent form to a patient and witness his or her signature. The nurse even may translate some of the physician's medical terminology for the patient, but she is not legally authorized "to explain the surgery or the critical procedure in lieu of the surgeon or physician."[26] If the patient tells the nurse that he doesn't understand what is to be done, the nurse should notify the physician that the patient does not understand and needs additional explanation. She certainly "should not proceed to get the patient's signature"[27] to a procedure he does not understand.

In situations where formal consent is not required (*e.g.,* when no surgery is planned), the position of the nurse is ambiguous. In such situations, a patient may have no legal right to information; hence, it could be argued that no one (physician or nurse) has a legal obligation to provide information. However, the absence of legal obligation is not the equivalent of a prohibition—particularly in the presence of a moral obligation to act.

> A person cannot absolve himself from the responsibility to act morally by transferring it to another person within the authority structure of an institution . . . Therefore, . . . the moral obligation to provide . . . information [rests] equally upon anyone who [possesses] the information, [has] the competence to disclose it, and [is] requested by the patient to disclose it.[28]

Accordingly, nurses do have a moral obligation truthfully to disclose information in answer to patients' queries if they are competent to do so. Does the scope of nursing include the presentation of information to patients and their families, that is, are nurses competent to answer questions? Nurses always have imparted information to patients in collaboration with physicians and, often, at the request of physicians. Therefore, it can be concluded that nurses in general are competent to disclose certain information to patients. However, we now must ask: Are nurses competent to release information to patients if the physician does not authorize it and, particularly, if he prohibits it? Inherent in this question are two other questions:

1. Does the medical prerogative include control of all information about patients? If not, what are the limits of this control?

2. Does nursing practice include independent judgments regarding the disclosure of accurate information to patients upon their request?

Clearly, the practice of medicine does not include absolute control over information regarding a patient. For example, the legal principle of privileged information between physician and patient precludes the indiscriminate release of private information about a patient—even when a physician is under oath in a court of law.[29] Moreover, the physician has a positive legal duty to release information to patients or their families under certain circumstances.[30] In addition, under some circumstances the physician has a legal obligation to release information about the patient to others (such as in the instance of gunshot wounds and reportable diseases) even though such disclosure may be uncomfortable, embarrassing or socially undesirable for the patient.[31]

However, a legal duty to protect patients' privacy or to provide information to patients does not in itself include a legal right to forbid the disclosure of such information by others. The right to disclose to others private information rests most properly with individuals. For example, a patient may release information to anyone or everyone if he chooses to do so. The physician has no moral or legal right to force a person to remain silent about his condition or to force a patient's family to withhold information from him. He may urge the family to do so, but he cannot coerce them.

The very nature of nursing practice necessarily includes a knowledge of personal and private information about others. Nurses, therefore, have moral obligations similar to physicians, obligations regarding the disclosure of private information about patients. In general, nurses' moral obligations to protect confidential information about patients are the same as those of physicians.[32] However, in most states, nurses rarely have the same legal protections (i.e., a legally defined right to withhold privileged information) as do physicians. Because, today, nurses are called to testify in court cases, this situation can cause severe problems. Debates presently are taking place about extension of the principle of privileged information to nurses and other health professionals.

Given the foregoing legal and moral considerations, we now can approach the question of whether the disclosure of sensitive, emotion-laden information to dying patients is strictly a medical decision. To answer this question, we must look to the nature of the information, to the personality of the patient and to the qualifications of the information-giver. The disclosure of diagnostic and prognostic information to a patient is not a physician's right, but rather his duty.[33] In addition, the duty of veracity pertains in most if not all circumstances. If something is one's right, one is free to choose to do it or to refrain from doing it.[34] A duty, on the other hand, is not permissive for the duty holder, that is, one is not morally (and sometimes legally) free to decide not to fulfill one's responsibilities. This point is significant in a situation in which a physician fails or refuses to perform his duty to answer truthfully a patient's questions about his or her condition.

The nature of the information to be conveyed also is a significant factor in determination of who has the duty or right to impart it. For example, a physician has a legal as well as a moral duty to explain a surgical procedure to a patient.[35] By virtue of his education, training, experience, and professional relationship to the patient, the physician is the person most qualified to explain a patient's medical condition, medical prognosis, and any proposed course of action.[36] However, there is a distinct difference between explaining the nature of an illness or treatment and answering a patient's questions about his possible or impending death. Medical expertise is not required. For example, a physician can and often does prefer that someone else impart this information to a patient, for example, a family member, a close friend, a clergyman or a nurse with whom the patient has established a close rapport.[37] That is, the physician, both legally and morally, is permitted to delegate this responsibility to others when it is preferable for whatever reason. Such a distinction directly infers that the imparting of this type of information is not reserved solely, necessarily or morally to medicine.

The question of whether a patient should be told about his impending death—particularly when he is requesting such information—is more a moral decision than it is a medical decision.[38] Physicians may believe that to lie or to withhold information from patients under these circumstances is in the patients' best interests, but their legal or moral right to do so is questionable. Even more questionable is a physician's authority to require others to lie or to withhold the truth. Clearly, it is not legitimate to forbid someone to respect another person's legal right. For example, if a physician fails or refuses to obtain informed consent from a patient for a surgical procedure, the nurse not only may refuse to explain the procedure and to persuade the patient to sign the consent form, she has a duty to refuse to do so.

Attempting to forbid another to respect a person's human rights is at least as reprehensible as attempting to force others to violate a person's civil or legal rights. A dying individual's right (if he chooses to exercise it) to adequate and accurate information, which will permit him to prepare himself spiritually, psychologically and socially for his own death, is derived directly from the right to self-determination. Although abridging this right may be seen by some to be in a patient's best interests, this rationale cannot be justified in the face of repeated and direct queries from that patient. Even though the law (in many instances) may not require disclosure, respect for the patient as a person does require it. Thus, it seems that a physician does not have the moral authority to suspend or negate a patient's human rights or to require that others including nurses do so. Neither physicians nor nurses may infringe on the legal or moral rights of others. In this sense, neither nurses nor physicians have a right to refuse to tell an inquiring patient that he is dying, because their right to choose to disclose or to choose not to disclose information is constrained by their positive duty to respect the patient's human rights.

However, this discussion cannot be construed to mean that the physician does not have the professional and institutional power to withhold information from patients or even to lie to them and to require that others do so.[39] In this context, the physician's power is not to be equated with either legal or moral authority; rather, it refers to the physician's ability to assure other people's compliance. In fact, in health care today, the physician's ability to withhold information is exercised widely and rarely is it challenged openly by nurses.[40]

Although some commentators such as Friedson maintain that the medical profession "has the authority to direct and evaluate the work of others without in turn being subject to formal direction and evaluation by them"[41] and that the physician's expertise entitles him to give orders to others,[42] such formulations should not be extended outside a strictly defined medical scope—and certainly may not be extended to matters of moral responsibility. Nevertheless, the physician through means of position power and coercive power generally will secure compliance in moral as well as medical decisions or assure disciplinary action against those who fail to comply.[43]

Although nurses have a moral duty to be honest in answering patients' questions and although patients have a moral right to ask questions of nurses and although there is no law expressly forbidding nurses to disclose information to patients, it is unlikely that nurses will do so (at least in any great numbers) as long as physicians have the professional and institutional power to coerce and punish them. Ideally, nurses and physicians should work together collaboratively and cooperatively and, in many instances, they do so, to the great benefit of patients and their families. However, until the entire profession of nursing adopts a mutually supportive stance and institutionalizes it through enabling legislation and agency policies, individual nurses will be placed in uncomfortable if not untenable positions when conflicts arise regarding professional prerogatives, moral and ethical duties and patients' rights.

SUMMARY AND CONCLUSIONS

The questions of whether, what, and who should impart information of a particular nature to patients are complex and do not lend themselves to simplistic or absolute responses. However, from this analysis one can conclude that:

1. Patients do not have a legal right in most instances to information about themselves unless medical or surgical treatment is proposed.

2. Patients have a human right to request information and to receive truthful replies to their queries.

3. Physicians have a non-transferable legal duty to provide information that is adequate for decision making when any course of medical or surgical treatment is proposed.

4. Physicians and nurses have a moral and legal duty to respect patient confidentiality.

5. Nurses and physicians have a moral and a legal duty to respect patient rights.

6. Neither physicians nor nurses have the moral authority to require others to violate a patient's legal or moral rights.

7. Neither physicians nor nurses have a right to refuse to tell an inquiring person that he is dying because their right to choose to disclose or to choose not to disclose is constrained by their positive duty to respect the patient's human rights. Family members, friends, and clergymen may share this duty because it is not the sole or even shared prerogative of either nursing or medicine.

8. Physicians have the power to coerce nurses in matters of ethical accountability, but they do not have the moral or legal authority to do so.

9. Patients are best served by cooperative, collaborative and respectful care from both physicians and nurses.

DENOUEMENT

In the case of Mr. R, Jean S did tell Mr. R the truth. Not only was Mr. R grateful to her, but he took steps to control his own care. With the help of his children and the information provided by Ms. S, he contacted the hospice organization in that city and died several months later in his own home. The physician was very angry with Jean S and lodged a charge of insubordination against her. The director of nursing supported her and marshalled various forces in her defense. For example, the hospital chaplain's office, the social work department and the patient and his family all supported the appropriate nature of Jean's intervention. The hospital's legal counsel advised the medical executive committee and the hospital administrator not to recommend disciplinary action against Jean S unless they were prepared to take the case to court. Moreover, several physicians on the medical executive committee thought that this particular physician had not handled the situation properly (one of them was a member of the executive board of the local hospice) and, therefore, were not inclined to support his actions. The director of nursing took great care to present the situation as one of what actually was in the best interests of this patient rather than as a power struggle between nursing and medicine. As a result, the decision could not be generalized to any other situations and institutional policies were not altered with regard to the disclosure of information to patients. However, Jean S and her career were salvaged. Her conduct was not censured and no disciplinary action was proposed. On the other hand, the physician's conduct was not censured and no significant changes in the prevailing situation in this institution were made. This solution may not have been ideal, but it did help many physicians to understand the difficult problems nurses sometimes face; provide at least tacit support for a nurse's disclosure of information in this one instance; and save face for both Jean S and the physician.

COMMENTARY: CASE STUDY XIV

M. Josephine Flaherty

In her analysis of this situation, Curtin has identified a number of issues that were involved and has presented background data that have implications for these issues.

It has been established that patients, as human beings with dignity, have the right to information about their own bodies and treatment of them. Whether this is a legal, moral, or humanitarian right seems less important than is the fact that it is a right that should not be denied. As has been noted, a patient may have a particular need for information, in situations such as this one in which death was imminent; this patient expressed a need to notify relatives and possibly, had he been aware that he was dying, he would have wanted to make certain personal arrangements in his life. All health professionals have responsibilities to share information with patients.

The nurse in this situation was in a difficult position because she recognized the patient's desire to be informed and his frustration at the obvious avoidance by his care-givers of response to his questions. She had witnessed the refusal of the patient's physician and the interns to be truthful to him. When she discussed this with the physician, he made it clear that he was not going to inform the patient and that he was instructing her not to give the patient any information.

Jean S's action in her consulting the head nurse was appropriate. The head nurse's response, however, was inadequate. As the senior nurse in the unit, she was responsible for the quality of nursing care and the coordination of it with other health care in the area. Although she was aware that neither was appropriate and acceptable for Mr. R in relation to his information needs, she apparently did nothing more to support her staff nurse than to tell her that her questions were not inappropriate; she did not confront the physician about his behavior or seek assistance from a higher authority. Thus she was not being faithful to her professional and ethical responsibilities to a patient in her unit and to her staff member who asked guidance and help; in addition, she was failing to work in a truly collegial relationship with the physician as another member of the health care team and to fulfill her institutional responsibility for the quality and coordination of care in her unit.

Jean S, as the primary nurse, talked with the family and informed them about the availability of hospice care and, in so doing, engendered the displeasure of the physician. The latter also disagreed that hospice care was appropriate for the patient.

In her decision to tell the truth to the patient about his condition, Jean S took a major risk because she knew that the physician would be angry. This resulted in his laying of a complaint of insubordination against her.

The physician's charge appeared to be motivated by the fact that a colleague exercised a professional judgment, and decided to share information with a patient in contravention of his, a physician's, order to her to say nothing. The physician appeared to be unaware of or to refuse to accept the reality and appropriateness of the nurse's professional responsibility to exercise judgment in the teaching of and sharing of information with patients and families and to work in collaboration with other members of the health care team; the nurse also has an advocacy role to protect the patient from unacceptable behavior by another health professional. All of these responsibilities are spelled out in American, Canadian, and International codes of ethics for nurses, in standards of nursing practice and in statements and position papers of the nursing profession.[44]

How a physician could lodge a complaint of insubordination against a nurse is unclear, because a nurse should be responsible and accountable to the nursing authority in the agency and not to a medical authority as such. It is not clear whether the physician actually wrote an order to the effect that the patient be told nothing about the true nature of his condition; had the physician been certain that his decision on this was correct, why did he not write an order accordingly and thus subject it to the scrutiny of his peers? The case study data indicate that at least some physicians on the medical executive committee believed that the physician had not handled the situation properly; the case study is silent, however, about whether these or other physicians made their opinions known in defense of Jean S, a primary nurse in their institution. The outcome of the situation suggests, however, that they did not do this.

It is interesting that the director of nursing supported her staff nurse and "marshalled various forces in her defense." There is no mention of whether the head nurse was conspicuously in support of her staff member, but it was noted that the chaplain's office, the social work department and the patient and his family supported the appropriate nature of Jean's actions. Even the legal counsel of the hospital apparently believed that the nurse's behavior would stand up in court. However, where were the nursing personnel in all of this?

Curtin reported that the director of nursing "took great care to present the situation as one of what was actually in the best interests of this patient rather than as a power struggle between nursing and medicine"; hence, the situation could not be generalized and "institutional policies were not altered with regard to disclosure of information to patients." Since details were not given about what were the institutional policies on this matter, the meaning of this is not clear. That the director of nursing emphasized the interests of the patient is commendable and appropriate. However, it is appalling that she failed to assert the role and responsibility of the nurse, particularly a primary nurse who presumably was a senior professional, to practice according to the standards for which she was accountable. It appears that the director failed to exercise her responsibility as a nursing leader to interpret the role of the nursing profession and to ensure that the conditions in her institution were conducive to acceptable nursing practice.

It is *no great credit* to the institution that "Jean S and her career were salvaged. . . . [that her] conduct was not censured and no disciplinary action was proposed" because her actions were not subject to censure or discipline. At the same time, it is to the *discredit* of the hospital that the physician's conduct was not censured when some of his colleagues believed that he had not acted properly, and it is to even greater discredit that no significant changes in the prevailing situation in the institution were made. One would wonder why the nursing department, the chaplain's office, the social work department, members of the medical executive committee and the patient and his family did not join forces to *ensure* that the situation was improved.

If, as Curtin suggested, the outcome of the situation did help "many physicians" to understand the difficult problems that nurses sometimes face, were they aware also of the problems that patients could face in their institution—largely because of the behavior of one or more members of their own profession? What did these physicians do about this? Why did they not work to have the situation changed?

Was "at least tacit support of a nurse's disclosure of information in this one instance" good enough? The answer clearly is "No," but what did the responsible and accountable health professionals in the situation do about this?

Finally, was it acceptable that there was saving of face for both Jean S and the physician? Why should it be necessary to "save face" for a nurse who was correct in decision making and actions in her professional practice? Indeed, she should have been commended and supported for her integrity, excellence in practice and courage of her convictions—her role-modeling of the behavior of a true professional.

Should there have been face-saving for a physician whose behavior was highly questionable at best and thoroughly irresponsible and unprofessional at worst? Will he continue to practice in this manner? If he does, will he and the hospital fulfill their responsibilities for the provision of excellent care of patients?

NOTES

1. *Shloendorf v. Society of New York Hospitals,* 105 N.E. 92 (N.Y. 1914).
2. *Natanson v. Kline,* 350 p. 2d, 354 p. 2d 670 (Kans. 1960).
3. *Salgo v. Leland Stanford Board of Trustees,* 317 p. 2d 170 (Cal. 1957).
4. Creighton, Helen. "More About Informed Consent," *Supervisor Nurse,* Vol. 9, No. 3 (March 1978) p. 85.
5. *Cf.* Yarling, R. "Ethical Analysis of a Nursing Problem," *Supervisor Nurse,* Vol. 9, No. 5 (May 1978) p. 41. California and Utah limit access to patients' attorneys; Illinois, Massachusetts, New Jersey, Louisiana, Mississippi, and Connecticut grant access to medical records in limited circumstances—often only after discharge from the hospital.
6. *Op. cit.,* Yarling, p. 41.
7. May, William F. "Normative Inquiry and Medical Ethics in Our Colleges and Universities," in David Smith and Linda Bernstein, eds. *No Rush to Judgment* (Indiana University Foundation, Bloomington, 1978) p. 338.
8. *Ibid.,* p. 355.
9. Plato. *Republic.* 38913-389D.
10. Aristotle. *Nichomachaen Ethics.* 4, 7, 1127.
11. *Summa Theologica* II-II 40, 3.
12. "De Mendacio" and "Contra Mendacio" in R. J. Defarrari, ed. *St. Augustine. Treatises on Various Subjects,* Vol. 14 (Fathers of the Church, New York, 1955) pp. 45–110 and pp. 111–179.

13. Kant, Immanuel. "On Lying" in Mary Gregor (trans.) *The Doctrine of Virtue: Part II of the Metaphysics of Morals and the Pref. to the Doctrine of Law* (Harper and Row, New York, 1964). Reprinted by the University of Pennsylvania Press, Philadelphia, 1971, pp. 92–96.

14. Bentham, Jeremy. "Division of Offenses," in *An Introduction to the Principles of Morals and Legislation,* 1823 (Hofner Library of Classics, No. 6, New York, 1948) pp. 204–308.

15. Bok, Sissella. "Truth Telling: Ethical Aspects" in Warren Reich, ed. *Encyclopedia of Bioethics,* Vol. 4 (The Free Press, New York, 1978) p. 1684.

16. Yarling, R. "Ethical Analysis of a Nursing Problem II," *Supervisor Nurse,* Vol. 9, No. 6 (June 1978) p. 29.

17. Fried, Charles. *An Anatomy of Values: Problems of Personal and Social Choice* (Harvard University Press, 1970) pp. 141–142.

18. *Ibid.*

19. *Ibid.,* p. 144.

20. *Op. cit.,* Bok, p. 1686.

21. Henderson, L. J. "Physician and Patient as a Social System," *New England Journal of Medicine,* Vol. 212 (1935) pp. 819–823.

22. McFadden, Charles. *Medical Ethics* (F. A. Davis Company, Philadelphia, 1967) pp. 388–413.

23. Cited in A. G. Bearn, D. A. K. Blank, and H. H. Hiatt, eds. *Medical Experimentation: Personal Integrity and Social Policy,* Vol. 5 of *Clinical Studies,* A North-Holland Frontiers Series (American Elsevier, New York, 1974) p. 22.

24. Fletcher, Joseph. "Medical Diagnosis: Our Right to Know the Truth," in *Morals and Medicine* (Beacon Press, Boston, 1960) pp. 34–64.

25. "Notes: Informed Consent and the Dying Patient," *The Yale Law Journal,* Vol. 83 (1974) pp. 1632–1664.

26. Creighton, *op. cit.,* p. 85.

27. *Ibid.,* p. 86.

28. Yarling, *op. cit.* (May 1978) p. 47.

29. Greenawalt, Kent. "Privacy" in Warren Reich, ed. *Encyclopedia of Bioethics,* Vol. 3 (The Free Press, New York, 1978) p. 1362.

30. See notes 1, 2, 3, and 25 above.

31. Greenawalt, *op. cit.*

32. International Council of Nurses. *ICN Code for Nurses—Ethical Concepts Applied to Nursing* (International Council of Nurses, Geneva, 1973).

33. *Cf.* Kelly, Gerald. *Medico-Moral Problems.* (The Catholic Hospital Association, St. Louis, Missouri, 1958) p. 42.

34. Bandman, Bertram. "Human Rights of Patients, Nurses and Other Health Professionals," in Elsie Bandman and Bertram Bandman, eds. *Bioethics and Human Rights* (Little, Brown, Boston, 1978) p. 322.

35. Creighton, *op. cit.,* p. 85.

36. *Ibid.,* p. 86.

37. Kelly, *op. cit.,* p. 42-45.

38. Freeman, Howard, Anville Brim and Greer Williams. "New Dimensions of Dying," Introduction to Orville Brim, Howard Freeman, Sol Levine and Norman Scotch, eds. *The Dying Patient.* (Russell Sage Foundation, New York, 1970) p. XV.

39. Rosenthal, Carolyn J., Victor W. Marshall, A. S. Macpherson and Susan E. French. *Nurses, Patients and Families.* Chapter 5 "Controlling Information" (Springer Publishing Company, New York, 1980) pp. 111–125.

40. *Ibid.,* p. 124.

41. Friedson, Eliot. *Professional Dominance* (Atherton Books, New York, 1970) p. 136.

42. Friedson, Eliot. *Profession of Medicine.* (Dodd, Mead, New York, 1970).

43. There are exceptions to this statement. For example, nurses and other health professionals have a legally protected right to refuse to participate in abortions or sterilizations. Moreover, in cases where a physician clearly is violating the law, the courts have held that nurses have a legal duty to intervene to protect the patient. *Cf.* "Legal Briefs"*RN Magazine,* January 1980.

44. See, for example, a) American Nurses' Association. *Code for Nurses with Interpretative Statements* (American Nurses' Association, Kansas City, Missouri, 1976).

b) College of Nurses of Ontario. *Standards of Nursing Practice for Registered Nurses and Registered Nursing Assistants* (College of Nurses of Ontario, Toronto, 1979).

c) _____ . *Guidelines for Ethical Behavior in Nursing* (College of Nurses of Ontario, Toronto, 1980).

d) International Council of Nurses. *ICN Code for Nurses—Ethical Concepts Applied to Nursing* (International Council of Nurses, Geneva, 1973).

Case Study XV: Nurse–Patient Conflict—Consent for Nursing Intervention

Leah Curtin

Mary Jones, an independent and intelligent twenty-seven-year-old primipara, entered the hospital at 11:00 PM in active labor; her membranes had ruptured at home. She was apprehensive, but self-possessed. According to routine procedures, she and her husband had signed all pre-admission forms, among which was a blanket consent form. Sixteen hours later, she delivered a healthy male infant.

Again, according to routine procedures, she was kept *N.P.O.* and catheterized immediately prior to delivery. Only two untoward events occurred: (1) Mrs. Jones' blood pressure was unstable after delivery and she remained in the recovery room for three hours until the pressure returned to and remained normal. (2) Mrs. Jones was transferred to the floor, no bed was ready for her and she remained on a stretcher in the hall for about three more hours. Mrs. Jones received nothing to eat or drink, either in the recovery room or while she was on the stretcher in the hall. During most of this time, she was asleep.

When Mrs. Jones finally was admitted to a room, she was given an initial bath and her vital signs and the fundus of her uterus were checked; everything was normal. However, the nurse forgot to place water at her bedside. Mrs. Jones went back to sleep until shortly after change of shifts when the night nurse came into her room, awakened her and asked her if she had voided. Mrs. Jones said no and pointed out that she had not had anything to drink. The nurse gave her some water and urged her to drink it. Mrs. Jones drank two glasses of water and fell asleep again. At 2:00 AM, the nurse returned to see if Mrs. Jones had voided. She had not. The nurse checked her to see if she was distended. She was not. The nurse urged her to drink more water and to go to the bathroom and to try to void. Mrs. Jones did so. At 3:00 AM the nurse came

341

to Mrs. Jones' room again and asked her if she had voided yet. Mrs. Jones said, "No, not yet." The nurse said, "Then I'll have to catheterize you." Mrs. Jones refused to be catheterized. The nurse threatened to call Mrs. Jones' obstetrician if she (Mrs. Jones) would not allow her (the nurse) to proceed with the catheterization. Mrs. Jones said, "Go ahead and call him, but I wouldn't bother him with something so silly if I were you."

The nurse left the room. It had been a busy night and she was tired and frustrated. Moreover, the nurse thought that she might be reprimanded if she did not follow the established policies. She did not call the physician, but she did call Orthopedics to ask the night nurse there to "lend" her an orderly for 15 minutes to help her to restrain an unruly patient. The nurse on the orthopedic floor complied, but she did not notify the night supervisor of this unusual request.

The nurse in charge of Mrs. Jones gathered the appropriate supplies, washed her hands, and returned to the patient's room—accompanied by the orderly. She again asked Mrs. Jones if she would consent to be catheterized. Mrs. Jones again refused. The nurse told the patient that catheterization of women who had not voided within 12 hours of surgery was a routine procedure and that the catheterization was in her best interests because she could suffer bladder damage if she were not catheterized. The patient responded, "I am not uncomfortable, I don't want to be catheterized and *I won't be catheterized*. All I need is a little more time." The nurse then told the orderly to restrain Mrs. Jones physically while she catheterized her. Mrs. Jones was very angry and she used passive resistance to fight them. Finally, the orderly managed to force Mrs. Jones' legs apart and the nurse proceeded with the catheterization—she drained 230 *cc* of urine from Mrs. Jones' bladder.

Were the nurse's actions justified? Was the nurse acting in the patient's best interests by forcing her to be catheterized? Is a nurse always obligated to follow routine policy? Is the use of force ever justified in the practice of nursing? Was it justified in this case? Did Mrs. Jones have a right to refuse to be catheterized? Was her refusal to undergo this procedure unreasonable? Did Mrs. Jones have an obligation to conform to the established routines and policies of the hospital? Did Mrs. Jones have an obligation to do what the nurse said was in her best interests?

ANALYSIS

When Mrs. Jones was admitted to the hospital, she entered into both a formal and implied contract with the hospital. At the very least, the formal contract consisted of a promise on the part of the hospital to provide her with the services that were necessary to her care. In return, Mrs. Jones and her husband promised to pay the hospital for the supplies used and services rendered. In addition, Mrs. Jones signed the blanket consent form that the hospital routinely required all patients to sign prior to admission. It is alleged that a blanket consent form authorizes the hospital and its employees to take whatever action is deemed necessary for the patient's welfare throughout the course of the hospitalization.

Presumably, Mrs. Jones entered this hospital voluntarily and there is no evidence that she was coerced in any way to sign the blanket consent form. However, the legal status of such consent forms is questionable at best; the moral force of them is even more questionable. Several factors should be considered by those who sign such a form, by institutions that require the signing of such a form and by professionals who would rely solely on such a consent form to authorize their actions—particularly in the face of a patient's refusal to submit:

1. Few people who are asked to sign blanket consent forms on admission to a hospital are entirely free of coercion. In this particular instance, Mrs. Jones "chose" to come to this hospital because it was the one in which her physician practiced obstetrics. In this sense, she was not free to choose from among any one of the several hospitals in her community that offered obstetrical services. If there had been no other hospital or no other hospital that offered obstetrical services, she still was not free for she had no alternatives. Moreover, Mrs. Jones was in active labor—her membranes had ruptured at home. Had she refused to sign the blanket consent form and consequently had been refused admittance to the hospital, she could not have known how much time was available to her to find another physician or another hospital. In addition, it can be assumed safely that both Mrs. Jones and her husband were under duress. That is, this was their first experience with childbirth; not only did they not know what to expect, but they also did not want to jeopardize either Mrs. Jones or their baby. On these grounds, the Jones' freedom could be seen as limited and their consent "coerced."

2. The legitimacy of any blanket consent form can be questioned. How can people give valid consent to as yet unexplained procedures in as yet undefined circumstances? How can the requirements for informed consent be met when the patient is uninformed?

3. Even if one accepts the validity of a blanket consent form, the authority granted to the hospital and its employees is limited on at least two counts: (a) such consent cannot be construed as permission to violate the civil or human rights of any person; (b) the consent given is provisional. That is, the hospital and its employees are authorized to act only if the procedure, surgery or treatment is deemed necessary to the patient's well-being.

4. Although blanket consent forms generally confer the right to make decisions about what is necessary to the patient's welfare on physicians or hospital employees in general, it is at least implied that such decisions must be reasonable and justifiable. Unreasonable and unjustifiable actions are not authorized by any consent form—blanket or otherwise.

5. Even though a person has signed a consent form, the permission given is not irrevocable. If a conscious, rational adult patient refuses any particular

procedure, treatment, or surgery, the hospital, its employees, and the physician have no authority to act unless a Court order is granted. If blanket consent forms are valid at all, they are valid only when the persons who sign them are incapable of further decision making or when a court of law has authorized a particular course of action.

Reflection on the above points leads one to conclude that while Mrs. Jones did have some obligations to the hospital and its employees, she did not have an obligation to submit to any procedure, surgery or treatment just because she had signed a blanket consent form. It also leads one to the conclusion that the nurse had no formal, legal or moral authority to act, even though she might have believed that her actions were in Mrs. Jones' best interests.

IMPLIED CONTRACTS

When a person enters a hospital, he also enters into a number of implied contracts with professionals and other employees who may render services to him. It is implied that, when asked, a patient will provide the truthful information that is necessary to the design and delivery of his care. For example, a person who knows that he is allergic to penicillin is expected to respond truthfully when asked if he is allergic to penicillin. If he does not, he must bear some of the responsibility for any untoward reactions that result from the administration of penicillin.

Implied contracts with health professionals also include the expectation that a patient will cooperate in his care and treatment. For example, a person who is admitted to a hospital for the treatment of diabetes is expected to follow the diet that is prescribed for him. Although a patient may persuade friends to bring him food secretly, he must bear at least some of the responsibility for the outcome of his actions.

In return, an implied contract with a health professional infers that a patient has a right to expect competent care. It also infers that he will be apprised of all relevant information, that his civil and human rights will be respected and that the professional will act in accord with his best interests. Moreover, the implied contract also infers that information about the patient will be kept confidential and that his informed consent will be sought for all procedures prior to their initiation.

If a patient refuses to cooperate with a health professional's reasonable request, the contract between them may be broken. If a health professional acts contrary to the patient's best interests, without consent, or in direct opposition to a patient's expressed wishes, the contract between them may be broken. However, the dissolution of the implied contract does not authorize the use of force by either party. For example, a nurse has no right to force a patient to undergo any procedure. A patient has no right to hit a nurse who refuses to comply with even a reasonable request.

Although written consent (other than the blanket consent form) rarely is required for nursing interventions, this should not be construed to mean that consent is not required. At the very least, consent is a necessary component of the implied contract between a patient and a nurse. Moreover, unconsented touching is forbidden by law. In addition, the nurse has a moral and ethical obligation to respect the bodily integrity of any patient. The previous reflections on the obligations of both parties to an implied contract lead one to the conclusion that Mrs. Jones did have some implied obligations to the nurse, but she had no implied obligation to submit to any procedure whether or not (as in this case) it was invasive. It also leads one to conclude that the nurse had no implied legal or moral authority to act even though she might have believed that her actions were in Mrs. Jones' best interests.

WAS MRS. JONES' REFUSAL UNREASONABLE?

Mrs. Jones had not voided in the twelve hours following the delivery of her son. However, she was not distended and stated that she was not uncomfortable. The fact that she had not voided could be related to the bladder's decreased sensitivity to fluid pressure or swelling of tissues around the bladder or urethra that was secondary to bruising that may have occurred during delivery. If this were the case, there could be an increased risk of urinary tract infection. In addition, bladder distention may increase risk of uterine relaxation by displacing the uterus or interfering with its contractibility. If this happens, hemorrhage may occur.

However, the absence of palpable distension and discomfort seem to indicate that Mrs. Jones' bladder was not distended. This observation was confirmed when Mrs. Jones' eventual catheterization yielded only 230 cc of urine. If Mrs. Jones were experiencing fluid retention in the tissues or if her kidneys were not functioning properly, catheterization would not help her. In fact, there do not seem to have been clinical signs   other than the fact that she had not voided in 12 hours—that indicated a necessity for catheterization. Is a catheterization warranted (particularly as it carries a certain risk of its own) when an observation is not confirmed by any other clinical sign? In addition, catheterization following childbirth should be undertaken only with meticulous attention to aseptic technique and should be performed carefully. In view of the fact that the patient was resisting her efforts actively, the nurse could have done the patient more harm than good. In short, the competence of the nurse's clinical decision was open to question.

It is at least possible that Mrs. Jones' evaluation of her own condition was correct. She had not had fluids for almost 24 hours. She was catheterized immediately prior to delivery. She was not experiencing discomfort. She thought she was dehydrated and that, given time and more fluids, she eventually could void on her own. Was it unreasonable for her to want to attempt to void on her own? In short, the patient's "clinical evaluation" of her own condition seemed at least as competent as the nurse's. Given these considerations, it could be concluded that Mrs. Jones' refusal was reasonable.

WAS THE USE OF FORCE JUSTIFIED?

The nurse in this case not only made a decision to catheterize the patient, she also decided to force her to undergo catheterization. Are nurses ever justified in the use of force and was this nurse justified in this instance? To answer this question, one must examine the derivation and scope of a nurse's authority.

A professional's authority to act is derived from three possible sources: the consent of the patient, position power, and expert power. In the context of health care, the first source (consent) almost always is a prerequisite to action.* Position power enables some action; *e.g.*, it enables a person to carry out the legitimate policies of an institution and to supervise the work of others. For a professional, position power includes the power granted by the state to practice the profession (licensure) and, in limited circumstances, it may include the power to use the state's authority to protect the lives of others until such time as a court order can be requested and granted/rejected. In most instances, however, the source of professional authority is expert power. It generally involves an ability to act or to influence action rather than a right to act. A professional earns an epistemological right to be believed and not a moral right to be obeyed. The use of professional authority (expert power) derives its force from persuasion not coercion—that is, its use requires not only consent but also cooperation.

An examination of the use of expert power outside the health care arena might help to clarify its source and use. For example, a man might want to build a home. He can go about it in several ways: (1) He can rely on his own knowledge and strength to design and build it. (2) He can turn the building of his house over to architects and building contractors. (3) He can seek the advice and assistance of architects and building contractors in the building of his house. Through long years of study and experience, these people have earned the right to be believed. The chances are that the final product will be improved if the man seeks their advice. However, the house is his—he can refuse to seek or accept their advice if he so desires. If he is a wise man, however, he will neither give the building of his house completely over to the architects and building contractors nor undertake the project alone. The experts know how to build a house, but only he knows the kind of a house that he wants.

---

*The exceptions include a court order; clear and present danger of harm to the patient or other persons or, at times, a reasonable inference that it may be present; and possibly the authorization of the patient's legal guardian.

The expert power exercised by health professionals does not differ significantly from that of the experts in this example. A person's body is his own. Health professionals can advise, counsel, inform, even persuade, but they should not coerce. The temptation to use coercion in health care is strong because the "product" involved may be someone's life or health. Health professionals know that a patient's ability to reason may be affected by lack of knowledge, pain, drugs, exhaustion, and fear. They also know full well that a wrong decision could have disastrous consequences. Certainly, these factors constitute a good rationale for health professionals' uncommon readiness to make decisions for patients, but it rarely provides sufficient rationale to act in the face of patient opposition.

However, the use of subtle and flagrant coercion not infrequently is rewarded with success. That is, the patient does what the professional wants him to do. Because people already are coerced by their conditions to seek professional intervention, they are more vulnerable to further coercion. Pain, institutionalization, and fear all reduce the patient's ability to resist a professional's will. Even if a patient remains adamant in his opposition and the professional proceeds in the face of this opposition, not infrequently the patient later will thank the professional for ordering the course of events. Add to this the many times that people (families, in particular) may tell the professional, "Do as you think best," and one can begin to see why professionals may come to think that their expert power includes the use of coercion. The fact is that all of these factors, reinforced by success, lead some health professionals to adopt the notion that their laudable ends (the health or well-being of a patient) justify whatever means (coercion) they deem necessary. They transform an epistemological right to be believed into a moral right to be obeyed. It was just such an authoritarian attitude that led the nurse in this case study to use physical force to catheterize the patient. Thus, the nurse violated Mrs. Jones' rights to bodily integrity, privacy and self-determination.

The use of force in the practice of nursing can be justified only if the person (patient) represents or can reasonably be believed to represent a clear and present danger to others or possibly to himself. The use of coercion in any form is undesirable and is unjustifiable in most circumstances. In almost all instances, health professionals derive their authority from expert power, not coercive power, and the line between persuasion and coercion should not be crossed.

DENOUEMENT

Mrs. Jones, justifiably incensed, complained to her physician and to the nursing office. The nurse involved in this case was reprimanded but not dismissed. One can hope that in the future this nurse will approach her professional obligations less dogmatically and her patients more respectfully. Perhaps she will have learned that the well-being of the whole human being who happens to be a patient is best served by cooperation not coercion, that policies are to be applied with discernment and that patients, too, have rights.

BIBLIOGRAPHY

Annas, George, "Who to Call When the Doctor is Sick," *Hastings Center Report,* Vol. 8, December 1978, pp. 18–29.

Barber, Bernard. *Informed Consent in Medical Therapy and Research.* Rutgers University Press, New Brunswick, New Jersey, 1980.

Burt, Robert A. *Taking Care of Strangers.* The Free Press, New York, 1979.

Geretz, Tom, "Conversations About Death and Power," *Hastings Center Report,* Vol. 10, November 4, 1980, pp. 19–21.

Graber, Glenn C. and Frank H. Marsh, "Ought a Patient Be Drugged to Stand Trial?" *Hastings Center Report,* Vol. 9, February 1979, pp. 8–10.

Hunt, Robert and John Arras, eds. *Ethical Issues in Modern Medicine.* Mayfield Publishing Company, Palo Alto, California, 1977, pp. 249–340.

Kass, Leon R., "The New Biology: What Price Relieving Man's Estate?" *Science,* Vol. 174, November 1971, pp. 779–788.

Kessler, C., "Contracts of Adhesion—Some Thoughts About Freedom of Contract," *Columbia Law Review,* Vol. 43, 1943, p. 629.

May, William F., "Code, Covenant, Contract or Philanthropy," *Hastings Center Report,* Vol. 5, December 1975, pp. 33–36.

Patient's Bill of Rights. American Hospital Association, Chicago, Illinois.

Pratt v. Davis, 118 Ill., App. 161, 166 (1905), Aff. 2d 244 Ill. 300, 79 N.E. 562 (1906) The issue of informed consent, as structured by the Illinois court, helped to define the relationship of patient and physician. The law enters the case only when a physician seeks to enforce his wishes on a non-consenting patient.

Ramsey, Paul. *The Patient as Person.* Yale University Press, New Haven, 1970.

Wellman, Carl. *Morals and Ethics.* Scott, Foresman and Company, Glenview, Illinois, 1975, pp. 294–297.

Index

N

T

U

V